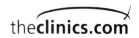

ENDOCRINOLOGY AND METABOLISM CLINICS

OF NORTH AMERICA

Thyroid Function and Disease

GUEST EDITOR
Kenneth D. Burman, MD

CONSULTING EDITOR
Derek LeRoith, MD, PhD

September 2007 • Volume 36 • Number 3

SAUNDERS

An Imprint of Elsevier, Inc.
PHILADELPHIA   LONDON   TORONTO   MONTREAL   SYDNEY   TOKYO

W.B. SAUNDERS COMPANY
A Division of Elsevier Inc.

1600 John F. Kennedy Boulevard • Suite 1800 • Philadelphia, Pennsylvania 19103-2899

http://www.theclinics.com

ENDOCRINOLOGY AND METABOLISM	Volume 36, Number 3
CLINICS OF NORTH AMERICA	ISSN 0889-8529
September 2007	ISBN-13: 978-1-4160-5066-7
Editor: Rachel Glover	ISBN-10: 1-4160-5066-3

The ideas and opinions expressed in *Endocrinology and Metabolism Clinics of North America* do not necessarily reflect those of the Publisher. The Publisher does not assume any responsibility for any injury and/or damage to persons or property arising out of or related to any use of the material contained in this periodical. The reader is advised to check the appropriate medical literature and the product information currently provided by the manufacturer of each drug to be administered to verify the dosage, the method and duration of administration, or contraindications. It is the responsibility of the treating physician or other health care professional, relying on independent experience and knowledge of the patient, to determine drug dosages and the best treatment for the patient. Mention of any product in this issue should not be construed as endorsement by the contributors, editors, or the Publisher of the product or manufacturers' claims.

Endocrinology and Metabolism Clinics of North America (ISSN 0889-8529) is published quarterly by Elsevier Inc., 360 Park Avenue South, New York, NY 10010-1710. Months of publication are March, June, September, and December. Business and editorial offices: 1600 John F. Kennedy Boulevard, Suite 1800, Philadelphia, PA 19103-2899. Customer Service Office: 6277 Sea Harbor Drive, Orlando, FL 32887-4800. Periodicals postage paid at New York, NY and additional mailing offices. Subscription prices are USD 193 per year for US individuals, USD 319 per year for US institutions, USD 99 per year for US students and residents, USD 242 per year for Canadian individuals, USD 383 per year for Canadian institutions, USD 264 per year for international individuals, USD 383 per year for international institutions and USD 138 per year for Canadian and foreign students/residents. To receive student/resident rate, orders must be accompanied by name of affiliated institution, date of term, and the *signature* of program/residency coordinator on institution letterhead. Orders will be billed at individual rate until proof of status is received. Foreign air speed delivery is included in all *Clinics* subscription prices. All prices are subject to change without notice. POSTMASTER: Send address changes to *Endocrinology and Metabolism Clinics of North America*, Elsevier Periodicals Customer Service, 6277 Sea Harbor Drive, Orlando, FL 32887-4800. **Customer Service: (+1) 800-654-2452 (US). From outside of the US, call (+1) 407-345-4000; e-mail: hhspcs@harcourt.com.**

Reprints. For copies of 100 or more, of articles in this publication, please contact the Commercial Rights Department, Elsevier Inc., 360 Park Avenue South, New York, NY 10010-1710; phone: (+1) 212-633-3813; fax: (+1) 212-462-1935; e-mail: reprints@elsevier.com.

Endocrinology and Metabolism Clinics of North America is covered in *Index Medicus, EMBASE/Excerpta Medica, Current Contents/Clinical Medicine, Current Contents/Life Sciences, Science Citation Index, ISI/BIOMED, BIOSIS,* and *Chemical Abstracts.*

Printed in the United States of America.

CONSULTING EDITOR

DEREK LEROITH, MD, PhD, Chief, Division of Endocrinology, Metabolism, and Bone Diseases, Mount Sinai School of Medicine, New York, New York

GUEST EDITOR

KENNETH D. BURMAN, MD, Chief, Endocrine Section, Washington Hospital Center; and Professor, Department of Medicine, Georgetown University, Washington, DC

CONTRIBUTORS

SUZANNE MYERS ADLER, MD, Fellow, Division of Endocrinology and Metabolism, Department of Medicine, Georgetown University School of Medicine; and Washington Center Hospital, Washington, DC

DOUGLAS W. BALL, MD, Associate Professor of Medicine and Oncology, Johns Hopkins University School of Medicine, Baltimore, Maryland

KENNETH D. BURMAN, MD, Chief, Endocrine Section, Washington Hospital Center; and Professor, Department of Medicine, Georgetown University, Washington, DC

MADHURI DEVDHAR, MD, Resident, Internal Medicine, Washington Hospital Center, Washington, DC

CATHERINE DINAUER, MD, Associate Research Scientist, Department of Pediatrics, Yale School of Medicine, New Haven, Connecticut

D. ROBERT DUFOUR, MD, Consultant, Pathology and Laboratory Medicine Service, Veterans Affairs Medical Center; and Emeritus Professor of Pathology, George Washington University Medical Center, Washington, DC

GARY L. FRANCIS, MD, PhD, Professor and Chair, Division of Endocrinology and Metabolism, Department of Pediatrics, Medical College of Virginia, Virginia Commonwealth University, Richmond, Virginia

HOSSEIN GHARIB, MD, MACP, MACE, Professor of Medicine, Mayo Clinic College of Medicine; and Consultant, Division of Endocrinology, Metabolism, and Nutrition, Mayo Clinic, Rochester, Minnesota; Former President, American Association of Clinical Endocrinologists, Jacksonville, Florida

STEVEN P. HODAK, MD, Clinical Assistant Professor of Medicine, University of Pittsburgh Center for Diabetes and Endocrinology, University of Pittsburgh Medical Center, Pittsburgh, Pennsylvania

PRIYA KUNDRA, MD, Endocrine Fellow, Endocrine Sections, Washington Hospital Center, Georgetown University Medical Center, Washington, DC

RÉBECCA LEBOEUF, MD, Assistant Professor of Medicine, Sherbrooke University, Centre Hopitalier Universitaire de Sherbrooke, Sherbrooke, Quebec, Canada

ANDREW J. MARTORELLA, MD, Assistant Professor of Medicine, Joan and Sanford I. Weill College of Medicine of Cornell University; and Assistant Attending, Memorial Sloan-Kettering Cancer Center, New York, New York

BINDU NAYAK, MD, Fellow, Division of Endocrinology and Metabolism, Georgetown University Hospital; and Washington Hospital Center, Washington, DC

YOLANDA C. OERTEL, MD, Director, FNA Service, Pathology Department, Washington Hospital Center; and Professor Emerita of Pathology, The George Washington University School of Medicine and Health Sciences, Washington, DC; Adjunct Professor of Pathology and Laboratory Medicine, MCP Hahnemann University School of Medicine, Philadelphia, Pennsylvania

YASSER H. OUSMAN, MD, Staff Endocrinologist, Washington Hospital Center, Washington, DC

ENRICO PAPINI, MD, FACE, Chief, Department of Endocrine and Metabolic Diseases, Regina Apostolorum Hospital, Albano Laziale; and President, Associazione Medici Endocrinologi, Rome, Italy

JOHN SHARRETTS, MD, MedStar Diabetes and Research Institute, Washington Center Hospital, Washington, DC

R. MICHAEL TUTTLE, MD, Associate Professor of Medicine, Joan and Sanford I Weill Medical College of Cornell University; and Associate Attending, Memorial Sloan-Kettering Cancer Center, New York, New York

DOUGLAS VAN NOSTRAND, MD, FACP, FACNP, Director, Division of Nuclear Medicine, Washington Hospital Center; and Professor of Medicine, Georgetown University Medical Center, Washington, DC

LEONARD WARTOFSKY, MD, MACP, Chairman, Department of Medicine, Washington Hospital Center; and Professor of Medicine, Georgetown University School of Medicine, Washington, DC; Professor of Medicine, Physiology, Anatomy, and Genetics, Uniformed Services University of the Health Sciences, Bethesda, Maryland

JASON A. WEXLER, MD, Division of Endocrinology, Washington Hospital Center, Washington, DC

CONTENTS

mastering this deceptively simple technique. The author shares technical hints learned over 30 years.

Papillary Thyroid Cancer: Monitoring and Therapy

R. Michael Tuttle, Rébecca Leboeuf, and Andrew J. Martorella

The last 10 years have seen a major paradigm shift in the management of thyroid cancer, with greater reliance on serum thyroglobulin and neck ultrasonography, and less emphasis on routine diagnostic whole-body radioactive iodine scanning for detection of recurrent disease. As our follow-up tests become more sensitive for detection of recurrent disease, we are finding many asymptomatic patients who have low-level persistent disease many years after initial therapy that may or may not benefit from additional testing and therapy. These difficult issues have been addressed by at least five different sets of guidelines published recently by various thyroid specialty organizations around the world. In this article, the authors compare and contrast the recommendations from the various guidelines in an attempt to define areas of consensus and explore possible reasons for differing recommendations.

Thyroid Cancer in Children

Catherine Dinauer and Gary L. Francis

In 1996, the authors were asked to review the subject of thyroid cancer in children. Over the subsequent decade, much has been learned about the treatment and outcome of these uncommon tumors. We now recognize quantitative and perhaps qualitative differences in genetic mutations and growth factor expression patterns in childhood thyroid cancers compared with those of adults. We also know that thyroid cancers induce a robust immune response in children that might contribute to their longevity. Patients under 10 years of age probably represent a unique subset of children at particularly high risk for persistent or recurrent disease; the management of these patients is under evaluation. We remain limited in our knowledge of how to stratify children into low- and high-risk categories for appropriate long-term follow-up and in our knowledge of how to treat children who have detectable serum thyroglobulin but negative imaging studies. In this article, the authors update our understanding of thyroid cancers in children with special emphasis on how these data relate to the current guidelines for management of thyroid cancer developed by the American Thyroid Association Taskforce. The limited data regarding management of children who have detectable serum thyroglobulin but negative whole-body scans are also reviewed.

Radioiodine in the Treatment of Thyroid Cancer

Douglas Van Nostrand and Leonard Wartofsky

This article presents an overview of the use of radioactive iodine (131-I) in the treatment of patients who have well differentiated thyroid cancer. We review definitions; staging; the two-principal methods for selection of a dosage of 131-I for ablation and treatment; the objectives of ablation and treatment; the indications for ablation and treatment; the recommendations for the use of 131-I for ablation and treatment contained in the Guidelines of the American Thyroid Association, the European Consensus, the Society of Nuclear Medicine, and the European Association of Nuclear Medicine; the dosage recommendations and selection of dosage for 131-I by the these organizations; and the Washington Hospital Center approach.

This article summarizes the clinical features and molecular pathogenesis of medullary thyroid cancer (MTC) and focuses on the current use of molecular, biochemical, and imaging disease markers as a basis for selection of appropriate therapy. Clinicians treating patients who have MTC face the following challenges: (1) distinguishing MTC as early as possible from benign nodular disease and differentiated thyroid cancer to choose the appropriate initial surgery, (2) managing low-level residual cancer in otherwise asymptomatic individuals, and (3) treating progressive metastatic disease. Early clinical trials using small molecules targeting Ret or vascular endothelial growth factor receptors suggest that such approaches could be effective and well tolerated. This article highlights early progress in targeted therapy of MTC and significant challenges in disease monitoring to appropriately select and evaluate patients being treated with these therapies.

Several agents are currently being tested that target thyroid molecular signaling and cancer cell biology. The pathways involved include but are not limited to the Ras pathway, vascular endothelial growth factor and epidermal growth factor receptors and antibodies, angiogenesis inhibitors, tyrosine kinase inhibitors, heat shock protein inhibitors, demethylating agents, histone deacetylase inhibitors, and gene therapy. Each of these targeted approaches holds promise for our future ability to treat patients with thyroid cancer unresponsive to traditional therapy.

FORTHCOMING ISSUES

RECENT ISSUES

THE CLINICS ARE NOW AVAILABLE ONLINE!

Access your subscription at:
http://www.theclinics.com

ENDOCRINOLOGY
AND METABOLISM
CLINICS
OF NORTH AMERICA

Endocrinol Metab Clin N Am
36 (2007) xi–xiii

Foreword

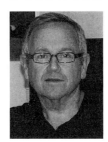

Derek LeRoith, MD, PhD
Consulting Editor

Thyroid dysfunction is extremely common, and this issue, by Guest Editor Kenneth Burman and the authors that have contributed articles, covers almost all the thyroid related conditions that internists and endocrinologists encounter.

Perhaps not well appreciated by practicing internists and some endocrinologists is the question of problems relating to laboratory testing for thyroid function. As described by Dufour, there are interfering substances, especially during acute illnesses, that give altered thyroid hormone levels, and heterophile antibodies, such as rheumatoid factor, that cause falsely high results with immunometric thyroid stimulating hormone (TSH), calcitonin, and thryoglobulin. Thus, until these problems have been resolved, physicians should be aware of these issues and request alternative techniques for measurement when a problem arises.

A comprehensive discussion on the etiology, diagnostic criteria, and therapy of hyperthyroidism is presented by Bindu Nayak and Steven Hodak. Although this condition is well described and the diagnostic and therapeutic approaches are fairly standard, it is critical to re-emphasize that the condition may present with very subtle signs and symptoms, and needs to be considered routinely in the differential diagnosis of many conditions.

Nonthyroidal illness syndrome equates to the alteration in thyroid function tests commonly seen in severely ill patients. Since the patients usually have normal thyroid function, it also goes by the name "eythroid sick syndrome". It is commonly associated with a low serum T3, normal free T4 and TSH, and elevated reversed T3 levels. Adler and Wartofsky explain the

doi:10.1016/j.ecl.2007.06.003

endo.theclinics.com

normal synthesis and control of thyroid hormones, and how they are affected in the "euthyroid sick syndrome." They also describe the acute illnesses and pharmacologic agents that cause these changes. Finally, they describe the theory that the changes in hormonal levels may be adaptive—a hypothesis that has led investigators to propose thyroid replacement for this situation. They correctly warn that this approach is controversial and not without danger.

Jason Wexler and John Sharretts discuss the effects of thyroid hormones on bone development and also on adult bone. Bone cells express receptors for TSH and thyroid hormones. As they describe, hypothyroidism leads to growth arrest, epiphyseal dysgenesis, delayed bone age, and short stature. On the other hand, juvenile hyperthyroidism causes accelerated growth, advanced bone maturity, and premature closure of the growth plate, which also leads to short stature. In adults, hypothyroidism and hyperthyroidism may lead to an increased risk for fractures caused by reduced bone mineral density, and this decrease may be reversed by appropriate treatment of these thyroid disorders. They also discuss the metastasis of thyroid cancer to bone, its diagnosis, and treatment that includes 131-I therapy, bisphosphonates, and other innovative new therapies.

In their article, Gharib and Papini present the current recommendations for a very common physical finding—the thyroid nodule. Thyroid nodules carry a risk of malignancy of about 5%, and the initial workup to exclude a thyrotoxic nodule is to measure a serum TSH level. Ultrasound (US) and fine needle aspiration (FNA) should be used routinely, since both small and large nodules, single nodules, and those within a multinodular gland may harbor malignancies. While a certain degree of controversy exists regarding the exact criteria for US–FNA, this article gives very practical suggestions regarding the criteria that indicate suspicious nodules. Oertel describes, in clear detail, the technique for FNA and stresses that too much suction leads to uninterpretable pathology results. The article also describes the pathologic results to be expected and their interpretation, and serves as a useful resource for those performing FNAs.

In the article by Tuttle, Leboeuf, and Martorella, the changing paradigm in the management and evaluation of thyroid cancer is presented. The use of neck ultrasound, very sensitive thyroglobulin assays (especially following rhTSH injection [rather than thyroid withdrawal]), and PET scanning are now routinely used in evaluation and radioactive iodine remnant ablation. However, these sensitive tests have also demonstrated that remnant disease, albeit minimal, is now more readily identified, leaving the physician and the patient uncertain as to whether and when progression of the cancer will be detected and require further management. Thyroid cancer is fortunately much less common in children than in adults, as discussed by Dinauer and Francis. Similar to the situation of differentiated tumors in adults, the life expectancy is only mildly reduced. Evaluation and treatment of these tumors as well as medullary thyroid cancer (MTC) are similarly dealt with in adults.

The use of radioactive iodine in the management of well-differentiated thyroid cancer (WDTC) is presented by Van Nostrand and Wartofsky. They strongly suggest that a team approach is essential, including the nuclear medicine physician and an endocrinologist, since dosing is critical for "ablation" of the remnant thyroid cancer following surgical removal and "treatment" of metastases. They also outline the criteria of staging and dosage determination by the American Thyroid Association as well as their European counterparts, and leave the reader with a clear understanding of the procedures needed for this type of therapy.

Douglas Ball, on the other hand, discusses MTC, a less common cause of cancer in comparison with follicular and papillary thyroid cancer. Only one quarter of all cases of MTC are inherited as part of the multiple endocrine neoplasia (MEN) 2 syndrome, or as familial MTC. The outcome for this type of cancer is worse than in differentiated thyroid cancers. Activating mutations of the ret oncogene are commonly found in the inherited and sporadic forms. Calcitonin and carcinoembryonic-antigen levels are used preoperatively and postoperatively with imaging techniques to determine further therapy. Chemotherapy has not proven extremely successful and agents that inactivate the ret tyrosine kinase or block vascular endothelial growth factor (VEGF) and epidermal growth factor (EGF) receptor activity are being tested with some promising results. Given the poor responses with conventional therapy, these new approaches afford some hope.

In the final article, Priya Kundra and Kenneth Burman explore the exciting research opportunities targeted to the molecular changes that occur in thyroid cancer; these include tyrosine kinase inhibitors, inhibitors of the Ras pathway, VEGF and EGF receptors and antibodies, angiogenesis inhibitors, tyrosine kinase inhibitors, heat shock protein inhibitors, demethylating agents, histone deacetylase inhibitors, and gene therapy. Many are in preclinical development, whereas others are in early clinical trials. Their promise lies in the ability to treat patients who have failed conventional therapy—an exciting and long-awaited approach.

In summary, a well organized and comprehensive issue on thyroid disorders with all the latest in relevant research and therapeutic modalities is presented; a tribute to the issue editor, Kenneth Burman.

Derek LeRoith, MD, PhD
Division of Endocrinology, Metabolism, and Bone Diseases
Mount Sinai School of Medicine
One Gustave L. Levy Place, Box 1055
Atran 4-36
New York, NY 10029, USA

E-mail address: derek.leroith@mssm.edu

Endocrinol Metab Clin N Am
36 (2007) xv–xvi

ENDOCRINOLOGY
AND METABOLISM
CLINICS
OF NORTH AMERICA

Preface

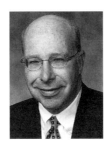

Kenneth D. Burman, MD
Guest Editor

It is a privilege for me to work with Dr. LeRoith to help organize and edit this issue of the *Endocrinology and Metabolism Clinics of North America,* discussing important, clinically relevant thyroid-related issues. A group of experienced, knowledgeable, and acclaimed authors have agreed to contribute articles that review their current approach to specific thyroid problems. The articles are arranged with an initial review of current thyroid physiology and testing procedures, followed by common thyroid problems that are encountered, such as the diagnosis, assessment, and treatment of hypothyroidism, hyperthyroidism, nonthyroidal illness, and the relationship between bone and thyroid pathophysiology and disease. We then focus on various types of thyroid cancer, starting out with a discussion of recent concepts and treatment regarding thyroid nodules, fine needle aspiration of the thyroid, and papillary thyroid cancer, first in adults and then in children. The proper use of radioiodine therapy is also discussed. Medullary thyroid cancer is less common than differentiated thyroid cancer, but presents new and interesting challenges. Lastly, there have been very important clinical developments regarding the use of targeted specific thyroid cancer agents for all types of thyroid cancer.

This issue of *Endocrinology and Metabolism Clinics of North America* should bring health care providers with varied interests and experience

doi:10.1016/j.ecl.2007.06.004

endo.theclinics.com

up-to-date on multiple thyroid problems; this is a tribute to the dedication of the authors, to whom I am grateful.

Kenneth D. Burman, MD
Endocrine Section
Washington Hospital Center
110 Irving Street NW
Washington, DC 20010, USA

Department of Medicine
Georgetown University
Washington, DC 20007, USA

E-mail address: kenneth.burman@medstar.net

ELSEVIER
SAUNDERS

Endocrinol Metab Clin N Am
36 (2007) 579–594

ENDOCRINOLOGY
AND METABOLISM
CLINICS
OF NORTH AMERICA

Laboratory Tests of Thyroid Function: Uses and Limitations

D. Robert Dufour, MD[a,b,*]

[a]Pathology and Laboratory Medicine Service, Veterans Affairs Medical Center,
50 Irving Street, NW, Washington, DC 20402, USA
[b]George Washington University Medical Center, 2300 Eye Street,
NW, Washington, DC 20037, USA

Laboratory tests are the most commonly used aids in the diagnosis and monitoring of individuals who have thyroid disease. In general, laboratory tests for thyroid evaluation are similar in accuracy and reliability to other laboratory tests. In some situations, thyroid tests can provide misleading or inaccurate information because, for the most part, test methods used in clinical laboratories do not use "definitive" methods for measuring compounds but instead use "comparative" methods. In almost all cases, solutions containing known amounts of the compounds of interest are analyzed, and some physical parameter of the solution (eg, amount of light absorbed) is measured. Samples from patients are then measured using the same method, and the signal obtained is compared with that from the known samples. This requires the assumption that the known and patient samples are similar in all other respects, save for the amount of the compound of interest. When this assumption is not valid, then the results are affected.

This article briefly summarizes the common methods of laboratory testing relating to thyroid disease and discusses specific information for individual tests on methods of analysis, their limitations, and situations where caution should be used in interpreting the results of thyroid tests. For a number of tests, the degree of inaccuracy varies with the specific method used in a given laboratory. Because laboratories generally do not have information on the clinical status of or medications taken by the patient at the time of testing, it is difficult for the laboratory to recognize when they are dealing with a sample that may produce misleading results. It is important for endocrinologists to be familiar with the methods used in the laboratories that they use and to contact the laboratory when test results seem to be

* 7311 Winterfield Terrace, Laurel, MD 20707.
  E-mail address: chemdoctorbob@earthlink.net

0889-8529/07/$ - see front matter. Published by Elsevier Inc.
doi:10.1016/j.ecl.2007.04.003

misleading. In many cases, the laboratory can perform additional tests or evaluate the sample for interferences.

Principles of laboratory testing used for thyroid testing

To measure the small amounts of thyroid hormones and peptides, simple chemical analyses generally do not have adequate sensitivity. Most thyroid tests are performed using one of two formats of immunoassay (Table 1). For thyroid hormones (and in one available assay for thyroglobulin), competitive immunoassays are used. In this format, a limited amount of antibody to thyroid hormone is incubated with the patient's serum, and a known amount of the same thyroid hormone is labeled. The labeled hormone and unlabeled hormone compete for binding by the antibody. The amount of label bound to the antibody is inversely proportional to the amount of hormone in the patient's serum. Competitive immunoassays are subject to interference by compounds that are similar in structure to the compound of interest; this is generally not a problem for thyroid hormones or thyroglobulin. Patients who have antibodies to the compound of interest (a common issue in thyroglobulin assays [1] and an occasional problem with thyroid hormone assays [2]) often have falsely increased results: As some of the labeled hormone becomes bound to the antibody in the serum, less is available to bind to the testing antibody, which leads to the false impression of high hormone levels.

A second format of immunoassay, often referred to as immunometric assay, is most commonly used to measure peptide hormones, such as thyroid-stimulating hormone (TSH), calcitonin, and thyroglobulin. In this format, a large amount of antibody to the hormone is bound to a solid support, and patient serum is added. After incubation, the support is washed to remove residual serum, and a second labeled antibody to the hormone is added. (Such assays are sometimes called "sandwich" assays; the two

Table 1
Features of immunoassay formats

Feature	Competitive	Sandwich
Most used for	Small molecules (T3, T4)	Larger molecules (TSH, calcitonin, thyroglobulin)
	Older assays for TSH, calcitonin, thyroglobulin	
Interferences by closely related compounds	Yes, significant	Rarely
Interferences by antibodies to compounds	Falsely increased	Usually decreased, rarely increased
Interferences by heterophile antibodies	Rare	Affects 0.1%–1% of samples

Abbreviation: TSH, thyroid-stimulating hormone.

antibodies represent the bread, and the hormone is the "filling" in the sandwich.) When the solid support is washed, the amount of labeled antibody remaining on the support should be directly proportional to the amount of hormone in serum.

Immunometric assays are generally much more specific for hormones than competitive assays; the use of two different antibodies, often reacting with different parts of the hormone, reduces the likelihood of interference from chemically similar compounds. There are other causes of interference in immunometric assays. Antibodies to the hormone can produce falsely low results with immunometric assays, a common problem in thyroglobulin measurement [3]. Human antibodies to the antibodies used in the assays may lead to attachment of the indicator antibody to the solid support, even in the absence of the hormone. This most commonly occurs with human antibodies to mouse proteins because mouse monoclonal antibodies are most widely used, although other antibodies that react with a variety of animal proteins (ie, "heterophile" antibodies) may also occur [4,5]. Rheumatoid factor is also a potential interference in immunometric assays. Although assay manufacturers add substances to reduce the potential for interference [6], it has been estimated that one to two samples per thousand have high enough antibody titers to cause falsely increased results [7]. This is most problematic for hormones that should be in low concentrations, such as thyroglobulin in a thyroidectomized patient or TSH in a hyperthyroid patient. Several approaches can be used when such interferences are suspected [8]. Commercial neutralizing reagents with extremely high amounts of mouse immunoglobulin can be preincubated with the patient serum. Serial dilution of the sample can document that the expected fall in results does not occur. Repeating the assay with a kit from a different manufacturer often shows significant differences in results because different assays have differing susceptibility to interference. When the results are incompatible with the clinical setting, the endocrinologist should contact the laboratory to ask whether the laboratory checked for such interferences and if not to request that one or more of the above steps be taken to evaluate for antibody interference.

Specific thyroid tests

Thyrotropin

Measurement of TSH has become the principal test for the evaluation of thyroid function in most circumstances. Assays for TSH have been classified in generations, based on the functional sensitivity of the assay (ie, the level at which the repeatability of measurement is ±20%). The National Academy of Clinical Biochemistry (NACB) guidelines recommend that laboratories use assays with third-generation functional sensitivity (0.02 mU/L) or better [9].

An unresolved issue is the upper limit of "normal" for TSH. Laboratories typically establish reference limits based on the central 95% of values seen in apparently healthy individuals; for TSH, such limits typically are around 0.4 to 0.5 mU/L for the lower limit and 4.5 to 5.5 mU/L for the upper limit. This approach has been called into question for several reasons. First, prospective studies of thyroid function have found that risk of subsequent hypothyroidism rises at TSH values higher than 2.0 mU/L [10]. Higher TSH values (within traditional reference limits) are typically found in persons who have risk factors for future thyroid disease, such as family history, presence of thyroid antibodies, pregnancy, or use of drugs affecting thyroid function (eg, amiodarone) [11,12]. This has led some investigators, including the authors of the NACB guidelines [9], to suggest that upper reference limits for TSH should be lowered to 2.5 mU/L. Not all individuals who have TSH values that are higher than this cutoff (or even those who have slightly higher values) develop overt hypothyroidism in long-term follow-up. Evaluation of clinical outcomes has suggested that treatment of subclinical hypothyroidism is not warranted until TSH exceeds 10 mU/L [12]. There thus seems to be a range of TSH values for which an alternative term, such as "borderline" or "at risk," might be more appropriate than the traditional interpretation of all values outside the reference limits as "abnormal."

TSH measurements have less-than-ideal agreement between different assays, which limits the ability to define arbitrary reference limits that should be used by all laboratories. For example, in a recent survey involving 2580 patients, the mean values for TSH using different assays, on a sample with "normal" TSH, ranged from 1.24 to 1.73 mU/L [13]. Because different manufacturers' assays use antibodies that recognize different epitopes of TSH and because multiple different forms of TSH are present in the circulation, it is difficult to reach agreement between assays. It is likely that, for use of a single common value for the upper reference limits, a process similar to the glycohemoglobin standardization program is required.

A number of conditions affect TSH or its measurement and may cause discordance between TSH levels and the clinical picture of the patient (Table 2). In acutely ill individuals, the range of TSH values seen in apparently euthyroid individuals changes markedly. A number of factors, such as cortisol, dopamine, and cytokines, affect TSH production. In one study of individuals subsequently shown to be euthyroid, 95% of TSH values were between 0.1 and 20 mU/L when the same individuals were acutely ill [14]. Only half of acutely ill individuals who had TSH values above 20 mU/L were found to have thyroid disease. A review of published studies found that TSH was predictive of thyroid disease only beyond these broadened "reference" values [15]. As a result, TSH levels must be interpreted with caution in hospitalized individuals unless values are below 0.1 or above 20 mU/L, and several groups have advised against routine testing of thyroid function in patients who have acute illness.

Table 2
Causes of misleading thyroid-stimulating hormone results

Condition	Effect
Acute illness	TSH central 95% reference interval widens to 0.1–20 mU/L
Central hypothyroidism	Abnormal forms predominate, with high immunoassay/ bioactivity ratio, leading to falsely high results
Heterophile antibodies	Falsely increased results; results differ between assays, nonlinear on dilution
	Neutralized by nonimmune mouse serum for assays using mouse antibodies
TSH autoantibodies	Falsely increased results; results differ between assays, nonlinear on dilution
	Not neutralized by mouse serum
	Removed by polyethylene glycol precipitation

Abbreviation: TSH, thyroid-stimulating hormone.

Abnormal forms of TSH may predominate in individuals who have central hypothyroidism. Decreased sialylation of TSH is common in central hypothyroidism and results in reduced bioactivity and increased TSH half-life [16,17]. Because TSH is typically measured by immunoassay, it is important to consider the effects of these changes on measured TSH. The ratio of bioactive to immunoreactive TSH is markedly reduced in central hypothyroidism; this results in TSH values that are seldom low but that typically fall within the reference range and that, in about 15% of cases, are elevated [18]. With successful treatment, TSH values typically fall below the lower reference limit or become undetectable.

Measurement of TSH can be subject to interference from heterophile antibodies and rheumatoid factor, producing falsely increased results. This is most commonly problematic in hyperthyroid individuals, in whom nonsuppressed TSH suggests TSH-producing tumors or thyroid hormone resistance. Greater degrees of interference can result in persistent TSH elevation despite successful treatment of patients who have hypothyroidism. Rarely, autoantibodies to TSH may occur or may develop after injections of bovine TSH. In one study, clinically significant interference occurred in only 2 of 300,000 samples tested [19]. TSH autoantibodies can cross the placenta, leading to a false impression of neonatal hypothyroidism [20]. One clue to the presence of either type of interference is relatively stable TSH values despite changing thyroid hormone levels. Another clue is discrepant results between different laboratories using different TSH assays; in the baby who had TSH antibodies that crossed the placenta, TSH values varied between 4 and 213 mU/L with four different assays [20]. If such interference is suspected clinically, the laboratory should be contacted to determine if it has evaluated for interfering substances and to request evaluation if it has not been performed.

Total thyroxine and triiodothyronine

In the 1970s and 1980s, most tests of thyroid hormone production evaluated total thyroid hormone concentration. Because well over 99% of T4 and T3 is bound to binding proteins (thyroxine-binding globulin [TBG], albumin, and transthyretin, also termed thyroxine-binding prealbumin), total thyroid hormone levels are affected by changes in binding protein levels or binding affinity. Assays for total thyroid hormone are now less frequently used, although they are still available in many laboratories. The major reasons for the decreased popularity of total thyroid hormone assays are the effects of binding protein changes and the lower sensitivity of total hormone assays for early thyroid dysfunction. Total thyroid hormone levels are more often abnormal due to binding protein changes than to thyroid dysfunction [9].

Assays for total thyroxine have reasonable comparability between methods from different manufacturers. In a study of 1528 laboratories, differences between methods were less than 10% from the result for total T4 for all but two methods [13]. Repeatability of results over time was excellent in another study using two mailings of fresh frozen serum 6 months apart [21]. For total T3, results in 926 laboratories were more than 10% from the actual result for 58% of methods and were more than 20% from the actual result for 33% of methods [13].

Changes in levels of binding proteins, particularly increases in TBG, are relatively common. Frequent causes of abnormal TBG levels are summarized in Table 3. With abnormal TBG, total thyroxine (T4) and triiodothyronine (T3) are affected. In the less common familial dysalbuminemic hyperthyroxinemia, total T4 is typically increased, whereas total T3 is not. In general, when there is an isolated abnormality in TBG, total thyroid values, when corrected for TBG levels by the use of T-uptake tests, reflect a euthyroid state. When hypo- or hyperthyroidism coexists with abnormal binding proteins, calculated free thyroxine index is often inappropriately normal [22]. Drugs that affect the binding of hormones to protein can also affect total thyroid hormone measurements; such drug effects are discussed under free T4 measurements.

Table 3
Factors affecting thyroxine-binding globulin levels

Factor	Increased	Decreased
Drugs	Estrogens, fluorouracil, opiates, methadone, mitotane, tamoxifen	Androgens, danazol, glucocorticoids, nicotinic acid
Liver disease	Acute, chronic hepatitis	Cirrhosis
Congenital disorders	Not reported	Rare deficiency
Renal disease	None	Nephrotic syndrome
Other conditions	Pregnancy	Malnutrition

Multiple abnormalities related to thyroid hormone binding protein levels and changes in binding affinity are common in patients who have acute illness. Levels of all binding proteins decrease in acute illness, and the affinity constant for TBG binding is reduced, leading to a disproportionate decrease in total thyroid hormone levels relative to changes in free thyroid hormones. Free fatty acid competes with thyroid hormone for binding sites on albumin; free fatty acid levels are commonly increased in acute illness as well. The NACB guidelines recommend the use of total T4 levels in persons who have acute illness [9]. Although one study found estimated free thyroid hormone levels calculated from total T4 and T-uptake to be normal in most acutely ill individuals [23], two other studies showed significant limitations of total T4 in acute illness. In one study, the calculated free thyroxine index was low in about 10% to 20% of cases, independent of the assay used [22]. In another study, calculated thyroid index based on total T4 levels was found to correlate with the reduced levels of all three binding proteins [24]. Total and free T3 levels are also typically decreased in individuals who have acute illness, regardless of method used.

Another cause for erroneous total thyroid hormone levels is autoantibodies to thyroid hormones. These are most commonly found in persons who have the major autoimmune thyroid disorders, Graves' disease and Hashimoto's thyroiditis. A recent review estimates the prevalence of antithyroid hormone antibodies in these disorders to be approximately 10%, although not all cause significant interference in thyroid hormone assays [2]. Typically, total thyroid hormone levels are increased, sometimes markedly, by such autoantibodies. The degree of elevation varies between different methods, and increases may involve T4, T3, or both. Naturally occurring antibodies that react with the conjugate used in at least one assay are also capable of interfering in thyroid uptake assays, causing falsely low results [25].

Free thyroxine and triiodothyronine

Assays for measurement of free thyroxine have become the most common direct test of thyroid gland function, replacing total thyroid hormone measurements in many laboratories. A recent review highlights some of the problems in the measurement of free thyroxine [26]. The measurement of the extremely small relative amount of free thyroid hormone in the presence of massive amounts of protein-bound hormone must make a number of assumptions. The assay must be highly specific for the free form of the hormone and must not measure any of the bound hormone (or, if it does, it must measure the same proportion in all samples, as in the materials used to calibrate the assay). There must be no other substances that change the affinity of binding proteins for thyroid hormone compared with binding in the calibrators. The intrinsic affinity constants of the binding proteins must be similar to that in the calibrators. The method should be unaffected by changes in the level of the binding proteins. A number of conditions exist that can affect these assumptions and thus the measurement of free thyroid hormones.

One problem with measurement of free thyroid hormones is that there is no definitive method to accurately measure only free thyroid hormone [27]. The definitive method for total thyroid hormone, isotope dilution mass spectrometry, has been applied, in combination with ultrafiltration, for the measurement of free thyroid hormone but has not been evaluated under a wide variety of conditions [28]. The gold standard comparative method, equilibrium dialysis, is known to produce higher results in persons who have acute illness [29] but is thought to provide reliable results under most other circumstances. Because there is no current definitive method, this assumption cannot be validated. The temperature at which the test is performed affects the equilibrium and the results [30], and drugs that alter binding protein affinity affect equilibrium dialysis results.

Few laboratories perform equilibrium dialysis, and most laboratories in North America and Europe typically use methods relying on one of two basic principles [31]. The first assays for free thyroid hormones to be widely available used analogs of thyroid hormone in a competitive format, so that the amount of analog bound to antibody would be inversely proportional to free thyroid hormone concentration. Analogs were originally small-molecular-weight compounds developed so that they did not bind to TBG; however, analogs bound to albumin to varying degrees. Most modern "analog" assays use labeled antibodies (in such assays, T3 is typically used to compete for binding sites on antibody with free T4 in the sample) or an analog fixed to a solid support that competes with free hormone in the sample for binding to a limited amount of a labeled antithyroid hormone antibody. Analog assays are typically used in assays from Bayer, Ortho, and Roche, which collectively are used by about half of laboratories [21]. The other common format uses a two-step approach. Samples are briefly incubated with a bound antibody to thyroid hormone; after washing, a labeled thyroid hormone is added to the bound antibody, and the amount of label remaining bound to the antibody after washing is inversely related to the amount of free thyroid hormone in the sample. Two-step methods are used in assays from Abbott, Beckman-Coulter, and Dade-Behring, and some assays from Diagnostics Production Corporation by the remaining half of laboratories.

The differences in methods lead to variability in results for the same sample between different laboratories. In 1744 laboratories performing free T4 measurement on a fresh frozen sample, different methods reported average free T4 results between 0.79 and 1.17 ng/dL; 38% of methods had average results that differed more than 10% from the average of all methods, and 8% had average results more than 20% different [13]. For most methods, results were comparable on two different mailings of the same sample 6 months apart [21]. For free T3, differences between methods were greater than those for free T4; 55% of methods had average results more

10% from the mean of all methods, whereas 27% of methods differed from the average results by more than 20% [13].

A number of situations can lead to misleading results for free T4. Although less information is available, it is likely that similar changes occur with assays for free T3 because the assay principles are similar. Although free T4 methods are designed to be unaffected by changes in TBG, all (nonequilibrium dialysis) assays are affected to some degree by abnormal TBG levels [32]. In an elegant study using titrated, equilibrated amounts of free thyroxine, extremes of TBG concentration correlated directly with measured free T4. For a number of competitive analog-type and two-step methods, there was little effect of commonly encountered abnormal levels of TBG on measured free T4 [33].

Most studies evaluating free T4 assays in acute illness were done with older methods that commonly produced low results. A number of changes that occur with acute illness could theoretically affect free T4 measurement. Decreases in binding protein levels occur. Changes in pH can alter binding affinities. Free fatty acids increase in many acutely ill individuals, and these can displace T4 from albumin and can affect its measurement in unpredictable ways. In one recent study involving bone marrow transplant recipients, equilibrium dialysis and two one-step methods gave increased results in 20% to 40% of samples, whereas two other one-step methods had results that were mostly within the healthy normal range but with 10% to 20% below normal results; total T4 was normal in 95% of those studies [32]. Although data are limited, immune extraction results were less likely to be abnormal in acute illness than with other methods, with only 10% of results below the lower reference limit [29]. Normal results for free T4 can, therefore, be considered reliable, but abnormal results may be due to problems with the assay method. Laboratories should evaluate the effects of acute illness on their method, and, when requested, should use a different method (preferably one with an artifact that changes results in the opposite direction) to evaluate abnormal results. Discordant results (ie, low by one method and high by another) are likely to represent artifacts of measurement, whereas concordant results by methods with artifacts that change free T4 in opposite directions likely represent thyroid dysfunction.

A number of drugs alter the binding of thyroid hormone to one or more of its binding proteins [34]; these are summarized in Table 4. Most of these effects are method independent and as a result can cause abnormal free thyroid hormone levels in all laboratories.

Calcitonin

Calcitonin measurement has evolved over time, with measurement methods changing from simple competitive immunoassays to sandwich assays. Because of varying levels of other calcitonin gene products, results from competitive assays tended to be up to 10 times those of sandwich assays. Most laboratories use sandwich assays for measurement of calcitonin,

Table 4
Drugs affecting thyroid hormone binding

Drug/Effect	Total T4/T3	Free T4/T3
Furosemide (high-dose intravenous administration), salicylates (displaces T4, effect short lived)	Decrease	Increase by ultrafiltration Decreased in assays with marked dilution
Phenytoin, carbamazepine (decrease binding, decreased thyroid-stimulating hormone response)	Decrease	Decrease in most assays long term, may increase short term, normal by ultrafiltration
Heparin (activates lipoprotein lipase, releasing free fatty acids from triglycerides)	No effect	Increases, degree of increase rises with time of storage, accentuated with high serum triglycerides

Abbreviations: T3, triiodothyronine; T4, thyroxine.

and upper reference limits are usually up to 10 ng/L; using older assays, calcitonin upper reference limits were often 100 ng/L or higher. Even with the use of sandwich assays, calcitonin results show significant differences between methods [35], which makes it difficult to generalize information about calcitonin measurements. Assays that use monoclonal antibodies seem less likely to produce increased calcitonin levels in patients who have nonthyroid conditions than are assays using polyclonal antibodies [36].

Common causes of increased calcitonin with older assays, other than medullary thyroid carcinoma, included renal disease and acute illness. At least some of the increase in calcitonin in these states was due to the presence of other preprocalcitonin cleavage products, such as procalcitonin. Few data exist on the ability of newer calcitonin assays to produce normal results in these conditions. One recent study found that although assays using monoclonal antibodies were significantly less likely to produce elevated results, abnormal results occurred in some individuals who had either condition [36]. Other conditions, such as Hashimoto thyroiditis, may be associated with elevated calcitonin levels [37]. The use of immunometric assays can cause falsely elevated results in patients who have heterophile antibodies, as with other immunometric tests such as TSH.

The utility of calcitonin as a preoperative test in persons who have thyroid nodules (and in nonnodular thyroid disease) remains controversial. Although the German Society for Endocrinology recommends routine screening for medullary thyroid cancer using calcitonin in persons who have nodular goiter (followed by pentagastrin stimulation in patients who have elevated calcitonin) [38], others have recommended against routine calcitonin measurement [39–41].

Thyroglobulin

Thyroglobulin measurement is commonly used to evaluate eradication of thyroid tissue after treatment of differentiated thyroid carcinoma. Before thyroidectomy, the major variables that affect thyroglobulin level are thyroid mass and thyroid injury. After thyroidectomy, and particularly after elimination of remnant thyroid tissue by radioactive iodine, thyroglobulin levels are highly specific for residual thyroid carcinoma.

Thyroglobulin circulates in multiple, slightly different forms, although the variability in thyroglobulin structure is less in thyroid carcinoma than in persons who have benign disease [42]. As with other assays, the multitude of forms leads to discrepant results between different methods, and in some cases results differ by more than 40% between different assays [43]. The optimal lower limit of detection for thyroglobulin is not known; assays that detect extremely low levels (<0.1 ng/mL) detect measurable thyroglobulin in most individuals who have thyroid cancer after radioactive iodine ablation, even in the absence of residual thyroid tissue by even the most sensitive imaging techniques [44].

Commercially available kits for the measurement of thyroglobulin use the immunometric assay format. Heterophile antibodies can cause falsely increased results for thyroglobulin. The major cause for interference in thyroglobulin assays is the presence of thyroglobulin autoantibodies; an estimated 25% of patients who have thyroid cancer are antithyroglobulin positive [1]. With immunometric assays, thyroglobulin is typically falsely decreased, and results may be undetectable. Although some studies have suggested that low titer antibodies may not significantly interfere or that results are reliable if recovery (ie, measurement of thyroglobulin after addition of a known amount of thyroglobulin to samples) is close to 100% [45], other studies have shown that these approaches are unreliable for identifying clinically significant interference, especially with the expected low values in persons after thyroidectomy [3].

A single laboratory (in Dr. Carole Spencer's laboratory at University of Southern California) provides a competitive immunoassay for thyroglobulin with comparison to previous samples for true comparison of changes in results. Because interferences from heterophile antibodies are much less in competitive immunoassays and because thyroglobulin antibodies tend to produce falsely increased results with this assay format, it is often possible to detect whether significant interference is present based on comparison of results between this assay and an immunometric assay result.

Thyroid peroxidase and thyroglobulin antibodies

The methods for measuring these thyroid antibodies have changed over the years. Almost all laboratories use immune absorption assays. These are similar in approach to immunometric assays. A solid support

containing the target of the antibodies is incubated with the patient serum, and a reproducible proportion of antibody present is captured on
the solid support. After washing, an antibody to human immunoglobulin,
labeled in some way, is added. The amount of label is directly proportional to the amount of antibody bound. Until recently, ELISAs were
the most common labels. Chemiluminescence, which has fewer interferences than enzyme assays, is becoming more commonly used. Results
are often reported as units of enzyme activity present (typically reported
as mU/L) or as a signal to cutoff ratio (the cutoff being the arbitrary
amount of "signal" necessary to call a result positive, arbitrarily set as
1.0). Although in most cases there is good correlation between the results
using immune absorption and older assay formats, which were reported
as the highest dilution of serum that produces a positive result, the results are not directly equivalent. In some cases, antibodies are present
in high titer but attach to antigen weakly; such samples produce low signals. With another pattern, low titer antibodies have strong antigen binding and produce high signals. High immune absorption results usually
represent high titer antibodies, whereas weakly positive results are more
likely to be low titer or false-positive results.

Results for antibody assays may differ with kits from different manufacturers. Part of the problem, as summarized in the NACB guidelines, is that
International Reference Preparations used to try to standardize results are
outdated, and these preparations are not used by all assay manufacturers
[9]. It is critical in interpreting results that the reference range reported by
the laboratory be used.

Thyroid peroxidase (TPO) antibodies detect the major antigen found in
older thyroid microsomal antibody assays. Because TPO exists in several
isoforms and degree of glycosylation, the form of TPO used can affect the
ability of the test to detect antibodies in the patient's serum and the degree
to which other antibodies cross-react. Moreover, different patients develop
antibodies to different forms of TPO or to different epitopes of the TPO
molecule, which may affect results. This is generally more of a problem
with low-avidity antibodies and with weakly positive test results. It also
contributes to differences in results between laboratories [46]. In one study
involving six methods, positive results with a new method correlated with
positive results in the five other methods in 87% to 97% of cases [47].

There is controversy over how cutoff values for distinguishing positive
and negative results for TPO antibodies should be determined. The
NACB guidelines suggest using young male patients who have TSH levels
between 0.5 and 2.0 mU/L. Using a "composite logarithmic gaussian distribution," Jensen and colleagues found a cutoff of 9.8 kIU/L compared with
24 kIU/L using the NACB criteria [48].

Thyroglobulin antibodies are of most use in predicting interferences in
thyroglobulin measurement to monitor differentiated thyroid cancer. Because of the large size of thyroglobulin and the presence of different forms

in the circulation, results from different assays may differ. Comparing results from different assays revealed concordance between a new method and five existing methods in 87% and 96% of samples [47].

Probably because of this, results of thyroglobulin antibody "titers" do not correlate with the degree of interference in thyroglobulin assays [49] and cannot therefore be used to "correct" thyroglobulin results for the presence of antibodies. Decreasing levels of thyroglobulin antibody, especially if they become negative after being positive, have been found to correlate with absence of residual thyroid cancer [1]; those with successful treatment lose antibodies an average of 3 years after treatment [50]. It is important for laboratories to use the same method when assessing changes in results, and changes in antibody titer should be made using frozen serum samples analyzed at the same time as new samples from the same patient [9]; however, few laboratories save samples to analyze in this fashion.

Summary

Laboratory tests of thyroid function have improved over the years, but issues remain with their performance. Standardized TSH reference limits will be difficult to establish until TSH assays agree better between laboratories. Immunometric TSH, calcitonin, and thyroglobulin assays are subject to interferences from heterophile antibodies, including rheumatoid factor, which can cause falsely high results that can lead to incorrect diagnoses. Tests of total and free thyroid hormones are subject to a variety of interferences, which are most problematic in persons with acute illness. Differences between methods remain a problem for all thyroid hormone assays.

Because of these issues, it is imperative that those who use the endocrine laboratory be familiar with the tests used for measuring thyroid hormones. Laboratories need to be familiar with the limitations of their assays and prepared to measure hormones by an alternative method in situations where interferences are possible and to interpret the results of tests performed by alternative methods. Until perfect laboratory methods are available, close cooperation between those who perform and those who use thyroid tests is necessary to assure accurate interpretation of test results and appropriate patient care.

References

[1] Spencer C, Takeuchi M, Kazarosyan M, et al. Serum thyroglobulin autoantibodies: prevalence, influence on serum thyroglobulin measurement, and prognostic significance in patients with differentiated thyroid carcinoma. J Clin Endocrinol Metab 1998;83:1121–7.

[2] Despres N, Grant A. Antibody interference in thyroid assays: a potential for clinical misinformation. Clin Chem 1998;44:440–54.

[3] Mariotti S, Barbesino G, Caturegli P, et al. Assay of thyroglobulin in serum with thyroglobulin autoantibodies: an unobtainable goal? J Clin Endocrinol Metab 1995;80: 468–72.

[4] Preissner C, O'Kane D, Singh R, et al. Phantoms in the assay tube: heterophile antibody interferences in serum thyroglobulin assays. J Clin Endocrinol Metab 2003;88:3069–74.

[5] Kricka L. Human anti-animal antibody interferences in immunological assays. Clin Chem 1999;45:942–56.

[6] Reinsberg J. Different efficacy of various blocking reagents to eliminate interferences by human antimouse antibodies with a two-site immunoassay. Clin Biochem 1996;29: 145–8.

[7] Ismail A, Walker P, Barth J, et al. Wrong biochemistry results: two case reports and observational study in 5310 patients on potentially misleading thyroid-stimulating hormone and gonadotropin immunoassay results. Clin Chem 2002;48:2023–9.

[8] Klee G. Interferences in hormone immunoassays. Clin Lab Med 2004;24:1–18.

[9] Demers L, Spencer C. Laboratory medicine practice guidelines: laboratory support for the diagnosis and monitoring of thyroid disease. Thyroid 2003;13:3–126.

[10] Vanderpump M, Tunbridge W, French J, et al. The incidence of thyroid disorders in the community: a twenty year follow up of the Wickham survey. Clin Endocrinol (Oxf) 1995; 43:55–68.

[11] Hollowell J, Staehling N, Flanders W, et al. Serum TSH, T(4), and thyroid antibodies in the United States population (1988 to 1994): National Health and Nutrition Examination Survey (NHANES III). J Clin Endocrinol Metab 2002;87:489–99.

[12] Surks M, Ortiz E, Daniels G, et al. Subclinical thyroid disease: scientific review and guidelines for diagnosis and management. JAMA 2004;291:228–38.

[13] Steele B, Wang E, Klee G, et al. Analytic bias of thyroid function tests: analysis of a College of American Pathologists fresh frozen serum pool by 3900 clinical laboratories. Arch Pathol Lab Med 2005;129:310–7.

[14] Spencer C, Elgen A, Shen D, et al. Specificity of sensitive assays of thyrotropin (TSH) used to screen for thyroid disease in hospitalized patients. Clin Chem 1987;33:1391–6.

[15] Attia J, Margetts P, Guyatt G. Diagnosis of thyroid disease in hospitalized patients: a systematic review. Arch Intern Med 1999;159:658–65.

[16] Persani L, Boragato S, Romoli R, et al. Changes in the degree of sialylation of carbohydrate chains modify the biological properties of circulating thyrotropin isoforms in various physiological and pathological states. J Clin Endocrinol Metab 1998;83:2486–92.

[17] Persani L, Ferretti E, Boragato S, et al. Circulating thyrotropin bioactivity in sporadic central hypothyroidism. J Clin Endocrinol Metab 2000;85:3631–5.

[18] McDermott M, Ridgeway E. Central hypothyroidism. Endocrinol Metab Clin North Am 1998;27:187–203.

[19] Sapin R, d'Herbomez M, Schlienger J, et al. Anti-thyrotropin antibody interference in thyrotropin assays. Clin Chem 1998;44:2557–9.

[20] Halsall D, Fahie-Wilson M, Hall S, et al. Macro thyrotropin-IgG complex causes factitious increases in thyroid-stimulating hormone screening tests in a neonate and mother. Clin Chem 2006;52:1968–9.

[21] Steele B, Wang E, Palmer-Toy D, et al. Total long-term within-laboratory precision of cortisol, ferritin, thyroxine, free thyroxine, and thyroid-stimulating hormone assays based on a college of American pathologists fresh frozen serum study: do available methods meet medical needs for precision? Arch Pathol Lab Med 2005;129:318–22.

[22] Faix J, Rosen H, Velazquez F. Indirect estimation of thyroid hormone-binding proteins to calculate free thyroxine index: comparison of nonisotopic methods that use labeled thyroxine ("T-uptake"). Clin Chem 1995;41:41–7.

[23] Konno N, Hirokawa J, Tsuji M, et al. Concentration of free thyroxin in serum during nonthyroidal illness: calculation or measurement? Clin Chem 1989;35:159–63.

[24] Csako G, Zweig M, Glickman J, et al. Direct and indirect techniques for free thyroxin compared in patients with nonthyroidal illness: II. Effect of prealbumin, albumin, and thyroxin-binding globulin. Clin Chem 1989;35:1655–62.

[25] Ritter D, Brown W, Nahm M, et al. Endogenous serum antibodies that interfere with a common thyroid hormone uptake assay: characterization and prevalence. Clin Chem 1994;40: 1940–3.
[26] Stockigt J. Free thyroid hormone measurement: a critical appraisal. Endocrinol Metab Clin North Am 2001;30:265–89.
[27] Holm S, Hansen S, Faber J, et al. Reference methods for the measurement of free thyroid hormones in blood: evaluation of potential reference methods for free thyroxine. Clin Biochem 2004;37:85–93.
[28] Soldin S, Soukhova N, Janicic N, et al. The measurement of free thyroxine by isotope dilution tandem mass spectrometry. Clin Chim Acta 2005;358:113–8.
[29] Wong T, Pekary A, Hoo G, et al. Comparison of methods for measuring free thyroxin in nonthyroidal illness. Clin Chem 1992;38:720–4.
[30] Ross H, Benraad T. Is free thyroxine accurately measurable at room temperature? Clin Chem 1992;38:880–6.
[31] Midgley J. Direct and indirect free thyroxine assay methods: theory and practice. Clin Chem 2001;47:1352–63.
[32] Sapin R, d'Herbomez M. Free thyroxine measured by equilibrium dialysis and nine immunoassays in sera with various serum thyroxine-binding capacities. Clin Chem 2003;49: 1531–5.
[33] Wang E, Nelson J, Weiss R, et al. Accuracy of free thyroxine measurements across natural ranges of thyroxine binding to serum proteins. Thyroid 2000;10:31–9.
[34] Surks M, Sievert R. Drugs and thyroid function. N Engl J Med 1995;333:1688–94.
[35] Martinetti A, Seregni E, Ferrari L, et al. Evaluation of circulating calcitonin: analytical aspects. Tumori 2003;89:566–8.
[36] Saller B, Gorges R, Reinhardt W, et al. Sensitive calcitonin measurement by two-site immunometric assays: implications for calcitonin screening in nodular thyroid disease. Clin Lab 2002;48:191–200.
[37] Karanikas G, Moameni A, Poetzi C, et al. Frequency and relevance of elevated calcitonin levels in patients with neoplastic and nonneoplastic thyroid disease and in healthy subjects. J Clin Endocrinol Metab 2004;89:515–9.
[38] Karges W, Dralle H, Raue F, et al. Calcitonin measurement to detect medullary thyroid carcinoma in nodular goiter: German evidence-based consensus recommendation. Exp Clin Endocrinol Diabetes 2004;112:52–8.
[39] American Association of Clinical Endocrinologists and Associazone Medici Endocrinologi medical guidelines for clinical practice for the diagnosis and management of thyroid nodules. Endocr Pract 2006;12:63–102.
[40] Castro M, Gharib H. Continuing controversies in the management of thyroid nodules. Ann Intern Med 2005;142:926–31.
[41] Hodak S, Burman K. The calcitonin conundrum: is it time for routine measurement of serum calcitonin in patients with thyroid nodules? J Clin Endocrinol Metab 2004;89: 511–4.
[42] Druetta L, Croizet K, Bornet H, et al. Analyses of the molecular forms of serum thyroglobulin from patients with Graves' disease, subacute thyroiditis or differentiated thyroid cancer by velocity sedimentation on sucrose gradient and Western blot. Eur J Endocrinol 1998;139: 498–507.
[43] Spencer C, Wang C. Thyroglobulin measurement: techniques, clinical benefits, and pitfalls. Endocrinol Metab Clin North Am 1995;24:841–63.
[44] Wunderlich G, Zophel K, Crook L, et al. A high-sensitivity enzyme-linked immunosorbent assay for serum thyroglobulin. Thyroid 2001;11:819–24.
[45] Bourrel F, Hoff M, Regis H, et al. Immunoradiometric assay of thyroglobulin in patients with differentiated thyroid carcinomas: need for thyroglobulin recovery tests. Clin Chem Lab Med 1998;36:725–30.

[46] Wood W, Hanke R. Comparability of method results and performance in a national external quality assessment scheme between 1993 and 2003 using thyroid associated antibodies as examples. Clin Lab 2004;50:209–21.

[47] Bohuslavizki K, vom Baur E, Weger B, et al. Evaluation of chemiluminescence immunoassays for detecting thyroglobulin (Tg) and thyroid peroxidase (TPO) autoantibodies using the IMMULITE 2000 system. Clin Lab 2000;46:22–31.

[48] Jensen E, Petersen P, Blaabjerg O, et al. Establishment of reference distributions and decision values for thyroid antibodies against thyroid peroxidase (TPOAb), thyroglobulin (TgAb) and the thyrotropin receptor (TRAb). Clin Chem Lab Med 2005;44:991–8.

[49] Cubero J, Rodriguez-Espinosa J, Gelpi C, et al. Thyroglobulin autoantibody levels below the cut-off for positivity can interfere with thyroglobulin measurement. Thyroid 2003;13:659–61.

[50] Chiovato L, Latrofa F, Braverman L, et al. Disappearance of humoral thyroid autoimmunity after complete removal of thyroid antigens. Ann Intern Med 2003;139:346–51.

ELSEVIER
SAUNDERS

Endocrinol Metab Clin N Am
36 (2007) 595–615

ENDOCRINOLOGY
AND METABOLISM
CLINICS
OF NORTH AMERICA

Hypothyroidism

Madhuri Devdhar, MD, Yasser H. Ousman, MD*,
Kenneth D. Burman, MD

*Washington Hospital Center, 110 Irving Street,
NW, Room 2A-72, Washington, DC 20010-2975 USA*

Hypothyroidism is one of the most common disorders encountered in an endocrine office practice. Hypothyroidism results from reduced thyroid hormone actions at the peripheral tissues. This reduction in thyroid hormone action is, in the vast majority of cases, secondary to reduced thyroid hormone synthesis and secretion by the thyroid gland. Occasionally, peripheral resistance to thyroid hormone is the culprit. The availability of sensitive biochemical tests and effective therapies has simplified the diagnosis and management of this endocrine condition. This article reviews the epidemiology, etiology, clinical presentation, diagnosis, and treatment of hypothyroidism. We emphasize some of the more recent issues, such as combination thyroid hormone therapy, management of hypothyroidism during pregnancy, and the management of subclinical hypothyroidism.

Epidemiology

Hypothyroidism is a relatively common disorder. The prevalence of hypothyroidism increases with age, and the disorder is nearly 10 times more common in females than in males. Hypothyroidism is particularly common in areas of iodine deficiency. Individuals who have thyroid peroxidase antibodies and those who have thyroid-stimulating hormone (TSH) values that are in the upper normal range are at increased risk for developing hypothyroidism.

The prevalence of overt hypothyroidism varies according to different surveys between 0.1 and 2% [1]. Subclinical hypothyroidism is more prevalent and can be seen in as many as 15% of older women. In the United States National Health and Nutrition Examination Survey (NHANES III), the

* Corresponding author.
E-mail address: yasser.ousman@medstar.net (Y.H. Ousman).

0889-8529/07/$ - see front matter © 2007 Elsevier Inc. All rights reserved.
doi:10.1016/j.ecl.2007.04.008
endo.theclinics.com

prevalence of overt hypothyroidism was found to be 0.3%;prevalence of sub-clinical hypothyroidism was found to be 4.3% [2].

Etiology

A summary of the most common causes of hypothyroidism is given in Box 1.

Resistance to thyroid hormones

Hypothyroidism may be transient or permanent, central, or primary. Central hypothyroidism can accompany disorders of the hypothalamic-pituitary axis, leading to reduced TSH secretion or reduced biological activity of TSH. As a result, there is reduction in thyroid stimulation by the TSH and, secondarily, reduced thyroid hormone synthesis and secretion.

Primary hypothyroidism refers to a defect in the thyroid gland resulting in reduced synthesis and secretion of thyroid hormones.

Central hypothyroidism

Central hypothyroidism is classically divided into secondary hypothyroidism, where the defect is in the pituitary gland, and tertiary hypothyroidism, where the defect is in the hypothalamus. From a practical point of view,

---

Box 1. Causes of hypothyroidism

Central hypothyroidism
Pituitary tumors, metastasis, hemorrhage, necrosis, aneurysms
Surgery, trauma
Infiltrative disorders
Infectious diseases
Chronic lymphocytic hypophysitis
Other brain tumors
Congenital abnormalities, defects in thyrotropin releasing
    hormone, TSH, or both

Primary hypothyroidism
Chronic autoimmune thyroiditis
Subacute, silent, postpartum thyroiditis
Iodine deficiency, iodine excess
Thyroid surgery, I-131 treatment, external irradiation
Infiltrative disorders
Drugs
Agenesis and dysgenesis of the thyroid

the end result is the same: a reduction in the release of biologically active TSH. A variety of disorders can cause central hypothyroidism. In clinical practice, pituitary adenomas are the most common. Less prevalent conditions include pituitary apoplexy and infiltrative disorders of the hypothalamus-pituitary axis, such as sarcoidosis, tuberculosis, and other granulomatous diseases. Depending on the extent of the damage incurred by the hypothalamus-pituitary axis, central hypothyroidism may be reversible or permanent. Although isolated deficiency of thyrotropin releasing hormone (TRH) or TSH is possible [3–5], more often the patient who has central hypothyroidism presents with deficiency of other pituitary hormones, and central hypothyroidism is only part of the larger clinical picture of hypopituitarism.

Primary hypothyroidism

Primary hypothyroidism is responsible for the majority of hypothyroid cases. The following discussion reviews the most common entities that result in primary hypothyroidism.

Chronic autoimmune (Hashimoto's) thyroiditis is the leading cause of primary hypothyroidism in iodine-sufficient areas. Clinically, patients who have Hashimoto's thyroiditis may present with or without goiter. Pathophysiologically, there is cell-mediated and antibody-mediated destruction of the thyroid gland [6]. Most patients have measurable autoantibodies against different components of the thyroid gland (thyroid peroxidase, thyroglobulin, TSH receptor, TSH blocking antibodies) [7–9]. Occasionally, a patient may present with thyrotoxicosis due to the presence of thyroid-stimulating autoantibodies (Hashitoxicosis) [10].

The prevalence is several times higher in women than in men. The prevalence of overt hypothyroidism varies from less than 1% to 2% of the population. Up to 15% of elderly women have thyroid autoantibodies [11]. Euthyroid individuals, who have detectable thyroid autoantibodies, are at increased risk for developing overt hypothyroidism.

Hypothyroidism due to autoimmune thyroiditis may be part of a polyglandular failure syndrome that may include autoimmune adrenal insufficiency, type 1 diabetes mellitus, hypogonadism, pernicious anemia, and vitiligo.

Iodine

Iodine deficiency is the most common cause of hypothyroidism [12]. Patients often have large goiters. Transient hypothyroidism may also result from iodine excess. This is referred to as the Wolff-Chaikoff effect. Most patients eventually escape this effect. Large amounts of iodine are found in radiographic contrast agents and in the drug amiodarone.

Thyroidectomy and radioactive iodine therapy of patients who have Graves disease, toxic thyroid nodules, or toxic multinodular goiters are common causes of hypothyroidism [13,14].

Postablative hypothyroidism develops several weeks after radioactive iodine therapy. Partial thyroidectomy may leave sufficient thyroid tissue behind to prevent the patient from taking thyroid hormone replacement [15]. Periodic monitoring of thyroid function tests is important after thyroidectomy and radioactive iodine therapy for early detection and treatment of hypothyroidism.

Hypothyroidism can occur after external radiation of the head and neck and after whole-body radiation. It usually takes several years for hypothyroidism to develop in these circumstances [16–18]. Given the relatively high incidence of hypothyroidism after head and neck irradiation, recipients of such therapy need periodic clinical and biochemical assessment of their thyroid function.

In addition to an increased risk of papillary thyroid cancer, children living in areas of radioactive fallout from the Chernobyl nuclear accident have a higher prevalence of thyroid autoantibodies [19] and may be at increased risk of developing hypothyroidism.

Amiodarone and lithium are among a number of drugs that can cause hypothyroidism. Both drugs are widely used in clinical practice. Thyroid function tests should be obtained before initiating therapy with these agents and periodically thereafter. Other incriminated drugs include perchlorate (rarely used clinically), ethionamide, interferon alfa, and interleukin-2. Thyroid function usually normalizes after discontinuation if these drugs.

Cases of primary hypothyroidism have occasionally been reported in patients who have infiltrative and infectious diseases such as fibrous thyroiditis of Riedel, sarcoidosis (which can also cause central hypothyroidism), hemochromatosis, leukemia, lymphoma, cystinosis, amyloid, scleroderma, and *Mycobacterium tuberculosis* and *Pneumocystis carinii* infection [20].

The antithyroid drugs propylthiouracil and methimazole are used to treat patients who have thyrotoxicosis. Overdosage can result in hypothyroidism.

Children and infants can present with hypothyroidism due to thyroid gland agenesis and dysgenesis and defects in thyroid hormone biosynthesis [21]. Treatment of thyrotoxic women during pregnancy with antithyroid drugs can result in hypothyroidism in the neonate.

Generalized resistance to thyroid hormone is a rare, autosomal recessive disorder caused by mutations in the tri-iodothyronine (T3) receptor gene [22]. The TSH level is usually normal. Thyroxine (T4) and T3 levels are elevated. Patients who have this disorder are usually euthyroid and do not require thyroid hormone replacement.

Transient hypothyroidism usually occurs in the setting of thyroiditis [23,24]. Common forms of thyroiditis include subacute thyroiditis, silent thyroiditis and postpartum thyroiditis, and consumptive hypothyroidism.

Subacute thyroiditis is usually preceded by a viral syndrome occurring a few weeks earlier. Patients typically present with tenderness in the anterior neck. An initial phase of hyperthyroidism is typical. This is followed by a hypothyroid phase that may last a few weeks to several months. There is return to a euthyroid state, but permanent hypothyroidism may develop [25].

Silent thyroiditis and post partum thyroiditis have a similar clinical course to subacute thyroiditis except for the absence of the prodromic syndrome. Postpartum thyroiditis is seen in 3% to 16% of postpartum women [26]. The disorder is more common in women who have type 1 diabetes and in those who have thyroid autoantibodies [26,27].

Consumptive hypothyroidism is a rare situation where hypothyroidism is the result of certain vascular and fibrotic tumors. A type 3 deiodinase present in these tumors metabolizes T4 and T3 into the inactive reverse T3 and T2, respectively [28].

Subclinical hypothyroidism

Subclinical hypothyroidism is the term used to define a state in which serum T4 and T3 levels are within normal limits, but there is underlying mild thyroid failure, as evidenced by a mild increase in serum TSH. The condition is sometimes designated as compensated, early, latent, mild, minimally symptomatic, and preclinical hypothyroidism [29,30].

The etiology of subclinical hypothyroidism is similar to that of overt hypothyroidism. Chronic autoimmune thyroiditis is the leading cause. In one study, chronic autoimmune thyroiditis was found in approximately 55% of patients who had mild thyroid failure [31]. Other common causes of subclinical hypothyroidism include thyroid ablation with radioactive iodine; partial thyroidectomy antithyroid drugs; external beam radiation; drugs such as amiodarone, lithium, or radiographic contrast agents; and inadequate T4 therapy for overt hypothyroidism (intentionally or due to poor patient compliance) [32].

Natural history

Mild thyroid failure represents an early stage of thyroid disease, and it has been shown that there is progression to overt hypothyroidism in approximately 4% to 18% of patients who have subclinical hypothyroidism every year [33,34]. The likelyhood of progression to overt hypothyroidism increases in the presence of antithyroid antibodies, serum TSH values greater than 20 $\mu U/mL$, positive history of radioiodine ablation therapy, history of external radiation therapy for nonthyroid malignancies, and chronic lithium treatment. One study found that a significant number of patients who had subclinical hypothyroidism recovered normal thyroid function, suggesting a transient form of thyroiditis as the probable etiology.

Symptoms

Patients who have subclinical hypothyroidism may be asymptomatic or may present with vague, nonspecific symptoms like fatigue; generalized weakness; depression; and memory, cognitive, and sleep disturbances. As in other thyroid disorders, there is a female preponderance. Women who have subclinical hypothyroidism may present with menstrual irregularities such as menorrhagia or fertility problems. Underlying maternal mild thyroid failure during pregnancy is an independent risk factor for adverse development in the offspring.

Cardiovascular system

Several epidemiologic studies have implicated subclinical hypothyroidism as a cardiovascular risk factor. The Rotterdam study [35] revealed an increased incidence of aortic atherosclerosis (odds ratio, 1.7) and myocardial infarction (odds ratio, 2.3) in women who had subclinical hypothyroidism [36]. Some studies have shown positive correlation between subclinical hypothyroidism and increased serum levels of total cholesterol and low-density-lipoprotein (LDL) cholesterol along with decreased high-density-lipoprotein cholesterol [37,38].

Subclinical hypothyroidism in the elderly population

A recent cross-sectional survey identified an independent association between the prevalence of subclinical thyroid dysfunction and deprivation that cannot be explained solely by the greater burden of chronic disease or consequent drug therapies in the elderly population [39]. One of the major difficulties in interpreting the results of these studies is related to the fact that thyroid function tests are not measured periodically. The TSH is sometimes obtained only at baseline with no further follow-up and therefore dose not take into accounts the possibility that a significant percentage of the study population might have progressed over time into overt hypothyroidism. Another important aspect is the fact that some studies included patients with varying degrees of TSH elevations.

Clinical presentation

The scope of thyroid hormone deficiency encompasses the different body systems and organs. The clinical presentation of a patient who has hypothyroidism depends on the severity of the condition. This depends on the degree of biochemical hypothyroidism. There is significant individual variation. Some patients present with mild symptoms in spite of having low levels of circulating thyroid hormones. Others who have less pronounced biochemical hypothyroidism may be more symptomatic. This is also true for patients who have thyrotoxicosis.

Many of the symptoms of hypothyroidism have poor sensitivity, and it is common for the physician to have patients referred for "thyroid dysfunction or thyroid imbalance" because of symptoms of fatigue, low energy, tiredness, weight gain, or memory changes. The increasing availability to the consumer of medical information, sometimes with excellent scientific value and sometimes with a commercial end in mind, leads some individuals to press the physician on the thyroid issue in spite of the fact that they have normal thyroid function.

In hypothyroidism, there is accumulation of matrix glycosaminoglycans in the interstitial fluids [40]. This is due to increased synthesis of hyaluronic acid. This and the metabolic change typical of the hypothyroid state explain many of the clinical symptoms and signs reported by individuals who have hypothyroidism.

Nutrition and metabolism

In hypothyroidism, there is slowing down of the body's metabolism. Basal metabolic rate and oxygen consumption are reduced. Reduced thermogenesis results in cold intolerance. Food intake and appetite are reduced, but body weight may increase due to water and salt retention and accumulation of fat. There is slowing down of the turnover of protein, biosynthesis of fatty acids, and lipolysis. Total and LDL cholesterol concentrations are increased due to reduced clearance of LDL cholesterol [41]. Serum triglycerides are normal or increased. A slight increase in HDL2 concentration may be seen. Plasma homocysteine level is increased [42]. The changes in lipid metabolism confer an atherogenic profile to the hypothyroid patient. Thyroid function screening should be performed in all patients who have hypercholesterolemia.

Hyponatremia is seen in patients who have profound hypothyroidism and is due to reduced renal free water excretion [43,44]. Serum creatinine is increased in many patients who have hypothyroidism [45].

Cardiovascular system

Reduction in myocardial contractility and heart rate results in reduced cardiac output and reduced exercise tolerance [46]. Systemic vascular resistance is increased, as is the diastolic blood pressure.

Hypothyroid patients can present with pericardial and pleural effusions. This accounts in part for the low voltage seen on the electrocardiographic tracings of these individuals.

Skin and appendages

Typical findings in hypothyroidism include dry, pale, sometimes yellow skin. Nonpitting edema is caused by the accumulation of glycosaminoglycans [47]. Hair is coarse and fragile. Nails are brittle. The presence of pretibial edema may be a clue to making the diagnosis of hypothyroidism. Sweating is reduced.

Nervous system

Sleepiness, slowing of thought processes, and memory changes are common features of hypothyroidism [48]. Functional imaging studies have shown reductions in cerebral blood flow and glucose metabolism that may account for the observed clinical changes.

A delay in the relaxation phase of deep tendon reflexes is an important bedside test when evaluating a patient suspected of having hypothyroidism. Hypothyroidism should be in the differential diagnosis of carpel tunnel syndrome.

Respiratory system

Hypoventilation and hypercapnia are serious complications of profound hypothyroidism. These changes are due to respiratory muscle weakness and inappropriate respiratory response to hypoxemia and hypercapnia [49,50]. Hypothyroidism may cause or worsen sleep apnea.

Gastrointestinal system

Constipation results from reduced intestinal motility and is a common symptom in patients who have hypothyroidism [51]. As with other autoimmune conditions, there is an increased risk of pernicious anemia and gastric atrophy in hypothyroidism.

Reproductive system

Oligo-amenorrhea or hypermenorrhea-menorrhagia can be present [52]. Patients who have primary hypothyroidism may have mild to moderate serum prolactin elevation due to increased prolactin secretion under the stimulatory effect of TRH. Hyperprolactinemia can result in hypogonadotropic hypogonadism. There is reduced fertility and increased risk of miscarriage.

Levels of total testosterone in men may be reduced in hypothyroidism due to areduction in the level of sex hormone–binding globulin. In these patients, the measurement of free or bioavailable testosterone is a better indicator of their gonadal status.

Hypothyroidism and pregnancy

Overt hypothyroidism is seen in about 1% to 2% of pregnant women [53]. Subclinical hypothyroidism is seen in another 2.5% [54]. Most cases of hypothyroidism during pregnancy have the same etiology as in hypothyroidism in general. In pregnancy, there is increased requirement of thyroid hormone [55] because of the increased rate of metabolism of thyroid hormones in the mother's body and transplacental transport of thyroid hormone, which is essential for the development and maturation of the different organs of the fetus [56,57]. As a result, women who have underlying thyroid disorders are more susceptible to becoming hypothyroid during pregnancy.

Some investigators recommend an automatic increase in thyroid hormone replacement dose early during pregnancy in women who have hypothyroidism. This issue is discussed later in this article.

Maternal hypothyroidism, overt and subclinical, during pregnancy is associated with a number of complications including, spontaneous abortion, pre-eclampsia, miscarriage, still birth, preterm delivery, and postpartum hemorrhage.

Negro and colleagues [58] demonstrated beneficial effects of levothyroxine treatment even in euthyroid pregnant women who had autoimmune thyroid disease. This study revealed that euthyroid women who have TPO antibodies may develop impaired thyroid function during pregnancy, and this is associated with an increased risk of miscarriage and premature deliveries. Therefore, in these women, treatment with thyroid hormone lowers the chances of miscarriage and premature delivery.

Normal thyroid function in the mother is critical for normal fetal brain development and for normal fetal neuropsychointellectual function. The fetal thyroid function begins at about 10 to 12 weeks of gestation, and the concentrations of free T4 and TSH reach mean adult values at about 36 weeks of gestation [59]. During the first and second trimester of pregnancy, when most of the development and maturation of the central nervous system occurs in the fetus, the thyroid hormone is solely derived from the mother [60]. Therefore, overt hypothyroidism in the mother during the early stages of pregnancy can lead to severe and permanent damage in the neuropsychointellectual function of the fetus, whereas hypothyroidism in the latter stages of pregnancy may lead to a less significant and partially reversible neurocognitive impairment [61].

Haddow and colleagues [62] showed that the IQ scores of offspring of women who had mildly elevated TSH during pregnancy were 4 points lower than those of offspring of matched, euthyroid women, indicating that mild thyroid failure during pregnancy may adversely affect the neurocognitive development of the fetus.

Diagnosis

The diagnosis of hypothyroidism is based on the combination of clinical context and laboratory tests. Imaging of the brain and pituitary gland is required for patients in whom central hypothyroidism is suspected.

In the majority of patients, making the diagnosis of hypothyroidism should not be complicated. A number of factors can affect the levels of TSH, total T4, and total T3; in particular, several medical conditions can increase or decrease the concentration of total T4 and total T3 through their effect on serum levels of thyroxine-binding globulin and albumin. Examples include estrogens, nephrotic syndrome, and other states of hypoproteinemia. The serum levels of free T4 remain normal in these circumstances and provide a better assessment of thyroid function.

We measure TSH, freeT4 (FT4), and total T3 (TT3) in patients who are suspected of having thyroid dysfunction. Some laboratories offer a thyroid panel that includes TSH, T3 resin uptake, and TT4. A free T4 "index" is calculated and offered as a substitute for a free T4. In addition, we may order thyroid peroxidase (TPO) and thyroglobulin antibodies in a subset of patients. Dynamic testing with TRH is seldom needed. Contrary to the situation in hyperthyroidism, radionuclide studies of the thyroid have much less of a role in hypothyroidism. In addition to its role in evaluating goiters and thyroid nodules, thyroid sonography can disclose the typical heterogeneous parenchymal echogenicity that characterizes Hashimoto's thyroiditis.

Patients who have primary hypothyroidism have elevated TSH and low FT4 and TT3. TPO antibodies are detectable in many patients who have Hashimoto's thyroiditis.

A repeatedly elevated TSH, between 4 and 15 mIU/mL, with normal FT4 and TT3 is suggestive of subclinical hypothyroidism. This is a good indication for obtaining TPO antibodies.

Routine measurement of thyroid function tests in hospitalized patients is not recommended due to the effect of nonthyroidal illness on thyroid function tests.

Patients who have central hypothyroidism have low FT4 and TT3. The TSH can be low, normal, or mildly elevated. If central hypothyroidism is suspected, the entire function of the hypothalamic-pituitary axis should be evaluated with the appropriate tests. If a diagnosis of central hypothyroidism is made, imaging of the brain and pituitary gland should be obtained (we prefer MRI as the initial study).

Several laboratory scenarios are worth mentioning here. Patients who are recovering from acute, nonthyroidal illness typically have a rebound in TSH level. T4 and T3 are usually normal in these patients. These patients should not be treated with thyroid hormone replacement, and their thyroid function should be re-evaluated after 2 to 3 weeks. Normalization of their thyroid function is the general rule.

Poor compliance with pharmacologic therapy can be encountered in patients who are taking thyroid hormone replacement. Some patients may not take their thyroid replacement pills for days and take several pills the day of their doctor's visit. An elevated TSH with high-normal or elevated FT4 is typical. No change in the levothyroxine dose is needed in this situation; rather, emphasis should be placed on compliance with therapy and repeat thyroid function in 3 to 4 weeks.

Treatment of hypothyroidism

Hypothyroidism can cause considerable morbidity. The treatment of hypothyroidism is, in principle, simple. Synthetic thyroxine is the preferred form of thyroid hormone replacement therapy. Hypothyroidism in the majority of patients is permanent and should be treated lifelong. The main exceptions are patients who have transient hypothyroidism due to subacute thyroiditis and patients who have drug-induced hypothyroidism. These patients should be treated during their hypothyroid phase.

The main goal of treatment is to restore the euthyroid state determined by measuring the serum thyrotropin levels, which should be maintained within the acceptable range. The other goals of therapy are to improve hypothyroid symptoms in these patients (although this could be highly individualized) and to decrease goiter size in patients who have goitrous autoimmune thyroiditis.

The choice of the starting dose of synthetic thyroxine should take into consideration factors such as age, presence of coronary artery disease and cardiac arrhythmias. Treatment can be started with a full replacement dose of 1.6 μg/kg/d in young and healthy adult patients who have no significant comorbidities [63], but in elderly patients or those who have significant underlying coronary artery disease, it is prudent to start thyroxine at a dose of 25 μg to 50 μg once daily. Because the plasma half-life of synthetic thyroxine is about 7 days, once-daily dosing results in a steady state being reached in about 6 weeks, with fairly stable serum T3 and T4 concentrations [63]. The dose of LT4 can then be increased by increments of 12.5 or 25 μg every 1 to 2 weeks until a normal TSH is achieved.

LT4 is a prohormone with little intrinsic activity. LT4 is converted by the peripheral tissues in the body to the active form T3, through which most of the actions of thyroid hormone are exerted. About 80% of T3 is obtained from the peripheral conversion of T4; the remaining 20% is obtained from direct thyroid secretion [64]. This is favorable in two ways: the patient's body controls the conversion of T4 to T3 and, there is a steady and adequate supply of T3 to the body.

T4 formulations

Several generic and branded formulations of LT4 are available, ranging from 25 μg to 300 μg in about 12 different strengths. There has been controversy regarding the bioavailability of these formulations. The US Food and Drug Administration in 2004 rejected a petition regarding the bioequivalence of levothyroxine sodium products and approved first-time generic levothyroxine sodium for the treatment of hypothyroidism. Nevertheless, current recommendations of the American Thyroid Association, The Endocrine Society, and American Association of Clinical Endocrinologists are to encourage patients to remain on the same levothyroxine formulation [65]. When patients must switch brands or use a generic, serum TSH should be checked 2 to 4 weeks later, and the dose should be modified accordingly.

Factors affecting T4 absorption

T4 is primarily absorbed in the jejunum, and about 70% of the dose administered is absorbed on an empty stomach [66]. Ideally, thyroxine should be taken on an empty stomach about 30 minutes before breakfast.

In one study evaluating the effect of food on the bioavailability of thyroxine, a breakfast containing bacon, eggs, toast, hash brown potatoes, and milk reduced thyroxine absorption by about 40% [67]. Calcium, iron in supplements, antacids, proton pump inhibitors, anticonvulsants, and food products increase the requirement of thyroxine by different mechanisms.

Monitoring of treatment

Adequacy of treatment is monitored by measurement of serum TSH levels. Serum TSH levels must be measured 4 to 6 weeks after commencing treatment and every 4 to 6 weeks thereafter until a normal TSH is reached. Although normal serum TSH levels range from 0.4 to 4 mU/L, many physicians prefer a target range of 0.5 to 3.0 mIU/L or 0.4 to 2.0 mIU/L, particularly in young and otherwise healthy patients. This is based on data form the NHANES III survey. Once target levels of serum TSH are reached, it is prudent to measure serum TSH and Free T4 levels once a year provided no other medications that may change the requirement of synthetic thyroxine are added. In addition, the patients may report amelioration of hypothyroid symptoms, which reflects adequacy of treatment, although this may be subjective and individualized.

If the patient has to be started on medications that are known to affect the absorption or metabolism of T4, serum TSH levels should be checked 4 to 6 weeks after the initiation of these medications to make sure that the dose of synthetic thyroxine is adequate. If necessary, the dose can be adjusted until the serum TSH levels are within the normal range.

Adverse effects of T4

An important adverse effect of treatment with synthetic thyroxine is hyperthyroidism due to over-replacement. It is estimated that more than one fifth of patients on treatment are clinically or subclinically thyrotoxic [68]. These patients have a suppressed (below 0.1) or low (between 01 and 0.4 mIU/L) TSH depending on the degree of over-replacement. In women over 65 years of age, a low serum TSH level is associated with a significantly increased risk of hip and vertebral fractures [69]. In the Framingham study, a TSH below 0.1 is associated with a threefold increased risk of atrial fibrillation in patients over the age of 60 years [70]. Rare adverse effects include allergy to the dye in the tablets.

Combination therapy with T3 and T4

Some patients who have hypothyroidism remain symptomatic in spite of replacement and normal serum TSH concentrations. For example, in a questionnaire-based study of patients who were taking thyroxin replacement, a significant percentage of patients reported an attenuated sense of psychosomatic well-being [71]. T4 normalizes FT4 and TSH levels in about 4 to 6 weeks, during which time symptoms may persist, whereas the onset of action of T3 is faster. Therefore, it was hypothesized that a combination of T3 and T4 may prove superior to treatment with T4 alone. Several controlled clinical trials compared treatment with T4 alone and combination treatment of T4 and T3. In only one study was there a significant improvement in mood, cognitive symptoms, and quality of life in favor of the T4 and T3 combination [72]. Other randomized controlled trials have failed to show similar findings [73–75]. In these studies, there was no improvement in psychologic or psychometric performance by objective tests, although in some of these studies, patients preferred a T3 plus T4 combination therapy for reasons unexplained objectively. A recent meta-analysis evaluated the results from 11 randomized control trials that included 1216 patients. The conclusion was that T4 and T3 combination was not superior to thyroxine monotherapy with respect to bodily pain, depression, anxiety, fatigue, quality of life, body weight, total serum cholesterol, triglyceride levels, low-density lipoprotein, and high-density lipoprotein [76]. Saravanan and colleagues [77] have shown that psychologic well-being correlates with free thyroxine but not free 3,5,3'-T3 levels in patients on thyroid hormone replacement. In addition to not improving general well being in patients who have hypothyroidism, T3 preparations result in wide-ranging fluctuations in serum T3 levels due to rapid gastrointestinal absorption and rapid onset of action. This can lead to arrhythmias, especially in elderly patients and in those who have underlying cardiac disease. Recent advances have shown that a slow-release preparation of T3 combined with T4 in the treatment of hypothyroidism avoids peaks in and fluctuating levels of serum T3, although larger-scale trials are warranted in this regard. Based on the current available literature, we do not recommend the use of T4 and T3 in combination to treat patients who have hypothyroidism.

Treatment of patients who have secondary or central hypothyroidism

In central hypothyroidism, TSH cannot be used as marker of adequate replacement therapy; instead, one should rely on the FT4 and sometimes Free T3 (FT3) concentrations. Typically, T4 and T3 levels are obtained before the daily dose of T4 is taken. We target FT4 and FT3 levels in the mid- to upper normal range.

Treatment of poorly compliant patients

The half life of thyroxine is 7 days. It can be given once weekly, which is beneficial in poorly compliant patients. A crossover trial of 12 patients showed that a single weekly dose achieved fairly good therapeutic results. Weekly dosing is contraindicated in patients who have coronary artery disease [78].

Management of hypothyroidism in pregnancy

Given the importance of maternal euthyroidism for normal neurocognitive development in the fetus, it is recommended that serial monitoring of serum TSH serum concentrations be performed in hypothyroid pregnant women and pregnant women susceptible to thyroid disease.

Based on the results of a study by Alexander and colleagues [53], it was recommended that for women who are being treated for hypothyroidism, the dose of levothyroxine be increased approximately by 30% as soon as the pregnancy is confirmed. Thereafter, serum thyrotropin levels should be monitored, and the levothyroxine dose should be adjusted accordingly. We recommend monitoring of thyroid function as soon as a pregnancy is confirmed and every 2 to 3 weeks thereafter with adjustment of thyroxine dose based on the results of thyroid function tests.

The target range of TSH during pregnancy is an area of controversy. Some clinicians recommend 0.4 to 4 mIU/L, whereas other clinicians recommend 0.4 to 2 mIU/L.

In recent articles, some investigators raised the question of the utility of administering thyroxine to pregnant women who have elevated levels of TPO antibodies but who otherwise have normal thyroid function tests. Such treatment is given to reduce the risk of miscarriage and premature deliveries that seems to be increased in these women. Further studies are needed in this regard [58,79].

Universal screening of pregnant women for subclinical hypothyroidism and hypothyroxinemia is not recommended because there is no evidence to justify the efficacy of screening and treatment and there have been no interventional studies to prove that this improves outcome [80–83]. Thyroid screening is recommended for high-risk pregnant women, such as those who have a personal history of thyroid or other autoimmune disorders or those who have a family history of thyroid disorders.

Treatment of subclinical hypothyroidism

There is debate on whether to treat subclinical hypothyroidism [84]. The question is whether subclinical hypothyroidism is associated with significant clinical impairment in affected patients, and if so, whether treatment with levothyroxine leads to better outcomes. There are conflicting data and controversial reports in this respect.

There is debate on what should be a "normal" reference range for TSH. The National Academy of Clinical Biochemistry guidelines state that "greater than 95% of healthy, euthyroid subjects have a serum TSH concentration between 0.4 and 2.5 mIU/L" [85]. The latest thyroid disease guidelines of the American Association of Clinical Endocrinologists recommend a reference TSH range of 0.3 to 3.0 mIU/L [86]. Recently, an expert panel met at a joint convention organized by the Endocrine Society, American Thyroid Association, and American Association of Clinical

Endocrinologists. The consensus was that there was good evidence that treatment of patients who have TSH levels above 4.5 mU/L prevents progression to overt hypothyroidism but that there was little convincing evidence that early treatment was beneficial [87]. Another school of thought upholds that there are enough data to support thyroid replacement in individuals who have subclinical hypothyroidism [88–91]. The strongest data in favor of treatment with thyroxine seem to be related to improvement in surrogate markers of cardiovascular disease, such as lipids, vascular resistance, and cardiovascular hemodynamics. Future studies should shed more light on this subject. Studies with hard end points, such as total mortality, cardiovascular mortality, and morbidity, will determine if thyroxine replacement should become the standard care for patients who have subclinical hypothyroidism. In general, treatment is strongly recommended in the following patients who have subclinical hypothyroidism: patients who have TSH levels higher than 10 mIU/L on repeated measurements, patients who have symptoms or signs (eg, goiter) associated with thyroid failure, patients who have convincing family history of thyroid disease, pregnant patients, patients who have a strong habit of tobacco use, or patients who have severe hyperlipidemia.

Myxedema coma

Myxedema coma is a term used to describe severe manifestations of hypothyroidism. It was first reported by Ord [92] in 1879 in London. It is a medical emergency. In the past, the overall mortality rate for myxedema coma was 60% to 70%. Early diagnosis and advances in intensive care and management have reduced the mortality to 20% to 25% [93].

Most patients who have myxedema coma are elderly women who have long-standing or uncontrolled hypothyroidism. Myxedema coma usually occurs during the winter months, suggesting that the low temperatures associated with winter may be a contributing factor for the clinical deterioration of underlying hypothyroidism. Myxedema coma can be precipitated by factors such as hypothermia, acute cardiovascular events such as myocardial infarction and stroke, infection, drugs that can compromise the central nervous system, trauma, and gastrointestinal bleeding.

Clinical features

The diagnosis of myxedema coma is mainly clinical. The presence of marked stupor, confusion, or coma and hypothermia in a patient with findings of hypothyroidism is strongly suggestive of myxedema coma. Treatment should not be delayed until the results of thyroid function tests are available. Physical examination is demonstrative of hypothyroidism: dry, coarse, scaly skin; sparse or coarse hair; nonpitting edema of the skin and soft tissues; macroglossia; hoarse voice; and delayed deep tendon reflexes. Other important clinical features of myxedema coma include hypoventilation, bradycardia, decreased cardiac contractility, decreased intestinal motility, paralytic ileus, and megacolon [94]. There is a high incidence of pericardial effusion that may contribute to the decreased cardiac contractility. Early detection of infections that may be the precipitating events for myxedema coma may be difficult because bradycardia and hypothermia are likely to mask the fever and tachycardia of infections.

Laboratory findings in myxedema coma

Elevated TSH, very low serum total T4, FT4, and TT3 concentrations confirm the diagnosis of myxedema coma. The TSH level in myxedema coma may underestimate the degree of biochemical hypothyroidism because many of these patients may have a nonthyroidal illness in addition to severe hypothyroidism, and this can lower the TSH. Other laboratory findings include anemia, hyponatremia, hypercholesterolemia, high serum lactate dehydrogenase, and creatine phosphokinase concentrations. Arterial blood gas may reveal hypoxemia, hypercapnia, and acidosis.

Management of myxedema coma

The patient who has myxedema coma should be managed in an intensive care setting under continuous monitoring. Special attention should be given to ventilatory support in these patients, and mechanical ventilation should be given as required. Hypothermia and hypotension should be corrected. Metabolic disturbances such as hyponatremia, hypoglycemia, and hypercalcemia, which can aggravate the altered mental status, should be corrected. A thorough search for all the precipitating factors for myxedema coma should be done. Cultures should be drawn, and chest radiographs should be taken to rule out infections. If present, they should be treated aggressively with adequate antibiotic therapy.

Glucocorticoid therapy

All patients in myxedema coma should be given stress-dose steroids for the first 24 to 48 hours because supplementation of thyroid hormones leads to increased metabolism and thereby increases the requirement of cortisol.

Thyroid hormone therapy

T4 alone or in combination with T3 is given. An intravenous route should initially be used. Switching to the oral route is possible when the patient's condition has improved.

The advantages of T4 are a smooth, slow, and steady onset of action. Disadvantages include the need for extrathyroidal conversion of T4 to T3, which may be reduced in patients who have serious illnesses. The onset of action of T4 is slower.

The advantages of T3 therapy include more rapid onset of action and no need for extrathyroidal conversion. T3 crosses the blood–brain barrier more readily than does T4 in baboons [95]. Disadvantages of T3 include rapid action and highly fluctuating serum levels, which may not be desirable in patients who have underlying coronary atherosclerosis.

A commonly used dosing regimen for T4 includes administration of an initial high dose of T4, between 300 to 600 μg. This is followed by maintenance doses of 50 to 100 μg daily [96]. T3 can be administered at a dose of 10 to 20 μg intravenously every 4 hours on the first day followed by gradual tapering over the next 2 days, after which oral administration of T3 or T4 is usually possible.

In a study of eight patients who had myxedema coma, age, the presence of cardiac comorbidities, and a high dose of thyroxine were found to be associated with worse outcome [97]. The small number of the study patients is a limiting factor. The study authors recommended avoiding large dose of thyroxine in the treatment of myxedema in elderly patients.

We usually administer intravenous thyroxine alone at an initial dose of 200 to 400 μg for 2 days followed by a physiologic dose thereafter. We always administer intravenous corticosteroids, in the form of hydrocortisone, 100 mg every 8 hours for the first 24 hours. The first dose of hydrocortisone should be given before thyroxine is administered. Any precipitating factor, such as infection or cardiovascular event, should be addressed and treated appropriately.

References

[1] Vanderpump MP. The epidemiology of thyroid diseases. In: Braverman LE, Utiger RD, editors. The thyroid: a fundamental and clinical text. 9th edition. Philadelphia: Lippincott Williams and Wilkins; 2004. p. 398–406.

[2] Hollowell JG, Staehling NW, Flanders WD, et al. Serum TSH, T(4), and thyroid antibodies in the United States population (1988 to 1994): National Health and Nutrition Examination Survey (NHANES III). J Clin Endocrinol Metab 2002;87:489–99.

[3] Doeker BM, Pfäffle RW, Pohlenz J, et al. Congenital central hypothyroidism due to a homozygous mutation in the thyrotropin beta-subunit gene follows an autosomal recessive inheritance. J Clin Endocrinol Metab 1998;83:1762–5.

[4] Gagné N, Parma J, Deal C, et al. Apparent congenital athyreosis contrasting with normal plasma thyroglobulin levels and associated with inactivating mutations in the thyrotropin receptor gene: are athyreosis and ectopic thyroid distinct entities? J Clin Endocrinol Metab 1998;83:1771–5.

[5] Collu R, Tang J, Castagne J, et al. A novel mechanism for isolated central hypothyroidism: inactivating mutations in he thyrotropin-releasing hormone receptor gene. J Clin Endocrinol Metab 1997;82:1561–5.

[6] Weetman AP, McGregor AM. Autoimmune thyroid disease: further developments in our understanding. Endocr Rev 1994;15:788–830.

[7] Mariotti S, Caturegli P, Piccolo P, et al. Antithyroid peroxidase autoantibodies in thyroid disease. J Clin Endocrinol Metab 1990;71:661–9.

[8] Nordyke RA, Gilbert FI Jr, Miyamoto LA, et al. The superiority of antimicrosomal over antithyroglobulin antibodies for detecting Hashimoto's thyroiditis. Arch Intern Med 1993;153:862–5.

[9] Endo T, Kaneshige M, Nakazato M, et al. Autoantibody against thyroid iodine transporter in the sera from patients with Hashimoto's thyroiditis possesses iodine transport inhibitory activity. Biochem Biophys Res Commun 1996;228:199–202.

[10] Bogner U, Hegedus L, Hansen JM, et al. Thyroid cytotoxic antibodies in atrophic and goitrous autoimmune thyroiditis. Eur J Endocrinol 1995;132:69–74.

[11] Tunbridge WM, Evered DC, Hall R, et al. The spectrum of thyroid disease in a community: the Whickham survey. Clin Endocrinol (Oxf) 1977;7:481–93.

[12] Andersson M, Takkouche B, Egli I, et al. Current global iodine status and progress over the last decade towards the elimination of iodine deficiency. Bull World Health Organ 2005;83: 518–25.

[13] Franklyn JA, Daykin J, Drolc Z, et al. Long-term follow-up of treatment of thyrotoxicosis by three different methods. Clin Endocrinol (Oxf) 1991;34:71–6.

[14] McHenry CR, Slusarczyk SJ. Hypothyroidism following hemithyroidectomy: incidence, risk factors, and management. Surgery 2000;128:994–8.

[15] Sridama V, McCormick M, Kaplan EL, et al. Long-term follow-up study of compensated low-dose 131I therapy for Graves' disease. N Engl J Med 1984;311:426–32.

[16] Hancock SL, Cox RS, McDougall IR. Thyroid diseases after treatment of Hodgkin's disease. N Engl J Med 1991;325:599–605.

[17] Mercado G, Adelstein DJ, Saxton JP, et al. Hypothyroidism: a frequent event after radiotherapy and after radiotherapy with chemotherapy for patients with head and neck carcinoma. Cancer 2001;92:2892–7.

[18] Tell R, Sjodin H, Lundell G, et al. Hypothyroidism after external radiotherapy for head and neck cancer. Int J Radiat Oncol Biol Phys 1997;39:303–8.

[19] Pacini F, Vorontsova T, Molinaro E, et al. Prevalence of thyroid autoantibodies in children and adolescents from Belarus exposed to the Chernobyl radioactive fallout. Lancet 1998;352: 763–6.

[20] Barsano CP. Other forms of primary hypothyroidism. In: Braverman LE, Utiger RD, editors. The thyroid: a fundamental and clinical text. 7th edition. Philadelphia: Lippincott-Raven; 1996. p. 768–78.

[21] Fisher DA, Klein AH. Thyroid development and disorders of thyroid function in the newborn. N Engl J Med 1981;304:702–12.

[22] Brucker-Davis F, Skarulis MC, Grace MB, et al. Genetic and clinical features of 42 kindreds with resistance to thyroid hormone. Ann Intern Med 1995;123:572–83.

[23] Lazarus JH. Silent thyroiditis and subacute thyroiditis. In: Braverman LE, Utiger RD, editors. The thyroid: a fundamental and clinical text. 7th edition. Philadelphia: Lippincott-Raven; 1996. p. 577–91.

[24] Pearce EN, Farwell AP, Braverman LE. Thyroiditis. N Engl J Med 2003;348:2646–55.

[25] Fatourechi V, Aniszewski JP, Fatourechi GZ, et al. Clinical features and outcome of subacute thyroiditis in an incidence cohort: Olmsted County, Minnesota, study. J Clin Endocrinol Metab 2003;88:2100–5.

[26] Gerstein HC. How common is postpartum thyroiditis? A methodologic overview of the literature. Arch Intern Med 1990;150:1397–400.

[27] Sakaihara M, Yamada H, Kato EH, et al. Postpartum thyroid dysfunction in women with normal thyroid function during pregnancy. Clin Endocrinol (Oxf) 2000;53:487–92.

[28] Ruppe MD, Huang SA, Jan de Beur SM. Consumptive hypothyroidism caused by paraneoplastic production of type 3 iodothyronine deiodinase. Thyroid 2005;15:1369–72.

[29] Wilson GR, Curry RW Jr. Subclinical thyroid disease. Am Fam Physician 2005;72:1517–24.

[30] Ayala A, Wartofsky L. Minimally symptomatic (subclinical) hypothyroidism. Endocrinologist 1997;7:44–50.

[31] Hamburger JI, Meier DA, Szpunar WE. Factitious elevation of thyrotropin in euthyroid patients [letter]. N Engl J Med 1985;313:267–8.

[32] Wartofsky L, Van Nostrand D, Burman KD. Overt and 'subclinical' hypothyroidism in women. Obstet Gynecol Surv 2006;61(8):535–42.

[33] Parle JV, Franklyn JA, Cross KW, et al. Prevalence and follow-up of abnormal thyrotrophin (TSH) concentrations in the elderly in the United Kingdom. Clin Endocrinol (Oxf) 1991;34: 77–83.

[34] Huber G, Mitrache C, Guglielmetti M, et al. Predictors of overt hypothyroidism and natural course: a long-term follow-up study in impending thyroid failure. 71st Annual Meeting of the American Thyroid Association. Portland (OR), 1998.

[35] Kahaly GJ. Cardiovascular and atherogenic aspects of subclinical hypothyroidism. Thyroid 2000;10:665–79.

[36] Hak AE, Pols HAP, Visser TJ, et al. Subclinical hypothyroidism is an independent risk factor for atherosclerosis and myocardial infarction in elderly women: the Rotterdam study. Ann Intern Med 2000;132:270–8.

[37] Bindels AJ, Westendorp RG, Frolich M, et al. The prevalence of subclinical hypothyroidism at different total plasma cholesterol levels in middle aged men and women: a need for case-finding? Clin Endocrinol 1999;50:217–20.

[38] Michalopoulou G, Alevizaki M, Piperingos G, et al. High serum cholesterol levels in persons with 'high normal' TSH levels: should one extend the definition of subclinical hypothyroidism. Eur J Endocrinol 1998;138:141–5.

[39] Wilson S, Parle JV, Roberts LM, et al. Prevalence of subclinical thyroid dysfunction and its relation to socioeconomic deprivation in the elderly: a community based cross-sectional survey. J Clin Endocrinol Metab 2006;12:4809–16.

[40] Smith TJ, Bahn RS, Gorman C. Connective tissue, glycosaminoglycans, and diseases of the thyroid. Endocr Rev 1989;10:366–92.

[41] O'Brien T, Dineen SF, O'Brien PC, et al. Hyperlipidemia in patients with primary and secondary hypothyroidism. Mayo Clin Proc 1993;68:860–6.

[42] Hussein WI, Green R, Jacobsen DW, et al. Normalization of hyperhomocysteinemia with L-thyroxine in hypothyroidism. Ann Intern Med 1999;131:348–51.

[43] DeRubertis FR Jr, Michelis MF, Bloom ME, et al. Impaired water excretion in myxedema. Am J Med 1971;51:41–53.

[44] Hanna FW, Scanlon MF. Hyponatraemia, hypothyroidism, and role of arginine-vasopressin. Lancet 1997;350:755–6.

[45] Kreisman SH, Hennessey JV. Consistent reversible elevations of serum creatinine levels in severe hypothyroidism. Arch Intern Med 1999;159:79–82.

[46] Klein I, Ojamaa K. Thyroid hormone and the cardiovascular system: from theory to practice. J Clin Endocrinol Metab 1994;78:1026–7.

[47] Heymann WR. Cutaneous manifestations of thyroid disease. J Am Acad Dermatol 1992;26: 885–902.

[48] Burmeister LA, Ganguli M, Dodge HH, et al. Hypothyroidism and cognition: preliminary evidence for a specific defect in memory. Thyroid 2001;11:1177–85.

[49] Siafakas NM, Salesiotou V, Filaditaki V. Respiratory muscle strength in hypothyroidism. Chest 1992;102:189–94.

[50] Ladenson PW, Goldenheim PD, Ridgeway EC. Prediction and reversal of blunted ventilatory responsiveness in patients with hypothyroidism. Am J Med 1988;84:877–83.

[51] Shafer RB, Prentiss RA, Bond JH. Gastrointestinal transit in thyroid disease. Gastroenterology 1984;86:852–5.

[52] Krassas GE, Pontikides N, Kaltsas T, et al. Disturbances of menstruation in hypothyroidism. Clin Endocrinol (Oxf) 1999;50:655–9.

[53] Alexander EK, Marqusee E, Lawrence J, et al. Timing and magnitude of increases in levothyroxine requirements during pregnancy in women with hypothyroidism. N Engl J Med 2004;351:241–9.

[54] Smallridge RC, et al. Thyroid function inside and outside of pregnancy: what do we know and what dont we know? Thyroid 2005;15:54–9.

[55] Burrow GN, Fisher DA, Larsen PR, et al. Maternal and fetal thyroid function. N Engl J Med 1994;331:1072–8.

[56] Glinoer D, Delange F. The potential repercussions of maternal, fetal, and neonatal hypothyroxinemia on the progeny. Thyroid 2000;10(10):871–87.

[57] Glinoer D. Potential consequences of maternal hypothyroidism on the offspring: evidence
and implications [Review] [17 refs] [Journal Article. Review]. Horm Res 2001;55(3):109–14.

[58] Negro R, Formoso G, Mangieri T, et al. Levothyroxine treatment in euthyroid pregnant
women with autoimmune thyroid disease: effects on obstetrical complications. J Clin Endocrinol Metab 2006;91(7):2587–91.

[59] Thorpe-Beeston JG, et al. Maturation of the secretion of thyroid hormone and thyroid-
stimulating hormone in the fetus. N Engl J Med 1991;324:532–6.

[60] Glinoer D. Management of hypo- and hyperthyroidism during pregnancy. Growth Horm
IGF Res 2003;13(Suppl A):S45–54.

[61] Kasatkina EP, Samsonova LN, Ivakhnenko VN, et al. Gestational hypothyroxinemia and
cognitive function in offspring. Neurosci Behav Physiol 2006;36(6):619–24.

[62] Haddow JE, Palomaki GE, Allan WC, et al. Maternal thyroid deficiency during pregnancy
and subsequent neuropsychological development of the child. N Engl J Med 1999;341:549–55.

[63] Fish LH, Schwartz HL, Cavanaugh J, et al. Replacement dose, metabolism, and bioavailability of levothyroxine in the treatment of hypothyroidism: role of triiodothyronine in pituitary feedback in humans. N Engl J Med 1987;316:764–70.

[64] Pilo A, Arvasi G, Vitek F, et al. Thyroidal and peripheral production of 3,5,3'-triiodothyro-
nine in humans by multicompartmental analysis. Am J Physiol 258:E715–26.

[65] Joint Statement on the U.S. Food and Drug Administration's decision regarding ioequiva-
lence of levothyroxine sodium by American Thyroid Association, The Endocrine Society,
and American Association of Clinical Endocrinologists.

[66] Hays MT, Nielsen KRK. Human thyroxine absorption: age, effects, and methodological
analyses. Thyroid 1994;4:55–64.

[67] Lamson MJ, Pamplin CL, Rolleri RL, et al. Quantitation of a substantial reduction in
levothyroxine absorption by food. Thyroid 2004;14:876.

[68] Canaris Gay J, Manowitz Neil R, Mayor Gilbert, et al. The Colorado thyroid disease prevalence study. Arch Intern Med 2000;160:526–34.

[69] Bauer Douglas C, Ettinger Bruce, et al. Risk for fracture in women with low serum levels of
thyroid-stimulating hormone. Ann Intern Med 2001;134:561–8.

[70] Sawin C, Geller A, Wolf PA, et al. Low serum thyrotropin concentrations as a risk factor for
atrial fibrillation in older persons [see comment] [Journal Article]. N Engl J Med 1994;
331(19):1249–52.

[71] Saravanan P, Chau WF, Roberts N, et al. Psychological well-being in patients on 'adequate'
doses of L-thyroxine: results of a large, controlled community-based questionnaire study.
Clin Endocrinol (Oxf) 2002;57:577–85.

[72] Bunevicius R, Kazanavicius G, Zalinkevicius R, et al. Effects of thyroxine as compared with thyroxine plus triiodothyronine in patients with hypothyroidism. N Engl J Med 1999;340:424–9.

[73] Walsh JP, Shiels L, Lim EM, et al. Combined thyroxine/liothyronine treatment does not
improve well-being, quality of life, or cognitive function compared to thyroxine alone: a
randomized controlled trial in patients with primary hypothyroidism. J Clin Endocrinol
Metab 2003;88:4543–50.

[74] Sawka AM, Gerstein HC, Marriot MJ, et al. Does a combination regimen of thyroxine (T4)
and 3,5,3'-triiodothyronine improve depressive symptoms better than T4 alone in patients
with hypothyroidism? Results of a double-blind, randomized, controlled trial. J Clin Endocrinol Metab 2003;88:4551–5.

[75] Clyde PW, Harari AE, Getka EJ, et al. Combined levothyroxine plus liothyronine compared
with levothyroxine alone in primary hypothyroidism: a randomized controlled trial. JAMA
2003;290:2952–8.

[76] Grozinsky-Glasberg S, Fraser A, Nahshoni E, et al. Thyroxine-triiodothyronine combination therapy versus thyroxine monotherapy for clinical hypothyroidism: meta-analysis of
randomized controlled trials. J Clin Endocrinol Metab 2006;91:2592–9.

[77] Saravanan P, Visser TJ, Dayan CM. Psychological well-being correlates with free thyroxine but not free 3,5,3'-triiodothyronine levels in patients on thyroid hormone replacement. J Clin Endocrinol Metab 2006;91(9):3389–93.
[78] Grebe SKG, Cooke RR, Ford HC, et al. Treatment of hypothyroidism with once weekly thyroxine. J Clin Endocrinol Metab 1997;82:870.
[79] Glinoer D. Miscarriage in women with positive anti-tpo antibodies: is thyroxine the answer? J Clin Endocrinol Metab 2006;91(7):2500–2.
[80] Pop VJ, Vulsma T. Maternal hypothyroxinaemia during (early) gestation. Lancet 2005;365: 1604–6.
[81] American College of Obstertricians and Gynecologists. ACOG practice bulletin. Clinical management guidelines for obstretician-gynecologists. No 37: thyroid disease in pregnancy. Obstet Gynecol 2002;100:387–96.
[82] Surks MI. Subclinical thyroid dysfunction: a joint statement on management from the American association of clinical endocrinologists, the American thyroid association and the endocrine society. J Clin Endocrinol Metab 2005;90:586–7.
[83] Spong CY. Subclinical hypothyroidism: should all pregnant women be screened? Obstet Gynecol 2005;105:235–6.
[84] Pinchera A. Subclinical thyroid disease: to treat or not to treat? Thyroid 2005;15:1–2.
[85] Baloch Z, Carayon P, Conte-Devolx B, et al. Guidelines committee, national academy of clinical biochemistry. Laboratory medicine practice guidelines: laboratory support for the diagnosis and monitoring of thyroid disease. Thyroid 2003;13:3–126.
[86] Baskin HJ, Cobin RH, Duick DS, et al. American association of clinical endocrinologists medical guidelines for clinical practice for the evaluation and treatment of hyperthyroidism and hypothyroidism. Endocr Pract 2002;8:457–69.
[87] Surks MI, Ortiz E, Daniels GH, et al. Subclinical thyroid disease: scientific review and guidelines for diagnosis and management. JAMA 2004;291:228–38.
[88] Jorde Rolf, Waterloo Knut, Storhaug Hilde, et al. Neuropsychological function and symptoms in subjects with subclinical hypothyroidism and the effect of thyroxine treatment. J Clin Endocrinol Metab 2006;91:145–53.
[89] Milionis HJ, Tambaki AP, Kanioglou CN, et al. Thyroid substitution therapy induces high density lipoprotein-associated platelet-activating factor acetylhydrolase in patients with subclinical hypothyroidism: a potential antiatherogenic effect. Thyroid 2005;15:455–60.
[90] Caraccio N, Natali A, Sironi A, et al. Muscle metabolism and exercise tolerance in subclinical hypothyroidism: a controlled trial of levothyroxine. J Clin Endocrinol Metab 2005;90: 4057–62.
[91] Brenta G, Mutti LA, Schnitman M, et al. Assessment of left ventricular diastolic function by radionuclide ventriculography at rest and exercise in subclinical hypothyroidism, and its response to thyroxine therapy. Am J Cardiol 2003;91:1327–30.
[92] Ord WM. On myxedema, a term proposed to the be applied to an essential condition in the cretinoid affection occasionally observed in middle-aged women. Med Chir Trans 1878;61: 57–78.
[93] Rodriguez I, Fluiters E, Perez-Mendez LF, et al. Factors associated with mortality of patients with myxoedema coma: prospective study in 11 cases treated in a single institution. J Endocrinol 2004;180(2):347–50.
[94] Solano FX Jr, Starling RC, Levey GS. Myxedema megacolon. Arch Intern Med 1985;145(2): 231.
[95] Chernow B, Burman KD, Johnson DL, et al. T3 may be a better agent than T4 in the critically ill hypothyroid patient: evaluation of transport across the blood-brain barrier in a primate model [Journal Article]. Crit Care Med 1983;11(2):99–104.
[96] Holvey DN, Goodner CJ, Nicoloff JT, et al. Treatment of myxedema coma with intravenous thyroxine. Arch Intern Med 1964;113:89–96.
[97] Yamamoto T, Fukuyama J, Fujiyoshi A. Factors associated with mortality of myxedema coma: report of eight cases and literature survey. Thyroid 1999;9(12):1167–74.

ELSEVIER
SAUNDERS

Endocrinol Metab Clin N Am
36 (2007) 617–656

ENDOCRINOLOGY
AND METABOLISM
CLINICS
OF NORTH AMERICA

Hyperthyroidism

Bindu Nayak, MD[a,b,*], Steven P. Hodak, MD[c]

[a]*Division of Endocrinology and Metabolism, Georgetown University Hospital, 4000 Reservoir
Road, Building D, Suite 232, Washington, DC 20007, USA*
[b]*Washington Hospital Center, 110 Irving Street NW, Washington, DC 20010, USA*
[c]*University of Pittsburgh Center for Diabetes and Endocrinology, University of Pittsburgh
Medical Center, Falk Medical Building, Suite 580, 3601 Fifth Avenue,
Pittsburgh, PA 15213, USA*

Thyrotoxicosis can range in severity from subclinical hyperthyroidism to life-threatening thyroid storm. Although the term *thyrotoxicosis* describes the state of increased circulating thyroid hormone without distinguishing the source of thyroid hormone excess, the term *hyperthyroidism* implies that the origin of surplus thyroid hormone arises directly from increased thyroid gland production of hormone [1]. In this article, the authors review the presentation, diagnosis, and management of various causes of thyrotoxicosis.

Epidemiology

According to data from the National Health and Nutrition Examination Survey III, which assessed thyroid hormone levels in a randomly selected group of people in the United States, the prevalence of hyperthyroidism was 1.2%, of which 0.7% was found to be subclinical hyperthyroidism [1].

The most common cause of thyrotoxicosis is Graves' disease. Other common causes are toxic multinodular goiter (TMNG), solitary toxic adenoma, and thyroiditis. Rare causes of thyrotoxicosis include thyroid-stimulating hormone (TSH)–secreting pituitary adenoma, struma ovarii, metastatic functioning differentiated thyroid cancer, and metastatic tumors within the thyroid gland causing destruction-induced thyrotoxicosis. Box 1 lists differential of causes of thyrotoxicosis.

---

* Corresponding author. Division of Endocrinology and Metabolism, Georgetown University Hospital, 4000 Reservoir Road, Building D, Suite 232, Washington, DC 20007.
E-mail address: bindumanuel@yahoo.com (B. Nayak).

0889-8529/07/$ - see front matter © 2007 Elsevier Inc. All rights reserved.
doi:10.1016/j.ecl.2007.06.002

Box 1. Causes of thyrotoxicosis

Graves' disease
TMNG
Solitary autonomous nodule (toxic adenoma)
Thyroiditis
    Subacute
    Lymphocytic/painless
    Drug-induced
Iodine-induced
    Amiodarone-induced
Thyrotoxicosis factitia

Rare causes of thyrotoxicosis
TSH-secreting pituitary adenoma
Trophoblastic tumors
    Hydatidiform mole
    Choriocarcinoma
Struma ovarii
Metastatic functioning differentiated thyroid cancer

Specific thyrotoxic states

Graves' disease

Graves' disease is caused by an activating autoantibody that targets the TSH receptor. Graves' disease is more common in women, with a female-to-male incidence ratio of approximately 7 to 10:1 [1,2]. Thyroid-stimulating antibodies (TSAb) bind to the TSH receptor, activating adenylate cyclase, causing increased production of thyroid hormone as well as increased thyroid growth and vascularity. Patients with hyperthyroidism attributable to Graves' disease may have TSAb and thyroid stimulation-blocking antibodies (TSBAb) simultaneously. Patients with hypothyroidism who are TSBAb-positive may also have detectable levels of TSAb. Rarely, Graves' disease can occur after a history of autoimmune hypothyroidism because of a shift in the balance of TSAb and TSBAb levels [3].

Physical examination findings of Graves' disease present in various organ systems. The patient with Graves' disease can have thyroid gland findings of goiter and bruit. Ophthalmic findings can include proptosis, ophthalmoplegia, and conjunctival irritation. Dermatologic findings in Graves' disease can include localized dermal myxedema and hair loss.

The proptosis and ophthalmoplegia seen in Graves' disease are attributable to infiltrative orbitopathy. The underlying pathophysiology of Graves' ophthalmopathy is uncertain. Thyroid-stimulating hormone receptor antibodies (TRAb) are thought to target the retro-orbital tissues by binding to a TSH receptor antigen, which initiates a subsequent T-cell inflammatory infiltrate. Fibroblasts stimulated by cytokines produce glycosaminoglycans causing ophthalmopathy as a result of mass effect in 20% to 40% of patients who have Graves' disease [4–6]. Although most cases of Graves' ophthalmopathy consist of mild ocular manifestations, 3% to 5% of cases are severe with symptoms of intense pain, double vision, or loss of vision. Graves' ophthalmopathy can also occur without concomitant hyperthyroidism. Up to 10% of patients with Graves' ophthalmopathy are euthyroid. Most patients with euthyroid Graves' ophthalmopathy have evidence of autoimmune thyroid disease, such as the presence of thyroid peroxidase antibodies or antibodies against the TSH receptor [7,8].

Most cases of Graves' ophthalmopathy do not require medical treatment. There are several settings in which treatment is clearly beneficial, however. In the 3% to 5% of patients with Graves' disease who develop severe ophthalmopathy, treatment options include glucocorticoids, orbital radiotherapy and orbital decompressive surgery. These may improve the associated symptoms of proptosis, chemosis, and vision loss. Systemic glucocorticoids are effective in treating Graves' ophthalmopathy by means of anti-inflammatory and immunosuppressive actions that cause inhibition of cytokine release, interference with the function of T and B lymphocytes, and a consequent reduction in glycosaminoglycan production by orbital fibroblasts [9]. Treatment of Graves' ophthalmopathy is discussed in the section on disease-specific treatment.

Graves' disease may also present with multiple dermatologic findings. Localized dermal myxedema can occur in 0.5% to 4.3% of patients with Graves' disease. The development of myxedema is almost always associated with preexisting Graves' ophthalmopathy. Up to 13% of patients with severe Graves' ophthalmopathy may develop myxedema [5]. Because myxedema of Graves' disease usually occurs in the anterior leg, it has been called "pretibial myxedema." It can occur in other areas as well, however, and tends to occur in areas that undergo trauma or in dependent areas. Myxedema can appear as asymmetric, raised, firm, pink-to-purple, brown plaques of nonpitting edema. The involved dermis contains an increased content of hyaluronic acid and chondroitin sulfates, presumed to be attributable to activation of fibroblasts by cytokines, interleukin-1α, and transforming growth factor-β [5].

Myxedema or thyroid dermopathy of the lower extremities may be subdivided into several types: myxedema may present as diffuse nonpitting edema presumed to be due to lymphatic compression and obstruction by dermal deposition of glycosaminoglycan. This is the most common form of myxedema and occurs in up to 43% of patients presenting with Graves' dermopathy. A plaque form of myxedema is also reported, consisting of raised plaques on a background of nonpitting edema. This occurs in up to 27% of myxedema cases. Nodular myxedema occurs in 18% of patients with myxedema and presents with sharply circumscribed tubular or nodular lesions.

The rarest form of myxedema is the elephantiasic variant. This occurs in 5% of myxedema cases and consists of nodular lesions that may be fungating or polypoid, along with significant lymphedema [5,10,11]. Treatment is not necessary for most cases of dermopathy when lesions are mild; however, more severe lesions that cause cosmetic concern can be treated with topical glucocorticoid therapy. Glucocorticoids of different potency have been used, ranging from midpotency steroids with 0.2% fluocinolone acetonide cream [12] to a high-potency topical steroid, clobetasol propionate [13]. The steroids are applied over the affected region and covered with an occlusive dressing, such as plastic film or DuoDERM (ConvaTec Ltd., Deeside, United Kingdom) for at least 12 hours daily. A trial treatment period of 4 to 6 weeks is recommended, with careful evaluation for unwanted side effects like atrophy, telangiectasia, or ecchymoses. With the elephantiasic form of dermopathy, compressive bandages provide benefit to alleviate fluid accumulation. Severity of disease is the greatest determinant of treatment outcomes. In a retrospective review of 178 patients with dermopathy of Graves' disease, patients with more severe disease received therapy with topical glucocorticoids or compression in some cases and patients with less severe disease received no medical therapy. Patients who did not receive any therapy had a higher rate of complete remission (34.7%) compared with those who received local therapy (18.7%) after an average follow-up period of 7.9 years [14].

Graves' disease may also present with thyroid acropachy, which consists of digital clubbing, soft tissue swelling of the hands and feet, and periosteal bone formation. Thyroid acropachy occurs in 0.1% to 1% of patients with Graves' disease and almost always occurs in patients with ophthalmopathy and myxedema. The most common manifestation of acropachy is clubbing of the distal fingers and toes [15].

Toxic multinodular goiter

TMNG is the second leading cause of thyrotoxicosis. TMNG generally arises in a multinodular thyroid gland that subsequently develops autonomously functioning nodules over time. The prevalence of TMNG varies inversely with iodine sufficiency, and TMNG is more prevalent in populations with greater iodine insufficiency.

The pathogenesis of TMNG may be attributable to somatic mutations in the TSH receptor gene, leading to constitutive receptor activation and upregulation of cyclic adenosine monophosphate (cAMP) signaling [16,17]. Only 60% of nodules in TMNG have these mutations, however, suggesting that other mechanisms are also involved [1].

TMNG usually presents in individuals older than 50 years of age who have had a long previous history of multinodular goiter [1]. The clinical presentation of the thyrotoxicosis is usually mild. Because of the presentation in older age groups, however, TMNG often presents with cardiovascular manifestations of thyrotoxicosis, such as palpitations, tachycardia, and atrial fibrillation. Diagnosis of TMNG is made through laboratory evaluation that demonstrates suppressed TSH and elevated levels of thyroxine (T_4) and triiodothyronine (T_3). Radioactive iodine uptake and scanning reveals normal to increased uptake and a heterogeneous pattern, with focal areas of increased uptake corresponding to the hyperfunctioning nodules [1].

Toxic adenoma

Hyperthyroidism may also occur as the result of a solitary autonomous nodule or "toxic adenoma." Like TMNG, the pathogenesis is thought to be attributable to a mutation in the TSH receptor gene, causing constitutive receptor activation. The course of the disease, like TMNG, generally evolves slowly, with frank nodule autonomy occurring only after the nodule has been present for many years. Unlike TMNG, which occurs in older patients, the clinical presentation of solitary toxic nodules usually occurs in the third and fourth decades [1]. Laboratory evaluation of a toxic adenoma demonstrates suppressed TSH and elevation of T_4 and T_3. Solitary toxic adenoma is one of the most frequent causes of isolated T_3 toxicosis, however. In this situation, T_4 may be normal with isolated elevation of T_3.

Imaging with ultrasound should reveal a nodule. Radioactive iodine uptake and scanning should demonstrate increased uptake over the nodule, with evidence of suppressed uptake throughout the remainder of the gland [1].

Thyroiditis

With few exceptions, thyroiditis is an inflammatory process that causes follicular disruption and release of follicular contents, including thyroglobulin and stored thyroid hormone. Release of stored thyroid hormone causes the transient thyrotoxicosis associated with these diseases. Thyroiditis is often categorized by the presence or absence of pain and thyroid tenderness. Multiple causes of painful and painless thyroiditis exist and may cause thyrotoxicosis. Box 2 lists various causes of thyroiditis. All listed forms of thyroiditis, except type I amiodarone induced thyroiditis (discussed below), cause hyperthyroidism through a disruptive rather than hypermetabolic process. Radioactive iodine scanning typically shows homogeneous low or absent tracer uptake in these cases.

Subacute "de Quervain's" thyroiditis

One of the most common causes of thyroid pain is subacute thyroiditis, also known as de Quervain's thyroiditis or granulomatous giant cell thyroiditis. In an incidence study based in Olmstead County in Minnesota, 160 cases of subacute thyroiditis were diagnosed over the course of 37 years, leading to an incidence rate of 4.9 cases per 100,000 population per year [18]. Subacute thyroiditis is often preceded by a viral infection and is

---

Box 2. Types of thyroiditis that cause thyrotoxicosis

Silent, lymphocytic, or painless thyroiditis
Postpartum thyroiditis
Subacute thyroiditis
Drug-induced thyroiditis
    Amiodarone
    Lithium
    α-interferon
    Interleukin-2

---

thought to be attributable to a subsequent autoimmune response. Markers of autoimmunity have been found during the acute phase of subacute thyroiditis, which can persist for many years after the episode. These support the role of aberrant autoimmunity in the pathogenesis of this disease [19].

Viruses implicated in pathogenesis of subacute thyroiditis include adenovirus, echovirus, influenza, coxsackie, and mumps virus [20]. The incidence of subacute thyroiditis is highest in summer, coincident with the peak of enterovirus season [21].

The inflammation of subacute thyroiditis is characterized by an infiltration of mononuclear cells in affected regions of the thyroid gland. Histopathologic examination can reveal the classic finding of a central core of colloid surrounded by multinucleated giant cells, which can progress to form a granuloma [22].

Anterior localized neck pain with or without fever is the hallmark of the clinical presentation of subacute thyroiditis. The pain may also radiate to the jaw or ear. Patients may report having hoarseness or dysphagia. Thyrotoxic symptoms, including palpitations, nervousness, and emotional lability, may also occur in up to 50% of patients [23]. Physical examination findings include a tender thyroid gland, with pain frequently localized to one side of the gland more than to the other side. Laboratory evaluation of subacute thyroiditis demonstrates suppressed TSH, elevated T_4 and T_3, elevation of the erythrocyte sedimentation rate, leukocytosis, and an elevated thyroglobulin level.

The course of subacute thyroiditis typically begins with an acute thyrotoxic phase as follicular destruction occurs, causing suppression of TSH. As follicular stores are depleted, the hyperthyroidism resolves. At this point, the patient typically becomes briefly euthyroid. If the follicular stores are sufficiently depleted and circulating thyroid hormone diminishes, TSH levels rise and a hypothyroid phase then ensues. If the thyroid has not been completely destroyed by the inflammation, thyroid hormone production resumes; at that point, TSH may return to the normal range. The entire cycle from onset of the hyperthyroid phase to resolution of the hypothyroidism is variable but usually ranges from 6 to 12 months [23]. Permanent hypothy-roidism has been reported to be relatively rare after subacute thyroiditis, oc-curring in approximately 5–15% of patients [18,24].

Silent, lymphocytic, or painless thyroiditis

Unlike subacute thyroiditis, silent thyroiditis is generally painless. The terms *sporadic* thyroiditis, *subacute lymphocytic* thyroiditis, and *painless* thy-roiditis are also used to describe this syndrome. No infectious cause has ever been definitively linked to silent thyroiditis. Silent thyroiditis is generally thought to be attributable to an acute exacerbation of underlying thyroid autoimmunity. The inflammatory infiltrate in this disease is generally char-acterized by a monotonous infiltrate of lymphocytes.

Silent thyroiditis usually occurs in the third to sixth decade with a female-to-male ratio of 1.5 to 2:1. As is the case with subacute thyroiditis, the course of the disease begins with thyrotoxicosis, followed by brief euthyroid-ism and a subsequent hypothyroid phase. Permanent hypothyroidism occur-ring immediately after painless thyroiditis has been variably reported between 5% and 20% [1,25].

Physical examination findings during silent thyroiditis include an enlarged thyroid gland in 50% to 60% of patients. Laboratory findings include suppression of TSH during the acute phase and the presence of autoantibodies to thyroperoxidase. Unlike subacute thyroiditis, the erythro-cyte sedimentation rate is generally normal.

Postpartum thyroiditis

Postpartum thyroiditis is also caused by exacerbation of underlying thy-roid autoimmunity. The immunologic resurgence that typically occurs after the relative immunosuppression of pregnancy is a key factor in the develop-ment of postpartum thyroiditis. The lymphocytic infiltrate and histopatho-logic findings in this disease are similar if not identical to those found in silent thyroiditis, suggesting that these two diseases have a closely related pathophysiology [26]. The prevalence of postpartum thyroiditis after normal pregnancy ranges between 1.1% and 16.7% in various studies, with a mean of approximately 7.2% [27]. The initial hyperthyroid phase can occur be-tween 2 and 10 months postpartum. Postpartum thyroiditis can also occur after miscarriage or termination of an early trimester pregnancy [28]. Only 33% of patients with postpartum thyroiditis experience symptomatic thyro-toxicosis. Thyrotoxicosis associated with postpartum thyroiditis generally lasts approximately 8 weeks. Patients may subsequently return to euthyroid-ism or develop a hypothyroid phase [29]. Permanent hypothyroidism occurs in 20% of women immediately after the onset of thyroiditis. Up to 60% of women develop permanent hypothyroidism within 3 to 10 years of follow-up [30]. Up to 70% of patients develop recurrent episodes of postpartum thyroiditis with subsequent pregnancies [31].

Most women with postpartum thyroiditis do not require treatment during the hyperthyroid or hypothyroid phase. Control of symptoms during the hyperthyroid phase with β-adrenergic blockade may be necessary but should always be used with appropriate caution in nursing mothers. Thyroid hormone replacement is rarely necessary for the treatment of the hypothyroid phase; however, it is considered safe during lactation when used at normal replacement doses.

Drug-induced thyroiditis

Several drugs can cause thyroiditis, including amiodarone, lithium, interferon-α, and interleukin-2. Amiodarone-induced thyroiditis is discussed elsewhere in this article. Lithium can cause thyrotoxicosis by inducing silent thyroiditis [32]. Use of α-interferon and interleukin-2 is associated with increased thyroid autoimmunity, which can result in hyperthyroidism or hypothyroidism [33]. In addition, α-interferon can cause thyrotoxicosis by inducing a destructive thyroiditis [34].

Iodine-induced thyrotoxicosis

Iodine-induced hyperthyroidism can cause thyrotoxicosis in iodine-deficient and iodine-sufficient populations. Iodine intoxication can occur after administration of radiographic contrast media or use of amiodarone and from dietary sources of iodine, such as kelp and seaweed.

Two major patterns of thyroid disorders predispose to development of iodine-induced hyperthyroidism in otherwise "normal" patients: nodular thyroid disease and the presence of indolent Graves' disease. These diseases are frequently clinically inapparent, with development of hyperthyroidism only after the iodine exposure occurs.

Amiodarone-induced thyrotoxicosis

Amiodarone is a widely used antiarrhythmia medication that contains approximately 37% iodide, or iodide 75 mg per 200-mg tablet [35]. Amiodarone is well known to produce both thyrotoxicosis and hypothyroidism.

Amiodarone-induced hypothyroidism (AIH) occurs with greater frequency in iodine-replete populations. AIT is more prevalent in iodine-insufficient populations and has been reported to have an incidence ranging from 1% to 23% [36]. In regions of Italy in which iodine intake is endemically low, the incidence of AIT was found to be 9.6%. The incidence of AIH in this same population was 5%. In iodine-replete regions, such as New England, a higher incidence of AIH up to 22%, compared with a 2% incidence of AIT, has been reported [37].

Amiodarone causes thyrotoxicosis through two mechanisms. Type I AIT is attributable to underlying latent autoimmunity that is exacerbated by the iodine load liberated by normal metabolism of amiodarone. Indolent TMNG and Graves' disease are the most common underlying etiologies in such cases.

Amiodarone can also induce a destructive thyroiditis that releases pre-stored thyroid hormone, leading to thyrotoxicosis. This is generally referred to as type II AIT. Recognition and differentiation of the type of AIT are important, because the choice of appropriate treatment is different for each type.

Thyroid-stimulating hormone–secreting pituitary adenoma

TSH-secreting pituitary adenoma is a rare cause of hyperthyroidism, occurring in less than 1% of all pituitary adenomas [38]. Laboratory evaluation typically demonstrates elevated serum T_4 and T_3, with inappropriately normal or modestly elevated serum TSH. Most of these patients present with a macroadenoma. The diagnosis is generally made by radiographic demonstration of a pituitary macroadenoma in the appropriate clinical setting [38]. Laboratory testing may assist in the identification of a TSH-secreting adenoma, however. Because the elaboration of TSH from such a tumor is attributable to thyrotroph autonomy, TSH does not easily suppress with exogenous administration of T_3. The T_3 suppression test has been performed by measuring TSH before and 48 hours after administration of T_3 at a dose of 300 μg at noon, with a normal response being a decline of the TSH value to less than 10% of the baseline TSH value [39,40]. A high ratio of the glycoprotein hormone α-subunit relative to the TSH level has also been used to differentiate TSH-secreting pituitary adenoma from thyroid hormone resistance syndrome. The α-subunit/TSH molar ratio can be calculated with the following formula: (α-subunit [μg/L]/TSH [mU/L]) × 10. Most patients with TSH-secreting pituitary adenomas have an α-subunit/TSH molar ratio greater than 1.0 [39]. Response to thyrotropin-releasing hormone (TRH) stimulation has also been used to evaluate TSH-secreting adenomas. Administration of TRH to patients with a TSH-secreting adenoma does not cause the typical rise in TSH associated with normal thyrotroph function. Because TRH is not currently available, however, this finding remains of academic interest only.

Thyroid hormone resistance

Thyroid hormone resistance is another rare cause of thyrotoxicosis. There have been more than 1000 published cases of resistance to thyroid hormone. Approximately 75% of these cases had a familial occurrence, with most demonstrating autosomal dominant inheritance. The disease has also been shown to occur sporadically in up to 21.3% of patients with thyroid hormone resistance [40].

As in the setting of TSH-secreting pituitary adenoma, thyroid hormone resistance presents with elevation of serum thyroid hormone levels and inappropriately normal or frankly elevated TSH. Resistance to thyroid hormone is always partial, with a variable extent of resistance among reported cases [41]. Resistance to thyroid hormone has been classified into two categories: generalized resistance to thyroid hormone (GRTH) and pituitary resistance to thyroid hormone (PRTH). In GRTH, all tissues in the body with thyroid hormone receptors are resistant to T_3 to a varying degree. Because this resistance is present in pituitary thyrotrophs, circulating levels of T_4 and T_3 must be elevated to produce normal pituitary feedback. This results in elevated circulating levels of thyroid hormone with a normal TSH level. Because the thyroid hormone resistance is present diffusely throughout most peripheral body tissues, elevated circulating levels of thyroid hormone do not cause clinical hyperthyroidism. PRTH presents with isolated pituitary resistance, with normal peripheral tissue thyroid hormone sensitivity. Higher levels of thyroid hormone are also required in this case to cause normal pituitary feedback. Because peripheral tissues are not resistant to thyroid hormone, patients with PRTH may develop clinical signs and symptoms of thyrotoxicosis [41].

The underlying pathophysiology of resistance to thyroid hormone is a mutation in one allele of the thyroid hormone receptor (TRβ). TRβ has two main receptor isoforms, TRβ1 and TRβ2. Although TRβ2 is mostly expressed in the hypothalamus and pituitary, TRβ1 is expressed in the liver and kidney. Many different mutations of the gene have been found. Testing for TRβ gene defects can be diagnostic [41].

Familial dysalbuminemic hyperthyroxinemia

Familial dysalbuminemic hyperthyroxinemia (FDH) is a cause of euthyroid hyperthyroxinemia. Patients with FDH are clinically euthyroid and have a normal TSH level; therefore, this is not a cause of true thyrotoxicosis. The pattern of thyroid hormone levels in this disorder is frequently mistaken for true hyperthyroidism, and thus warrants mention.

FDH is attributable to variant serum albumin that has preferential affinity for T_4, leading to elevated T_4 levels. The disorder is inherited in an autosomal dominant manner and has a prevalence of 0.17% [42]. Laboratory evaluation demonstrates elevated total T_4, normal TSH, normal T_3, and elevated or normal free T_4 [43]. The pattern of laboratory findings is similar to that caused by estrogen and other medications or drugs that increase the quantity of thyroid-binding globulin.

Clinically, patients with FDH are euthyroid. In the setting of an elevated total T_4 level with a normal free T_4 value and normal TSH serum concentration, FDH can be considered. Diagnosis of FDH can be confirmed with an in vitro test to demonstrate an abnormal increase in the binding of T_4 to serum albumin [44].

Thyrotoxicosis factitia

Thyrotoxicosis can also be caused by extrathyroidal sources of thyroid hormone. Thyrotoxicosis factitia, the ingestion of exogenous thyroid hormone, is the most common cause of extrathyroidal thyrotoxicosis. Thyrotoxicosis factitia can be seen, in mild forms, with the treatment of thyroid cancer when suppressive doses of levothyroxine are given. Surreptitious use of thyroid hormone is also another common cause of thyrotoxicosis factitia when people intentionally take thyroid hormone when they do not need it, such as may occur in psychiatric illness or in people who desire to lose weight and have access to the medication. Epidemics of thyrotoxicosis factitia have occurred regionally when bovine thyroid material was found in ground beef at a local slaughtering plant [45]. Diagnosis of thyrotoxicosis factitia can be difficult in patients who do not admit to use of exogenous thyroid hormone. Laboratory values reveal elevated T_3 and T_4, along with suppressed TSH. Radioactive iodine uptake reveals low uptake indistinguishable from the findings in thyroiditis. In this situation, a serum thyroglobulin level can be revealing because it is high in thyroiditis and thyrotoxicosis attributable to any other cause but is low in thyrotoxicosis factitia. Treatment for thyrotoxicosis factitia is simply discontinuation of the thyroid hormone. For patients who have taken excessive amounts or who are at risk for cardiovascular complications, more aggressive measures may be taken. In patients who have had a recent massive ingestion of thyroid hormone, measures to decrease absorption, such as activated charcoal or gastric lavage, may be used. Cholestyramine has also been used in this situation to decrease thyroid hormone levels rapidly by binding thyroid hormone in the enterohepatic circulation and increasing fecal excretion [46].

Struma ovarii

Struma ovarii is another rare cause of thyrotoxicosis. Struma ovarii is an ovarian tumor usually consisting of cystic teratoma with differentiation into thyroid tissue. The incidence of struma ovarii is low: 0.3% to 1% of all ovarian tumors are struma ovarii, whereas 2% to 4% of ovarian teratomas are struma ovarii. These ovarian tumors are benign in 95% of cases and associated with thyrotoxicosis in 5% to 8% of cases [47–49]. Clinically, women with struma ovarii may present with an abdominal mass. When thyrotoxicosis accompanies struma ovarii, women may have overt symptoms of thyrotoxicosis or subclinical thyrotoxicosis. In addition to a suppressed TSH level and elevated T_3 and T_4 levels, thyroglobulin is also elevated. Although nuclear medicine imaging with ^{123}I or ^{131}I does not reveal uptake in the neck, whole-body imaging reveals uptake in the pelvis [50]. Treatment of struma ovarii consists of surgical resection of the tumor with oophorectomy and salpingectomy or with total abdominal hysterectomy and bilateral or unilateral oophorectomy depending on the extent of capsular invasion and the desire for preserved fertility. Thyrotoxicosis associated with struma ovarii can be treated with thionamide therapy to achieve euthyroidism before surgery [51].

Metastatic thyroid carcinoma causing thyrotoxicosis

Thyrotoxicosis in the setting of metastatic thyroid cancer is an unusual occurrence. Thyrotoxicosis is usually related to the amount of functional differentiated thyroid cancer cells. Most cases of thyrotoxicosis caused by metastatic thyroid cancer have been reported with follicular cancer [52]. Patients are typically diagnosed with thyrotoxicosis at the time of cancer diagnosis. Diagnosis may be difficult after thyroidectomy for thyroid cancer when Levothyroxine (LT_4) suppressive therapy is ongoing. In this setting, a suppressed TSH level may be attributed to LT_4 suppression therapy. Differentiation of a suppressed TSH level attributable to LT_4 suppression versus functioning metastatic differentiated thyroid cancer can be made with withdrawal of LT4 for several weeks, however. After LT_4 withdrawal for several weeks, TSH does not increase appropriately when there is metastatic functioning thyroid cancer [53]. Imaging with ^{131}I whole-body scanning reveals low uptake in the thyroid bed, with increased uptake by the functioning metastatic tissue. Treatment for metastatic functioning thyroid cancer is similar to treatment for nonfunctioning metastatic thyroid cancer [54].

Clinical presentation of thyrotoxicosis

Thyrotoxicosis causes a hypermetabolic state resulting in an imbalance of energy metabolism in which energy production exceeds energy expenditure. This may cause increased heat production, resulting in perspiration, heat intolerance, and even fever. Despite the fact that this hypermetabolic state results in greater energy expenditure, symptoms of thyrotoxicosis can frequently and paradoxically include generalized weakness attributable to the cardiorespiratory effects of thyrotoxicosis and fatigue attributable to associated myopathy [10].

Thyrotoxicosis also causes neuropsychiatric changes resulting in restlessness, agitation, anxiety, emotional lability, psychosis, and even coma [55]. Behavioral studies reveal poor performance in memory and concentration testing proportional to the degree of thyrotoxicosis [56].

Gastrointestinal manifestations of thyrotoxicosis include increased frequency of bowel movements caused by increased motor contraction of the small bowel, resulting in more rapid transit of intestinal contents [10]. Thyrotoxicosis can affect the menstrual cycle in women, resulting in oligomenorrhea or amenorrhea. The etiology of the menstrual irregularity is unclear but may be attributable to the effects of thyroid hormone on gonadotropin-releasing hormone (GnRH) signaling, causing disruption of normal luteinizing hormone (LH)/follicle-stimulating hormone (FSH) pulsatility [1].

An increase in total estrogens can occur in hyperthyroidism as the result of an increase in sex hormone–binding globulin. The increased levels of sex hormone–binding globulin cause a decrease in metabolic clearance of estradiol and also cause an increase in conversion of androstenedione to estrone and estradione [57,58]. Approximately 10% of male patients with hyperthyroidism may experience symptoms of decreased libido or gynecomastia and development of spider angiomas as a result of these changes [10].

Thyroid hormone exerts effects on the systemic vasculature as well as on the heart itself. Thyroid hormone decreases systemic vascular resistance through a direct vasodilatory action on the smooth muscle, which is mediated by endothelial release of nitric oxide and other endothelial-derived vasodilators [59]. T_3 exerts its effects directly on the heart through genomic mechanisms influencing production of myofibrillary proteins, sarcoplasmic reticulum phospholamban, calcium-activated ATPase, and various plasma membrane transporters. In addition, T_3 acts through nongenomic pathways, altering the performance of sodium, potassium, and calcium channels. The manifestations of these changes include increased heart rate, cardiac contractility, and cardiac output [60,61].

Tachycardia is the most common cardiovascular sign of thyrotoxicosis. Thyrotoxic patients may also experience palpitations attributable to increased force of cardiac contraction [1]. Physical findings in thyrotoxicosis can include a strong apical impulse, increased pulse pressure, and a hyperdynamic precordium. Heart sounds can include the "Means-Lerman scratch" heard at the apex, which is thought to be attributable to the hyperdynamic precordium rubbing against the pleura [1,10].

Thyrotoxic patients can experience chest pain that may mimic ischemic angina pectoris. Because thyrotoxicosis can also lead to increased myocardial oxygen demand, coronary artery spasm, and frank coronary ischemia, ischemic heart disease should always be considered in a thyrotoxic patient presenting with chest pain.

Older individuals may present with atypical clinical manifestations of thyrotoxicosis. "Apathetic hyperthyroidism" is a common presentation in the elderly and is characterized by weight loss, weakness, palpitations, dizziness, or memory loss and physical findings of sinus tachycardia or atrial fibrillation [10]. Typical hyperadrenergic symptoms of thyrotoxicosis may be veiled by such medications as beta-blockers, which are frequently used in elderly patients for treatment of common diseases like hypertension or heart disease.

Laboratory diagnosis

A suppressed TSH level (<0.05 µU/mL) in combination with an elevated serum free T_4 level occurs in 95% of patients with clinically evident thyrotoxicosis. Although a TSH assessment alone may be appropriate for routine screening in an asymptomatic patient, the suspicion of thyrotoxicosis

warrants the additional assessment of T_4 and T_3. In cases in which subclinical hyperthyroidism is suspected, TSH measurement may be used as a first
diagnostic step, with subsequent T_4 and T_3 assessment if TSH is suppressed
[10,62]. Free hormone concentrations are preferable in the diagnosis of thyrotoxicosis because of the possible interference of protein binding with total
thyroid hormone levels [63].

Laboratory measurement of total T_3 and total T_4 reflects mainly protein-
bound hormone concentrations. Therefore, conditions that affect protein
binding alter measured total thyroid hormone levels. T_4-binding globulin
can be elevated in infectious hepatitis, during pregnancy, and in patients
taking estrogens or opiates. Also, many drugs interfere with protein binding,
including heparin, phenytoin, diazepam, nonsteroidal anti-inflammatory
drugs, furosemide, carbamazepine, and salicylates [10,52,64]. Genetic
abnormalities leading to abnormal protein binding, such as FDH, also
lead to protein-binding abnormalities. These protein-binding abnormalities
affect the index tests (free T_4 index and free T_3 index) and may give inaccurate values when changes in protein binding are present. For these reasons,
free T_4 assays are preferred over index tests [63].

Thyroid-stimulating hormone receptor antibodies

The measurement of TRAb may occasionally be helpful in the diagnosis
and management of Graves' disease. The routine assay to detect TRAb is
the TSH-binding inhibitor immunoglobulin (TBII) assay. The TBII assay
measures all antibodies to the TSH receptor and is not specific for antibodies that only cause thyroid stimulation. A second generation of this
assay using recombinant TSH receptor has been developed and has a reported sensitivity of 98.6% [65]. Assays also exist for direct measurement
of TSAb and TBAb, although it is unclear whether direct measurement of
these assays provides diagnostic information superior to that provided by
measurement of TRAb alone [66,67].

TRAb measurements are particularly useful in the prediction of postpartum Graves' thyrotoxicosis and neonatal thyrotoxicosis. In a prospective
study of 71 pregnant women with no previous diagnosis of a thyroid disorder who were found to have antithyroid microsomal antibody during early
pregnancy, TBII and TSAb were measured. Seven of 71 patients were found
to have positive TSAb activity during early pregnancy. Five (71%) of 7 patients with positive TSAb activity developed postpartum thyrotoxicosis, suggesting that detection of TSAb during early pregnancy can predict a higher
risk of developing Graves' thyrotoxicosis in the postpartum period [68].

The utility of using thyroid antibodies as a predictor of neonatal thyrotoxicosis was demonstrated in a study of 108 neonates born to mothers
with Graves' disease. Clinical overt thyrotoxicosis was predicted in 83%
of neonates when maternal TBII activity was greater than 8 U/mL and
TSAb activity was greater than 1.0 TSH microUEq [69]. In another study

assessing TBII levels in 44 pregnant women with active Graves' disease, neo-natal thyrotoxicosis was seen in 4 (8%) patients. Maternal TBII levels at de-livery for these 4 neonates exceeded 70% inhibition of tracer [70].

Thyroxine/triiodothyronine ratio

The ratio of T_4 to T_3 frequently has a characteristic pattern in different thyrotoxic states. Evaluation of the T_4/T_3 ratio may be a useful tool in the initial diagnosis of thyrotoxicosis when radioactive iodine uptake testing is not readily available or is contraindicated. Approximately 2% of thyro-toxic patients in the United States have an increase in serum free T_3 and nor-mal T_4. This is referred to as "T_3 toxicosis" [62,71]. Graves' disease and toxic nodular goiter typically present with increased T_3 production, with a T_3/T_4 ratio greater than 20 [72,73]. With thyrotoxicosis caused by thyroid-itis, iodine exposure, or exogenous levothyroxine intake, however, T_4 is the predominant hormone and the T_3/T_4 ratio is usually less than 20 [62].

Other laboratory findings

Thyrotoxicosis may also cause hyperglycemia, hypercalcemia, elevated alkaline phosphatase, leukocytosis, and elevated liver enzymes. The hyper-glycemia is typically mild and is caused by catecholamine-induced inhibition of insulin release and increased glycogenolysis. Mild hypercalcemia and elevated alkaline phosphatase occur as well because of direct TSH stimula-tion of osteoblastic bone resorption mediated by the NF-kB-RANKL path-way [55,64,74–76].

Imaging

Multiple imaging modalities may assist in the determination of the etiol-ogy of thyrotoxicosis. These include thyroid nuclear imaging studies and anatomic studies like thyroid ultrasound. The specific application of these imaging modalities in various etiologies of thyrotoxicosis is reviewed below.

Nuclear medicine scanning

A key diagnostic tool in the evaluation of thyrotoxicosis is radioactive iodine uptake and scanning. Radioactive iodine uptake and scanning uses a ra-dioactive isotope of iodine, typically ^{123}I or [131]I. After ingestion of the tracer, subsequently emitted γ-radiation allows external detection, scintigraphic im-aging, and calculation of fractional iodine uptake by the thyroid gland. The amount of radiation delivered to the thyroid by ^{123}I is approximately 1% of that delivered by the same amount of [131]I. For the purposes of scanning and computing uptake, an approximate dose of ^{131}I up to 5 μCi (0.19 MBq) or of ^{123}I up to 300 μCi (11.11 MBq) is given orally. Because of the potential for a high radiation dose to the gland with small amounts of ^{131}I, ^{123}I is frequently preferred for routine thyroid scanning. After administration of the isotope, relatively acute and delayed uptake data are acquired. Generally, uptake at 6 and 24 hours is obtained after dosing [1,77]. The normal values for the 24-hour radioiodine uptake range between 5% and 25%, and the average 6-hour uptake reference range is between 5% and 15% [78].

Radioactive iodine scanning can help to define the etiology of thyrotoxicosis; in the setting of hyperthyroidism, increased fractional uptake typically indicates de novo synthesis of thyroid hormone, whereas decreased uptake generally indicates that new hormone synthesis is not the underlying cause of the thyrotoxicosis. The differential diagnosis of thyrotoxicosis may be divided into categories based on whether increased or decreased uptake of radiotracer is observed during thyroid scanning.

Clinical syndromes associated with increased uptake

As previously noted, increased nuclear tracer uptake may be seen in TMNG, toxic solitary nodule, or Graves' disease. Graves' disease and TMNG have also been rarely reported in combination as part of the Marine-Lenhart syndrome [79].

Graves' disease generally demonstrates homogeneous uptake throughout the gland. With markedly increased thyroid hormone synthesis and turnover in Graves' disease, there can be a paradoxic finding of elevated uptake at 4 or 6 hours after radioiodine dosing but a normal uptake at 24 hours as a result of accelerated clearance of the radioactive iodine.

TMNG generally has a heterogeneous pattern of uptake with hyperfunctioning nodules that demonstrate increased radionuclide uptake on scan. These nodules appear on a background of partially or completely suppressed uptake in the uninvolved areas of the thyroid gland. Solitary toxic nodules have a radioactive iodine scan pattern demonstrating increased uptake in the hyperfunctioning nodule and decreased uptake in the remainder of the gland. When the uptake in the uninvolved parts of the thyroid is completely suppressed, such a nodule is frequently referred to as an autonomous or "hot" nodule. If the uninvolved parts of the thyroid are not completely suppressed, the nodule is frequently referred to as a "warm" nodule to differentiate this type of radiographic pattern.

Increased uptake on radioactive iodine scanning can be observed in conditions other than hyperthyroidism. Increased radioactive iodine uptake may be present with significant iodine deficiency. Iodine deficiency is typically confirmed by the presence of urinary iodine excretion < 100 μg/d. With chronic iodine deficiency, there is an increase in iodine uptake by the thyroid gland to compensate for the low circulating iodine concentration [80]. This may result in the finding of increased uptake on a radioactive iodine scan despite biochemical euthyroidism or hypothyroidism.

Paradoxically, increased radioactive iodine uptake may also be found in Hashimoto's thyroiditis. This finding usually occurs with early or relatively mild disease when elevated serum TSH levels stimulate the activity of the sodium-iodide symporter, leading to increased uptake on a radioactive iodine scan. Because Hashimoto's thyroiditis blocks normal thyroid peroxidase function, such increased uptake does not result in increased thyroid hormone synthesis [78].

Radioactive iodine uptake may also be increased in conditions associated with excessive thyroid hormone loss. The increase in uptake occurs as the thyroid gland increases synthesis of hormone to compensate for extrathyroidal hormone loss [1]. Urinary loss of binding protein in nephritic syndromes may induce such a compensatory increase in thyroid hormone synthesis. Gastrointestinal loss of thyroid hormone attributable to chronic diarrhea or ingestion of agents, such as bile acid resins, that interfere with thyroid hormone reabsorption from the intestinal tract may also cause increased uptake on radionuclide imaging.

Clinical syndromes associated with decreased uptake

Thyrotoxic conditions typically associated with decreased radioactive iodine uptake include exogenous thyroid hormone intake, thyroiditis, and iodine intoxication. The main cause of the decreased isotope uptake in all these conditions is suppression of TSH. Iodine intoxication also causes direct effects on the thyroid that decrease uptake.

In the initial phase of thyroiditis, inflammation destroys thyroid tissue, which releases stored thyroid hormone and causes thyrotoxicosis. This leads to suppression of TSH and a decrease of new hormone synthesis, causing low uptake on radioactive iodine uptake scanning. During the recovery phase of thyroiditis, the thyroid gland can enter a "rebound" phase during which thyroid hormone production is increased, with evidence of increased radioactive iodine uptake [77]. Following thyroid function tests over the course of thyroiditis should prevent confusion and allow appropriate interpretation of the observed uptake pattern over the course of typical thyroiditis.

Iodine-rich agents, such as amiodarone, radiographic contrast agents, or increased oral iodine intake from kelp or other seaweed, are a frequent cause of iodine intoxication. Iodine intoxication decreases radioiodine uptake because of intrathyroidal iodine pooling. The high concentration of unlabeled iodine competes with the radioactive iodine for organification and cellular transport, preventing significant tracer uptake. Acute exposure to sufficient iodine also induces a decrease in thyroid iodide trapping, further limiting or preventing thyroid uptake of circulating iodine [77,80]. This is the mechanism underlying the Wolff-Chaikoff effect.

Technetium-99m pertechnetate imaging

Technetium-99m (Tc-99m) may also be used for thyroid scanning, because technetium, like iodide, is actively trapped in the thyroid follicular cell. Tc-99m scanning may be quite useful in differentiating among the many etiologies of thyrotoxicosis that can cause increased or decreased uptake. One of the main advantages of Tc-99 scanning is the relatively rapid turn-around time of the study. The Tc-99m scan takes approximately 20 to 30 minutes to complete as opposed to radioactive iodine scanning, which usually requires imaging at 6 and 24 hours. This scan allows rapid distinction between hypermetabolic high-uptake states, such as Graves' disease or toxic nodular disease, and typically low-uptake states, such as thyroiditis. Tc-99 has limitations, however. Tc-99m is not organified and is only briefly retained within the thyroid. Therefore, the Tc-99m scan is not useful for detecting organification defects. In addition, discordant results have been found in comparing Tc-99m imaging of nodules in comparison to radioiodine imaging. Most often, discordance occurs when the Tc-99m scan shows a hyperfunctioning or warm nodule and radioiodine scan shows a normal or cold nodule. In one study, 40 (33%) of 122 cases had discordant findings between Tc-99m scans and ^{123}I radioiodine scans. Many of the discordant results occurred with a functioning nodule on the Tc-99m scan and a hypofunctioning nodule on the ^{123}I scan [81]. Also, thyroid uptake of pertechnetate cannot be used for assessing uptake for the purpose of calculating an ablative dose of [131]I.

Thyroid ultrasonography in the evaluation of hyperthyroidism

Thyroid sonography may be useful in the diagnostic evaluation of thyrotoxicosis. Sonographic assessment can identify thyroid nodules and goiter that may not be readily apparent on examination. Additionally, sonographic Doppler flow assessment may provide particularly useful information about several thyrotoxic states. Kurita and colleagues [82] used an index measurement of thyroid blood flow per unit area to distinguish between Graves' disease and thyrotoxicosis caused by nonhypermetabolic destructive thyroiditis. Using a thyroid blood flow area of 8% or greater had a sensitivity of 95% and a specificity of 90% for the prediction of Graves' disease.

In the setting of AIT, ultrasound may be particularly helpful. Ultrasound can detect the presence of nodules and goiter that may favor the diagnosis of type I AIT. Color flow Doppler sonography can also aid in the differentiation of type I AIT and type II AIT. Type I AIT is attributable to an underlying hypermetabolic state and typically demonstrates normal to increased blood flow that is readily apparent with Doppler imaging. Type II AIT, which is a type of destructive thyroiditis, generally presents with markedly decreased blood flow, however [83].

Treatment of hyperthyroidism

Management of thyrotoxicosis is tailored to its specific etiology. Hyperthyroidism caused by thyroid autonomy typically involves the use of antithyroidal drugs that exert multiple effects on thyroid hormone synthesis and release. β-adrenergic receptor blockers are also useful to mitigate the increased adrenergic tone caused by hyperthyroidism that is responsible for many of the symptoms associated with thyrotoxicosis.

Thionamides

Thionamides are the most commonly used antithyroid medication. This class of medication was first introduced in 1943 by Astwood [84]. Two classes of thionamides exist: thiouracils and imidazoles. Methimazole and carbimazole constitute the imidazole group, whereas propylthiouracil (PTU) is the only thiouracil. Once ingested, carbimazole is rapidly metabolized to methimazole. Carbimazole is not available in the United States but is used commonly in Europe [85]. Thionamides act to halt synthesis of thyroid hormone by interfering with thyroid peroxidase–mediated oxidation of iodide, iodine organification, and iodotyrosine coupling. Also, thionamides inhibit the thyroperoxidase-catalyzed coupling process through which iodotyrosine residues are combined to form T_4 and T_3. PTU, but not methimazole or carbimazole, also possesses the extrathyroidal action of blocking peripheral conversion of T_4 to T_3 in peripheral tissues through inhibition of type 1 deiodinase [85]. In cases of thyroid storm or severe thyrotoxicosis, this added benefit may be useful.

In addition to inhibiting organification of thyroid hormone, thionamides may have an inhibitory effect on the immune system [86]. Various in vitro and in vivo studies show that thionamides have important immunosuppressive effects, including decreasing immune-related molecules, such as intracellular adhesion molecule 1 and soluble interleukin-2, as well as decreasing antithyrotropin receptor antibodies over time [86–88]. Antithyroid drugs may also decrease human leukocyte antigen (HLA) class II expression and induce apoptosis of intrathyroidal lymphocytes [89,90].

Studies using high doses of thionamides in combination with thyroid hormone replacement have been conducted on the basis of the hypothesis that the additional immunomodulatory effect of high-dose thionamide treatment would convey a benefit beyond that of standard thionamide treatment alone. Romaldini and colleagues [91] showed that the recurrence rate was 25% among those who received combined therapy compared with a recurrence rate of 55% among those who were treated with a thionamide alone. These results have not been duplicated by numerous subsequent studies using combined therapy, however [92–94]. Therefore, the use of combination treatment with thionamides and thyroid hormone replacement is not currently recommended.

Methimazole and PTU have different pharmacologic properties that warrant consideration when a thionamide is selected for use in the treatment of hyperthyroidism. The serum half-life of methimazole is 6 to 8 hours, whereas the half-life of PTU is 1 to 2 hours. These short half-lives would suggest that the thionamides should be administered in divided daily doses. Several studies have shown that methimazole is effective in treating hyperthyroidism when given once daily, however [95–97]. In contrast, PTU is not as effective when given as a single daily dose [98]. Several factors may contribute to methimazole's increased efficacy. Methimazole interferes with iodine organification more effectively by irreversibly inhibiting thyroid peroxidase, whereas PTU causes reversible inhibition [99]. Also, in addition to its longer serum half-life, methimazole has been found to provide measurable intrathyroidal concentrations lasting up to 20 hours and more durable inhibition of organification compared with PTU [100,101].

Once-daily dosing with methimazole also significantly improves patient compliance. In a study of 22 hyperthyroid patients randomized to receive methimazole (30 mg/d) or PTU (100 mg every 8 hours), compliance in the methimazole group was 83.3%, whereas compliance in the PTU group was 53.3% [96]. Because of its effectiveness and improved compliance, the once-daily methimazole regimen is often preferred for the treatment of hyperthyroidism.

When treating thyrotoxicosis that is not life threatening, the usual starting dose of PTU is 300 mg/d in three divided doses, whereas the starting dose of methimazole is 15 to 30 mg/d in a single dose.

Although administration of thionamides is typically by mouth, rectal and parenteral routes of administration have been reported. Rectal formulations of thionamides have been administered as enemas or suppositories. Several case reports described different formulations. Walter and colleagues [102] used an enema formulation of PTU made up of 8 50-mg tablets dissolved in Fleet's mineral oil (C.B. Fleet Company, Inc., Lynchburg, Virginia) (60 mL) or in Fleet's Phospho-soda (C.B. Fleet Company, Inc., Lynchburgh, Virginia) (60 mL). Nabil and colleagues [103] used a suppository formulation of methimazole at a rate of 1200 mg dissolved in water (12 mL) with two drops of Span80 (Merck Schuchardt OHG, Hohenbrunn, Germany), mixed with cocoa butter (52 mL). Yeung and colleagues [104] used an enema preparation of PTU (12 50-mg tablets) dissolved in sterile water (90 mL) and administered by means of a Foley catheter inserted into the rectum, with the balloon inflated to prevent leakage. Jongjaroenprasert and colleagues [105] compared the use of a suppository preparation of, PTU (200 mg) dissolved in a polyethylene glycol base with an enema preparation of PTU (8 50-mg tablets) dissolved in sterile water (90 mL). The enema preparation provided better bioavailability than the suppository form; however, both preparations had comparable therapeutic effect.

Like rectal formulations of thionamides, parenteral formulations of thionamides are not commercially available. Methimazole has been shown to have similar pharmacokinetics for oral and intravenous use in normal subjects and subjects with hyperthyroidism, however [106]. The authors have previously reported successful use of a parenteral preparation of methimazole made by reconstituting methimazole powder (500 mg) with sterile 0.9% sodium chloride solution to a final volume of 50 mL [107]. The solution (10 mg/mL) was then filtered through a 0.22-μm filter and subsequently administered as a slow intravenous push over 2 minutes, followed by a saline flush. This method of administration is of great value as a therapy of last resort if oral and rectal administration of thionamides is not possible.

Side effects of thionamide therapy

Common adverse side effects associated with antithyroid drug use are abnormal sense of taste, pruritus, arthralgias, and urticaria, which occur in approximately 1% to 5% of cases [108]. For cutaneous reactions, antihistamine therapy may eliminate symptoms and allow continued use of the medication. Alternatively, switching to another thionamide may be necessary. Up to 50% of patients have cross-reactivity between methimazole or carbimazole and PTU. In such cases, discontinuation of thionamide therapy and preparation for definitive treatment with radioactive iodine is usually required. Other agents, such as lithium, potassium perchlorate, and inorganic iodine, have been used as a bridge to ablative therapy in such cases and are discussed elsewhere in this article.

Agranulocytosis is a rare but potential fatal complication of thionamide therapy that typically occurs within the first 3 months of treatment [109]. Agranulocytosis may arise idiosyncratically at any time during treatment; thus, appropriate vigilance is required. The incidence of agranulocytosis with methimazole and PTU ranges between 0.2% and 0.5%. In a large 26-year retrospective study assessing the incidence of antithyroid drug–induced agranulocytosis in 30,798 patients, 109 (0.35%) presented with thionamide-induced agranulocytosis, defined as an absolute granulocyte count less than 500 per cubic millimeter [110]. The number of reported cases of agranulocytosis in patients receiving moderate doses of methimazole may be lower. In a case series of 50 patients with antithyroid drug–induced agranulocytosis, this side effect only occurred with methimazole doses of greater than 30 mg/d [111]. This suggests a direct relation between the incidence of agranulocytosis and dose of methimazole. No correlation between the incidence of agranulocytosis and dose of PTU has been observed [112].

Agranulocytosis attributable to antithyroid drug therapy most commonly presents with fever and sore throat, which may progress quickly to sepsis. *Pseudomonas aeruginosa* has been reported as the most common isolate from the blood of patients with thionamide-induced agranulocytosis [113]. When a patient presents with agranulocytosis and fever, appropriate broad-spectrum intravenous antibiotic therapy to include *P aeruginosa* coverage should be started.

Routine monitoring of the blood cell counts to check for agranulocytosis in patients receiving thionamide therapy has not been considered cost-effective; therefore, it is not generally recommended or necessary. It should always be emphasized to patients that agranulocytosis is a relatively rare complication of thionamide therapy; however, fever and sore throat are common illnesses that occur frequently. The occurrence of fever, sore throat, or viral syndrome in a patient being treated with thionamides requires urgent evaluation, including assessment of the complete blood cell count to exclude the potentially lethal complication of agranulocytosis. In most cases, however, agranulocytosis is not found to be the cause of such symptoms.

Another rare but serious side effect of antithyroid drug therapy is hepatotoxicity, which is reported in 0.1% to 0.2% of treated patients. Methimazole-induced hepatotoxicity presents as a cholestatic process. Alternatively, PTU-related hepatotoxicity evolves as an allergic hepatitis with markers of hepatocellular injury [114].

Vasculitis is another uncommon but potentially serious side effect of antithyroid drug therapy. It is typically associated with the presence of serologic markers, including antineutrophil cytoplasmic antibodies and antimyeloperoxidase antineutrophil cytoplasmic antibodies. In addition, some patients may acquire antineutrophil cytoplasmic antibody positivity, which is associated with arthritis, skin ulcerations, vasculitic rash, possibly sinusitis or hemoptysis, and acute renal insufficiency [114].

β-Adrenergic receptor blockade

Management of symptoms is also a key element in the treatment of thyrotoxicosis. Controlling the cardiovascular and hyperadrenergic manifestations of thyrotoxicosis is best achieved through β-adrenergic receptor blockade. Beta-blocker use in the management of thyrotoxicosis was first reported in 1966 with the agent pronethalol [115]. In the United States, propranolol soon became the most commonly used beta-blocker. Relatively large doses of propranolol are typically needed because of more rapid metabolism induced by thyrotoxicosis. Evidence also suggests that the number of cardiac β-adrenergic receptors is increased in thyrotoxic states [62]. In addition to its effect on β-adrenergic receptors, propranolol in doses greater than 160 mg/d can decrease T_3 levels by up to 30%. This reduction is caused by inhibition of 5′-monodeiodinase, which develops slowly over the first 7 to 10 days of treatment. Because of the increased requirement for propranolol during thyrotoxicosis and its short half-life, multiple large daily doses or use of the long-acting preparation may be required. To facilitate compliance, longer acting cardioselective β-adrenergic receptor antagonists may be used alternatively. Atenolol can be used with doses ranging between 50 and 200 mg/d; however, twice-daily dosing may be required in some instances to accomplish adequate control [116]. Metoprolol, dosed at 100 to 200 mg/d, or nadolol, dosed at 40 to 80 mg/d, can also be used [85].

Less commonly used medications to treat thyrotoxicosis

Many other medications have direct antithyroid effects or other actions that make them useful in the treatment of thyrotoxicosis. These agents are useful in the management of severe thyrotoxicosis or in cases in which side effects to a particular class of medication, such as thionamides, prevent its use.

Iodine

Inorganic iodine therapy may be particularly useful for the acute management of more severe thyrotoxicosis. Iodine has several helpful means of action in the treatment of thyrotoxicosis. At high concentrations, iodine blocks release of prestored hormone, decreases iodide transport, and prevents oxidation in follicular cells. At lower concentrations, iodide can accelerate thyroid metabolism. Inhibition of thyroid metabolism by iodide is known as the Wolff-Chaikoff effect and is only transient. The thyroid gland begins to escape iodine inhibition after approximately 48 hours as the iodide transport system adapts to the higher concentration of iodide by modulating the activity of the sodium-iodide symporter [117]. Within 1 to 2 weeks, complete escape from inhibition occurs. The addition of thionamides during iodine therapy is typically necessary to prevent recurrent thyrotoxicosis after this loss of the Wolff-Chaikoff effect. In severe cases of thyrotoxicosis, thionamide therapy should be administered at least 1 hour before iodine treatment to inhibit possible exacerbation of the hyperthyroidism that may occur if iodine is given alone [118].

Oral formulations of inorganic iodine include a saturated solution of potassium iodide (SSKI) and Lugol's solution. Three to 5 drops of Lugol's solution are required daily (assuming 20 drops per mL and a concentration of 8 mg per drop) or 1 drop of SSKI daily (assuming 20 drops per mL and a concentration of 38 mg per drop) [85].

The oral iodinated contrast agents iopanoic acid and sodium ipodate have also been used for control of severe thyrotoxicosis. These agents have several novel effects, including inhibition of types 1 and 2 $5'$-monodeiodinase and inhibition of T_3 and T_4 binding to cellular receptors [55,119]. These agents are no longer marketed commercially, however, and are now unavailable for use. Parenteral formulations of iodine, including sodium iodide, are also effective in the management of thyrotoxicosis but are no longer available in the United States.

Potassium perchlorate

Potassium perchlorate is an indispensable agent for the treatment of AIT. Perchlorate may also be valuable as a second-line agent in patients who are intolerant of thionamide therapy. Long-term use of perchlorate is generally limited by the rare risk of side effects, such as aplastic anemia. Perchlorate is best used in this setting as a bridge to definitive ablative therapy with radioactive iodine or thyroidectomy. The use of potassium perchlorate is discussed further in the section on the treatment of amiodarone-induced thyrotoxicosis below.

Lithium

Lithium can be used when thionamide therapy is contraindicated because of an adverse reaction or toxicity; it can also be used in combination with PTU or methimazole [120]. Lithium has several effects on the thyroid gland that make it useful for treatment of thyrotoxicosis: lithium directly decreases thyroid hormone secretion and also inhibits coupling of the iodotyrosine residues that form iodothyronines (T_4 and T_3) [121]. For treatment of thyrotoxicosis, the dose for lithium is 300 mg administered every 8 hours. Serum lithium concentration should be monitored. To avoid toxicity during lithium treatment, the serum lithium level should remain less than 1 mEq/L.

Cholestyramine

Cholestyramine is an anion exchange resin that has been shown to decrease reabsorption of thyroid hormone from the enterohepatic circulation. It has been successfully used as a therapeutic agent for management of thyrotoxicosis [122]. Thyroid hormone metabolism occurs mainly in the liver, where thyroid hormone is conjugated to sulfates and glucuronides. Subsequently, these conjugation products are excreted in the bile. A fraction of conjugated thyroid hormone is deconjugated in the bowel, and the liberated hormone is subsequently reabsorbed. In the thyrotoxic state, enterohepatic circulation of thyroid hormone increases. Cholestyramine functions by binding thyroid hormone in the intestine, decreasing its reabsorption. Cholestyramine administered orally at a rate of 4 g four times daily, in combination with methimazole or PTU, has been found to cause a more rapid decline in thyroid hormone levels than thionamide therapy alone [122–124].

Radioactive iodine

Radioactive iodine thyroid ablation is the most widely used definitive treatment for thyrotoxicosis attributable to Graves' disease or TMNG in the United States. Thyroid ablation allows discontinuation of thionamide treatment and eliminates concern about the worrisome side effects, such as agranulocytosis, hepatotoxicity, or vasculitis, associated with these medications.

The major long-term side effect of radioactive iodine therapy is permanent hypothyroidism. Short-term side effects after treatment include radiation thyroiditis, which can present as anterior neck tenderness, as well as gastritis and sialadenitis.

Many studies have reviewed the incidence of secondary malignancy in patients who have received radioactive iodine therapy. Holm and colleagues [125] evaluated the risk of leukemia in a group of 10,552 patients treated with ^{131}I for hyperthyroidism over an average period of 15 years and found no increase in the risk of leukemia or malignant lymphoma. In this study, patients who received ^{131}I therapy for hyperthyroidism had a slightly greater (6%) overall cancer risk than that expected in the general population. In another study of 7417 patients treated with radioactive iodine for hyperthyroidism, Franklyn and colleagues [126] found a decrease in the relative risk of overall cancer mortality in treated patients. There was a significant increase in the incidence and mortality of thyroid cancer (standardized incidence ratio of 3.25, 95% confidence interval: 1.69–6.25) and of cancers of the small bowel (standardized incidence ratio of 4.81, 95% confidence interval: 2.16–10.72), although the absolute risk of these cancers was small.

Overall, the risk of increased secondary malignancies after treatment with radioactive iodine for hyperthyroidism is relatively small and not consistently demonstrated by all studies. Moreover, some of the malignancies reported were thyroidal in origin. These malignancies should be unexpected in individuals in whom minimal, if any, detectable residual thyroid tissue remained following treatment with [131]I. These studies may instead reflect an increased incidence of de novo thyroid malignancy in patients who did not receive completely ablative therapy and in whom significant amounts of remnant thyroid tissue remained. Further, some of the studies noted do not have an appropriate long-term control group. In summary, it is believed that ^{131}I therapy is relatively safe and effective. It is reasonable to bear in mind these suggestions regarding a mild possible increase in the rate of certain malignancies. However, individual circumstances must be considered for each patient and these data should not unduly influence the decision to utilize radioactive iodine therapy for the treatment of hyperthyroidism.

To achieve successful treatment of hyperthyroidism in the best possible manner, an ablative approach to radioactive iodine treatment is recommended, with a goal of rendering the patient hypothyroid. Giving lower doses of radioactive iodine in an attempt to achieve euthyroidism but to avoid hypothyroidism may fail to cure the hyperthyroidism and necessitate repeated treatments [127–129]. An estimate of the dose needed to deliver an activity sufficient for complete gland ablation requires consideration of thyroid gland weight and the 24-hour radioactive iodine uptake. One commonly used formula to calculate the required dose using these parameters is presented in Fig. 1 [130]. Higher doses of radioactive iodine may be required in some patients with a larger gland size and 24-hour uptake values of greater than 70% as well as in patients who have received pretreatment with antithyroid drugs for more than 4 months.

The administration of radioactive iodine to a thyrotoxic patient poses a minor risk of acute exacerbation of hyperthyroidism. This has rarely been reported to cause life-threatening thyrotoxicosis. McDermott and colleagues [131] calculated the frequency of hyperthyroidism exacerbation after radioactive iodine treatment. In this series, 10 (0.34%) of 2975 patients treated developed thyroid storm. An additional 26 patients (0.88%) had exacerbations of thyrotoxicosis that did not meet the criteria for thyroid storm.

Pretreatment with thionamides has been used to reduce the risk of such posttreatment thyrotoxicosis. Retrospective studies have shown that the

$$\frac{100\text{-}200 \ \mu Ci \ X \ \text{thyroid gland weight (g)}}{24 \ \text{hour RAIU (\%)}}$$

Fig. 1. Calculation of ^{131}I dose based on goiter size and radioactive iodine uptake (RAIU).

efficacy of radioactive iodine therapy is reduced after treatment with PTU [132,133]. Pretreatment with methimazole and carbimazole does not seem to reduce the effect of radioactive iodine therapy as long as the agents are discontinued 3 to 5 days before treatment [134,135]. In a prospective randomized trial, 32 hyperthyroid patients received ^{131}I therapy without pretreatment and 29 patients received ^{131}I therapy with methimazole pretreatment of at a rate of 30 mg/d. After 1 year, the success rate of the treatment was similar in both groups: 86.2% in the group that had methimazole pretreatment and 84.4% in the group that did not have pretreatment [134]. Other retrospective studies have demonstrated similar findings [136].

The response to radioactive iodine treatment is not immediate, and patients often require continued antithyroid drug treatment until hypothyroidism begins to develop. Usually, patients become hypothyroid after ablative doses of radioactive iodine within 2 to 3 months of treatment. Persistent hyperthyroidism 6 months after therapy may require retreatment with radioactive iodine to achieve complete ablation [130].

Thyrotoxicosis frequently causes emotional lability and anxiety that may prevent appropriate informed consent during formulation of a treatment plan. Pretreatment with thionamides and establishment of euthyroidism may improve comprehension of treatment options and rational decision making. This should always be considered during treatment of a thyrotoxic patient.

Disease-specific treatment

Graves' disease

Antithyroid drugs to decrease thyroid hormone production and β-adrenergic receptor blockade to control peripheral manifestations of thyrotoxicosis are the most effective medical means of controlling thyrotoxicosis associated with Graves' disease. Once the patient is euthyroid, treatment options include continued use of antithyroid drugs or definitive treatment with radioactive iodine or surgery.

The use of antithyroid medication in an effort to attain permanent remission of Graves' disease is more common in Europe than in the United States. If antithyroid medication is used to attain remission, the dose needed to control the disease is usually relatively low. Methimazole at a dose of 5 to 10 mg/d or PTU at a dose of 100 to 200 mg/d is typically sufficient. After 12 to 18 months of treatment, the antithyroid medication can be discontinued or tapered. Subsequently, close follow-up is required to assess relapse, which usually arises in the first 3 to 6 months after cessation of the antithyroid medication [137]. The overall recurrence rate after discontinuation of antithyroid medication is approximately 50% to 60% [138]. If a patient has recurrence after cessation of antithyroid drug therapy, radioiodine treatment or surgery should be considered.

Radioiodine treatment, as discussed previously, is effective for treatment of Graves' disease and has few side effects. In addition, no significant long-term sequelae other than hypothyroidism have been noted over the past 60 years of its use in clinical practice. The surgical option for treatment of Graves' disease is subtotal or total thyroidectomy. Although this represents the most invasive treatment option, several situations favor surgical management of Graves' disease (Table 1).

Treatment of Graves' ophthalmopathy

Intravenous and oral glucocorticoids have been used to treat severe Graves' ophthalmopathy. Oral regimens, typically employing prednisone at doses of 60 to 100 mg/d for several months, have demonstrated improvement of ophthalmopathy in approximately 60% of cases [139]. Some studies suggest that intravenous glucocorticoids may be more effective than oral glucocorticoids for the treatment of severe eye disease [140]. Multiple case reports suggest that intravenous steroid therapy for treatment of Graves' ophthalmopathy may increase the risk of complications, such as liver injury and significant loss of bone density. The decision to use this mode of therapy should be carefully considered. Patients receiving intravenous steroid therapy for treatment of Graves' ophthalmopathy should be carefully screened for the presence of liver disease before therapy and closely monitored through its completion [140].

Glucocorticoid treatment of marked Graves' ophthalmopathy is also beneficial after radioactive iodine ablation. Destruction of thyroid tissue by radioactive iodine causes release of thyroid antigens and further activation of T and B lymphocytes. This frequently leads to worsened

Table 1
General indications for surgery in preference to radioactive iodine for the treatment of hyperthyroidism attributable to Graves' disease or toxic thyroid nodule(s)

Absolute indications
Suspicious or biopsy-proven malignant nodules
Comorbidity also requiring surgery (eg, hyperparathyroidism)
Inability to use radioactive iodine ablation
Pregnancy or lactation
Children <16 years of age
Severe intolerance to antithyroid medication
Large compressive/obstructive goiter
Relative indications
Severe Graves' ophthalmopathy
Poorly controlled Graves' disease requiring definitive treatment
Patients desiring pregnancy within 6 to 12 months of treatment
Patients unable to continue close follow-up
Patients incompletely treated by initial attempt at radioactive iodine ablation

Adapted from Grodski S, Stalberg P, Robinson BG, et al. Surgery versus radioiodine therapy as definitive management for Graves' disease: the role of patient preference. Thyroid 2007;17(2):158; with permission.

ophthalmopathy. Two randomized, prospective, controlled trials by Barta-lena and colleagues [141] and Tallstedt and colleagues [142] showed a pro-gression of ophthalmopathy with radioiodine administration. The study by Bartalena and colleagues [141] also demonstrated that treatment with high-dose steroids at the time of radioactive iodine ablation significantly mitigated this effect. The study assessed 443 patients with Graves' hyperthy-roidism who received treatment with radioactive iodine alone or with radio-active iodine followed by a course of prednisone (0.4–0.5 mg/kg of body weight daily) starting 2 to 3 days after radioactive iodine therapy and continuing for 1 month, followed by a taper over 2 months. Bartalena and colleagues [141] demonstrated that 23 (15%) of 150 patients treated without steroids had new onset or worsening of preexisting ophthalmopathy 2 to 6 months after treatment. In the group that received prednisone, 50 (57%) of 75 patients with ophthalmopathy at the start of the study had improvement and no patients developed progression. The use of gluco-corticoid treatment has subsequently become a standard of care for patients with Graves' ophthalmopathy treated with radioactive iodine who have active eye disease [139].

Smokers have been shown to have up to a fourfold risk for developing Graves' eye disease [143]. Smokers with Graves' disease are also at increased risk for progression of orbitopathy after radioactive iodine ablation. Also, in comparison to nonsmokers with Graves' disease, they may be less responsive to glucocorticoid treatment to prevent worsening of eye disease after radioac-tive iodine ablation. In a study of patients with mild Graves' ophthalmopathy, the combination of radioactive iodine therapy and a short course of oral pred-nisone was associated with improvement of ophthalmopathy in 37 (64%) of 58 nonsmokers, whereas only 13 (15%) of 87 smokers had improvement [144].

Ophthalmologic evaluation to identify patients at increased risk for com-plications of Graves' eye disease can be a valuable resource when radioac-tive iodine therapy for Graves' disease is being considered. Smokers and all patients with significant Graves' ophthalmopathy should receive oph-thalmologic evaluation and be considered for appropriate steroid therapy at the time of radioactive iodine treatment.

Toxic multinodular goiter and solitary toxic adenoma

TMNG and solitary adenoma are caused by defects in the TSH receptor, resulting in constitutive activation and autonomous nodule function. Anti-thyroid drug therapy may be used to normalize thyroid function but does not provide definitive therapy. Recurrent hyperthyroidism is virtually cer-tain if antithyroid drug therapy is discontinued. Thionamides do not prevent the growth of autonomous nodules, and extended use of thionamides may place the patient at risk for toxicity, as discussed previously [145]. Radioac-tive iodine ablation of the thyroid and thyroidectomy are the most common treatments offering durable cure of these conditions.

Radioactive iodine ablation is generally the preferred method of definitive treatment for TMNG and toxic adenoma. Because the thyroid tends to be larger and the radioactive uptake lower in these diseases, however, the dose required for ablation is typically larger than that needed to treat Graves' disease [1]. To prevent recurrence, the dose given should be sufficient to cause complete thyroid ablation and permanent hypothyroidism. The usual dose given varies between 15 and 30 mCi depending on size of the gland and 24-hour radioactive iodine uptake of the gland [145]. The recurrence rate of hyperthyroidism after radioactive iodine treatment is approximately 20% [130]. If recurrence of hyperthyroidism occurs after radioactive iodine treatment, a second course of radioactive iodine or thyroidectomy should be considered. Thyroidectomy as a first-line mode of therapy for TMNG and solitary toxic adenoma may offer advantages in certain situations, as listed in Table 1.

Thyroiditis

Treatment of subacute thyroiditis is usually supportive and involves management of pain with nonsteroidal anti-inflammatory drugs and control of hyperadrenergic symptoms with beta-blockade. If pain is persistent with maximum nonsteroidal therapy, glucocorticoid therapy can be initiated with prednisone at doses of 40 mg/d for 7 to 10 days, followed by a tapered dose over 1 to 2 weeks [1,130]. Silent thyroiditis and postpartum thyroiditis do not present with pain. In these cases, treatment is aimed at controlling symptoms as needed with beta-blockade only.

Amiodarone-induced thyrotoxicosis

Treatment of type I AIT can begin with antithyroid drugs and beta-blockers for mild to moderate disease. For more severe thyrotoxicosis, treatment with potassium perchlorate in combination with thionamides is usually necessary. Thionamides and potassium perchlorate work by complementary means. Potassium perchlorate inhibits iodine uptake by the thyroid gland by means of direct inhibition of the sodium iodide symporter, whereas thionamides inhibit organification and synthesis of hormone within the thyroid gland. Potassium perchlorate at a dose of 500 mg administered twice daily and methimazole at a dose of 30 to 50 mg administered daily normalize thyroid hormone levels, with an average treatment course of 4 weeks [146,147]. Potential side effects of aplastic anemia and nephritic syndrome have been rarely reported with extended use of potassium perchlorate [148]. For this reason, limiting the course of treatment is recommended. Several studies have found that with a treatment time of 1 month and a potassium perchlorate dose of no greater than 1 g/d, aplastic anemia and nephritic syndrome did not occur [146,147,149]. When medical treatment is not effective in controlling thyrotoxicosis, thyroidectomy should be considered.

Because type II AIT is essentially a form of destructive thyroiditis with thyrotoxicosis because of release of stored hormone, thionamide therapy and treatment with potassium perchlorate is not effective. Type II AIT is self-limiting; it usually lasts from 1 to 3 months and resolves once intrathyroidal stores of thyroid hormone are depleted. It generally resolves without treatment but may present with severe symptoms that do require intervention. This is of particular concern in patients treated with amiodarone because they usually have significant underlying cardiac disease and may not tolerate any significant degree of thyrotoxicosis. Treatment with glucocorticoids effectively controls the hyperthyroidism associated with type II AIT and has been shown to normalize thyroid function rapidly, as assessed by measurement of free T_3, and inflammation, as indicated by interleukin-6 levels [146,150].

Hyperthyroidism and pregnancy

Hyperthyroidism during pregnancy can be deleterious to the fetus as well as to the mother; therefore, both patients need to be considered. Fetal complications include intrauterine growth retardation, prematurity, stillbirth, low birth weight, and neonatal hyperthyroidism. Maternal complications include obstetric complications, such as eclampsia, miscarriage, and placenta abruptio, as well as systemic complications, including congestive heart failure or thyroid storm [151].

The prevalence of true hyperthyroidism during pregnancy is approximately 0.1% to 0.4%. Normal variation of thyroid function indices during pregnancy frequently includes significant suppression of TSH and elevation of total T_4 and total T_3. During a normal first trimester of pregnancy, 18% of completely asymptomatic women have a TSH value less than the lower limit of normal. Of these, 50% have a TSH value that is completely suppressed and undetectable [152]. Peak suppression of maternal TSH directly corresponds to the peak human chorionic gonadotropin (HCG) concentration. This may be particularly confusing in multiparous pregnancies and in pregnancies complicated by hyperemesis gravidarum, because HCG is increased in both situations. Thirty percent to 50% of women with hyperemesis gravidarum develop biochemical evidence of hyperthyroidism and may also develop clinical symptoms. A missense mutation in the TSH receptor has been implicated in formation of a supersensitive TSH receptor that amplifies the response to HCG in hyperemesis gravidarum and may be responsible for the development of thyrotoxicosis [153].

Familial gestational hyperthyroidism is a rare cause of hyperthyroidism in pregnancy; it occurs as the result of a mutation of the thyrotropin receptor that renders it more sensitive to HCG. In this situation, gestational hyperthyroidism occurs with normal serum HCG concentrations [154].

These confounding factors often obscure the differentiation between true hyperthyroidism and normal gravid physiologic changes in the thyroid axis

[155,156]. True thyrotoxicosis should be suspected in pregnancy when TSH is less than 0.1. This is especially true if TSH suppression continues past 20 weeks of gestation; by that time, normal thyrotoxicosis of pregnancy generally resolves spontaneously [152].

Graves' disease accounts for up to 85% of all pregnancy-related hyperthyroidism [152,157]. The presentation may be somewhat atypical, however. Unless they predate the pregnancy, autoimmune sequelae typical of Graves' disease, such as orbitopathy and dermopathy, are rare because of the autoimmune suppression that occurs during normal pregnancy [1]. Goiter may be present and may suggest Graves' disease. Studies using ultrasound have documented thyroid size increases of 13% to 30% in normal pregnancies as well, however [158].

Treatment of thyrotoxicosis in pregnancy

Treatment of thyrotoxicosis during pregnancy can decrease associated complications [159]. The primary treatment for hyperthyroidism during pregnancy is antithyroid drug therapy with thionamides. PTU and methimazole cross the placenta and can be concentrated in the fetal thyroid gland. Use of methimazole during pregnancy has been associated with a scalp defect known as aplasia cutis, choanal and esophageal atresia, and minor facial dysmorphisms in newborns. Use of PTU has not been associated with these defects. To explain this observation, it has been suggested that methimazole crosses the placenta more easily than PTU [159–162]. This has not been supported by transplacental kinetic studies in term uterine tissue from women without thyroid disease after cesarean delivery [163]. The authors prefer PTU over methimazole for treatment of hyperthyroidism during pregnancy. If PTU is not tolerated, methimazole should be substituted, especially after first-trimester organogenesis is complete. Even with the use of PTU at daily doses as low as 100 to 300 mg, decreases in serum T_4 concentration with elevation in TSH have been observed in neonates [159,164]. Therefore, the lowest possible dose of PTU necessary to treat hyperthyroidism is recommended. In general, daily doses of PTU should be 200 mg or less. The authors suggest treating Graves' disease during pregnancy with a goal of maintaining maternal total T_4 in the upper to middle normal range and have adopted expert recommendations for using a pregnancy normal reference range for total T_4 that is 1.5 times the nongravid reference limit to guide therapy [152].

Graves' disease may spontaneously resolve as pregnancy progresses into the third trimester, and thionamides may be safely discontinued in up to 30% of patients. Routine assessment of maternal thyroid function every 2 to 4 weeks is therefore essential when following a pregnancy complicated by Graves' disease. Such vigilance prevents unnecessary use of thionamides and possible maternal or fetal hypothyroidism caused by overtreatment.

If doses of PTU greater than 600 mg/d or doses of methimazole greater than 40 mg/d are required to control thyrotoxicosis, consideration of thyroidectomy may be reasonable [1]. Surgery is also an alternative option if antithyroid drug therapy is contraindicated or if emergent treatment is needed for other reasons, such as acute obstruction attributable to enlarging goiter or medical noncompliance. Pregnant thyrotoxic patients being prepared for surgery may require β-adrenergic blockade. Inorganic iodine treatment may also be needed for up to 2 weeks before surgery to normalize thyroid function and to prevent the occurrence of thyroid storm during thyroidectomy [152].

It is frequently suggested that surgery should be performed in the second trimester [165]. No prospective data are present to guide this decision, however. In fact, at least one series suggests that surgery during the first trimester does not increase the risk of spontaneous abortion [166]. Therefore, risks related to delay of treatment versus the risk of the treatment itself should always be carefully considered.

When maternal hyperthyroidism is present, close fetal monitoring to evaluate the presence of fetal hyperthyroidism as well as to guard against the possible development of fetal hypothyroidism from overtreatment is essential. Ultrasonographic evaluation to assess the presence of fetal goiter, fetal growth rate, and monitoring of the fetal heart rate is the most commonly used means of observation. Fetal hyperthyroidism occurs in approximately 1% of pregnancies associated with maternal Graves' disease [158]. Fetal thyrotoxicosis occurs as a result of transplacental passage of maternal TRAb, causing stimulation of the fetal thyroid gland. If a fetal goiter is present along with fetal tachycardia, fetal thyrotoxicosis should be suspected. Treatment of fetal thyrotoxicosis is accomplished indirectly through maternal administration of thionamides. After optimizing treatment for 2 weeks with thionamide therapy and monitoring of maternal thyroid function tests, fetal ultrasound should be evaluated for resolution of goiter and tachycardia [167]. Persistence of fetal goiter may be attributable to continued fetal hyperthyroidism or hypothyroidism resulting from the use of thionamide therapy. Evaluation of maternal thyroid function tests may assist in deciphering the underlying cause of fetal goiter in such cases. If maternal total T_4 or free T_4 values are in the middle normal to lower range, the fetal goiter is likely attributable to hypothyroidism caused by overtreatment with thionamides. Persistent fetal goiter attributable to hyperthyroidism is more likely if maternal total and free T_4 values remain elevated, especially if this is associated with fetal tachycardia. In both cases, if fetal goiter does not improve with appropriate adjustment of thionamide therapy, more aggressive diagnostic and therapeutic measures may be needed. Periumbilical blood sampling to ascertain true fetal thyroid status and intra-amniotic levothyroxine therapy to treat persistent hypothyroidism have been successfully used for management of complicated fetal thyroid dysfunction in pregnancy [168,169].

Summary

Thyrotoxicosis is a condition resulting from elevated levels of thyroid hormone. Diagnosis and differentiation of the etiologies of thyrotoxicosis are aided by laboratory evaluation with thyroid function tests as well as TRAb in certain circumstances. Imaging with ultrasound and nuclear medicine scans, including radioactive iodine scans as well as Tc-99m scans, can aid in determining the etiology of thyrotoxicosis. Treatment modalities include medical treatment with thionamides, β-adrenergic receptor blockade, and iodine as well as with alternative agents, such as lithium, potassium perchlorate, and cholestyramine, in certain circumstances. Definitive therapy with radioactive iodine or surgery is recommended for Graves' disease, TMNG, and toxic adenoma.

References

[1] Larsen PR, Davies TF, et al. Thyrotoxicosis. In: Larsen PR, Kronenberg HM, Melmed S, et al, editors. Williams' textbook of endocrinology. 10th edition. Philadelphia: WB Saunders Co; 2002. p. 374–421.

[2] Turnbridge WMG, Evered DC, Hall R. The spectrum of thyroid disease in a community. Clin Endocrinol (Oxf) 1977;7:483–93.

[3] Takasu N, Yamada T, Sato A, et al. Graves' disease following hyperthyroidism due to Hashimoto's disease: studies of eight cases. Clin Endocrinol (Oxf) 1990;33(6):687–98.

[4] Marcocci C, Bartalena L, Bogazzi F, et al. Studies on the occurrence of ophthalmopathy in Graves' disease. Acta Endocrinol (Copenh) 1989;120(4):473–8.

[5] Fatourechi V. Pretibial myxedema: pathophysiology and treatment options. Am J Clin Dermatol 2005;6(5):295–309.

[6] Bahn RS. Understanding the immunology of Graves' ophthalmopathy: is it an autoimmune disease? Endocrinol Metab Clin North Am 2000;29:287–96.

[7] Salvi M, Zhang Z-G, Haegert D. Patients with endocrine ophthalmopathy not associated with overt thyroid disease have multiple thyroid immunological abnormalities. J Clin Endocrinol Metab 1990;70:89–94.

[8] Prabhakar B, Bahn RS, Smith TJ. Current perspective on the pathogenesis of Graves' disease and ophthalmopathy. Endocr Rev 2003;24(6):802–35.

[9] Smith TJ. Dexamethasone regulation of glycosaminoglycan synthesis cultured human fibroblasts: similar effects of glucocorticoid and thyroid hormone therapy. J Clin Invest 1984;64:2157–63.

[10] Dabon-Almirante CL, Surks M. Clinical and laboratory diagnosis of thyrotoxicosis. Endocrinol Metab Clin North Am 1998;27(1):25–35.

[11] Bull RH, Coburn PR, Mortimer PS. Pretibial myxedema: a manifestation of lymphoedema? Lancet 1993;341:403–4.

[12] Kriss JP, Pleshakov V, Rosenblum A, et al. Therapy with occlusive dressings of pretibial myxedema with fluocinolone acetonide. J Clin Endocrinol Metab 1967;27:595–604.

[13] Volden G. Successful treatment of chronic skin diseases with clobetasol propionate and a hydrocolloid occlusive dressing. Acta Derm Venereol 1992;72:69–71.

[14] Schwartz KM, Fatourechi V, Ahmed D, et al. Dermopathy of Graves' disease (pretibial myxedema). J Clin Endocrinol Metab 2002;87(2):438–46.

[15] Jabbour SA. Cutaneous manifestations of endocrine disorders. Am J Clin Dermatol 2003; 4(5):315–31.

[16] Tonacchera M, Agretti P, Chiovato L, et al. Activating thyrotropin receptor mutations are present in nonadenomatous hyperfunctioning nodules of toxic or autonomous multinodular goiter. J Clin Endocrinol Metab 2000;85:2270–4.

[17] Tonacchera M, VanSande J, Cetani F, et al. Functional characteristics of three new germline mutations of the thyrotropin receptor gene causing autosomal dominant toxic thyroid hyperplasia. J Clin Endocrinol Metab 1996;81:547–54.

[18] Fatourechi V, Aniszewski JP, Jacobsen SJ, et al. Clinical features and outcome of subacute thyroiditis in an incidence cohort: Olmstead County, Minnesota, study. J Clin Endocrinol Metab 2003;88(5):2100–5.

[19] Weetman AP, Smallridge RC, Nutman TB, et al. Persistent thyroid autoimmunity after subacute thyroiditis. J Clin Lab Immunol 1987;23:1–6.

[20] Stancek D, Stancekova-Gressnerova M, Janotka M, et al. Isolation and some serological and epidemiological data on the viruses recovered from patients with subacute thyroiditis de Quervain. Med Microbiol Immunol 1975;161:133–44.

[21] Martino E, Buratti L, Bartalena L, et al. High prevalence of subacute thyroiditis during summer season in Italy. J Endocrinol Invest 1987;10:321–3.

[22] Farwell AP. Subacute thyroiditis and acute infectious thyroiditis. In: Braverman LE, Utiger RD, editors. Werner's and Ingbar's the thyroid. 9th edition. Philadelphia: Lipincott, Williams, Wilkins; 2005. p. 536–47.

[23] Pearce EN, Farwell AP, Braverman LE. Thyroiditis. N Engl J Med 2003;348(26):2646–55.

[24] Lio S, Pontecorvi A, Caruso M, et al. Transitory subclinical and permanent hypothyroidism in the course of subacute thyroiditis (de Quervain). Acta Endocrinol 1984; 106:67–70.

[25] Nikolai TF, Coombs GJ, McKenzie AK, et al. Lymphocytic thyroiditis with spontaneously resolving hyperthyroidism (silent thyroiditis) and subacute thyroiditis: long-term follow-up. Arch Intern Med 1982;142:2281–3.

[26] Lazarus JH. Sporadic and postpartum thyroiditis. In: Braverman LE, Utiger RD, editors. Werner's and Ingbar's the thyroid. 9th edition. Philadelphia: Lipincott, Williams, Wilkins; 2005. p. 524–35.

[27] Stagnaro-Green A. Postpartum thyroiditis. J Clin Endocrinol Metab 2002;87(9):4042–7.

[28] Marqusee E, Hill J, Mandel S. Thyroiditis after pregnancy loss. J Clin Endocrinol Metab 1997;82(8):2455–7.

[29] Walfish PG, Meyerson J, Papsin F, et al. Prevalence and characteristics of post-partum thyroid dysfunction: results of a survey from Toronto, Canada. J Endocrinol Invest 1992;15: 265–72.

[30] Lucas A, Pizarro E, Granada ML, et al. Postpartum thyroiditis: long-term follow-up. Thyroid 2005;15(10):1177–81.

[31] Lazarus JH, Ammari F, Oretti R, et al. Clinical aspects of recurrent postpartum thyroiditis. Br J Gen Pract 1997;47(418):305–8.

[32] Miller KK, Daniels GH. Association between lithium use and thyrotoxicosis caused by silent thyroiditis. Clin Endocrinol (Oxf) 2001;55:501–8.

[33] Ronnblom LE, Alm GV, Oberg KE. Autoimmunity after alpha-interferon therapy for malignant carcinoid tumors. Ann Intern Med 1991;115:178–83.

[34] Wong V, Fu AX, George J, et al. Thyrotoxicosis induced by alpha-interferon therapy in chronic viral hepatitis. Clin Endocrinol (Oxf) 2002;56:793–8.

[35] Kennedy RL. Amiodarone and the thyroid. Clin Chem 1989;35:1882–7.

[36] Harjai KJ, Licata AA. Effects of amiodarone on thyroid function. Ann Intern Med 1997; 126(1):63–73.

[37] Martino E, Safran M, Haffajee C, et al. Environmental iodine intake and thyroid dysfunction during chronic amiodarone therapy. Ann Intern Med 1984;101(1):28–34.

[38] Usui T, Shoichiro I, Toshiaki S. Clinical and molecular features of a TSH-secreting pituitary macroadenoma. Pituitary 2005;8:127–34.

[39] Brucker-Davis F, Oldfield EH, Skarulis MC, et al. Thyrotropin-secreting pituitary tumors: diagnostic criteria, thyroid hormone sensitivity, and treatment outcome in 25 patients followed at the National Institutes of Health. J Clin Endocrinol Metab 1999;84(2):476–86.

[40] Refetoff S. Resistance to thyroid hormone. In: Braverman LE, Utiger RE, editors. Werner's and Ingbar's the thyroid: a fundamental and clinical text. 9th edition. Philadelphia: Lippincott, Williams, and Wilkins; 2005. p. 1109–29.

[41] Olateju T, Vanderpump M. Thyroid hormone resistance. Ann Clin Biochem 2006;43: 431–40.

[42] Arevalo G. Prevalence of familial dysalbuminemic hyperthyroxinemia in serum samples received for thyroid testing. Clin Chem 1991;37(8):1430–1.

[43] Jensen IW, Faber J. Familial dysalbuminemic hyperthyroxinemia. Acta Med Scand 1987; 221:469–73.

[44] Stockigt SA, Dyer SA, Mohr VS, et al. Specific methods to identify plasma binding abnormalities in euthyroid hyperthyroxinemia. J Clin Endocrinol Metab 1986;62:230–3.

[45] Hedberg CW, Fishbein DB, Janssen RS, et al. An outbreak of thyrotoxicosis caused by the consumption of bovine thyroid gland in ground beef. N Engl J Med 1987;316:993–8.

[46] Shakir KM, Michaels RD, Hays JH. The use of bile acid sequestrants to lower serum thyroid hormones in iatrogenic hyperthyroidism. Ann Intern Med 1993;118(2):112–3.

[47] Ayhan A, Yanik F, Tuncer R, et al. Struma ovarii. Int J Gynecol Obstet 1993;42(2):143–6.

[48] Grandet PJ, Remi MH. Struma ovarii with hyperthyroidism. Clin Nucl Med 2000;25(10): 763–5.

[49] Dardik RB, Dardik M, Westra W, et al. Malignant struma ovarii: two case reports and a review of the literature. Gynecol Oncol 1999;73:447–51.

[50] Joja I, Asakawa T, Mitsumori A, et al. I-123 uptake in nonfunctional struma ovarii. Clin Nucl Med 1998;23:10–2.

[51] Nahn PA, Robinson E, Strassman M. Conservative therapy for malignant struma ovarii: a case report. J Reprod Med 2002;47:943–5.

[52] Leiter L, Sieldin SM, Marinelli LD. Adenocarcinoma of the thyroid with hyperthyroidism and functional metastases. J Clin Endocrinol 1946;6:247–51.

[53] Burman KD. Special presentations of thyroid cancer in pregnancy, renal failure, thyrotoxicosis, and struma ovarii. In: Wartofsky L, Van Nostrand D, editors. Thyroid cancer: a comprehensive guide to clinical management. Totowa (NJ): Humana Press; 2006. p. 387–92.

[54] Pearce EN. Thyrotoxicosis of extrathyroid origin. In: Braverman LE, Utiger RD, editors. Werner's and Ingbar's the thyroid. 9th edition. Philadelphia: Lippincott, Williams, Wilkins; 2005. p. 548–51.

[55] Wartofsky L. Thyrotoxic storm. In: Braverman LE, Utiger RD, editors. Werner's and Ingbar's the thyroid. 9th edition. Philadelphia: Lippincott, Williams & Wilkins; 2005. p. 660–4, 652–7.

[56] MacCrimmon DJ, Wallace J, Goldberg WM, et al. Emotional disturbance and cognitive deficits in hyperthyroidism. Psychosom Med 1979;41(4):331–40.

[57] Ridgway EC, Longcope C, Maloof F. Metabolic clearance and blood production rates of estradiol in hyperthyroidism. J Clin Endocrinol Metab 1975;41(3):491–7.

[58] Ridgway EC, Maloof F, Longcope C. Androgen and oestrogen dynamics in hyperthyroidism. J Endocrinol 1982;95:105–15.

[59] Ojamaa K, Klemperer JD, Klein I. Acute effects of thyroid hormone on vascular smooth muscle. Thyroid 1996;6(5):505–12.

[60] Klein I, Ojama K. Thyroid hormone and the cardiovascular system. N Engl J Med 2001; 344(7):501–8.

[61] Klein I, Ojamaa K. Thyrotoxicosis and the heart. Endocrinol Metab Clin North Am 1998; 27(1):51–61.

[62] Ladenson P. Diagnosis of thyrotoxicosis. In: Braverman LE, Utiger RD, editors. Werner's and Ingbar's the thyroid. 9th edition. Philadelphia: Lippincott, Williams & Wilkins; 2005. p. 660–4.

[63] Baloch Z, Caryon P, Conte-Devolx B, et al. Laboratory medicine practice guidelines: laboratory support for the diagnosis and monitoring of thyroid disease. Thyroid 2003;13(1):3–126.

[64] Pimental L, Hansen K. Thyroid disease in the emergency department: a clinical and laboratory review. J Emerg Med 2005;28:201–9.

[65] Costagliola S, Morgenthaler NG, Hoermann R, et al. Second generation assay for thyrotropin receptor antibodies has superior diagnostic sensitivity for Graves' disease. J Clin Endocrinol Metab 1999;84(1):90–7.

[66] Quadbeck B, Hoermann R, Hahn S, et al. Binding, stimulating and blocking TSH receptor antibodies to the thyrotropin receptor as predictors of relapse of Graves' disease after withdrawal of antithyroid treatment. Horm Metab Res 2005;37:745–50.

[67] Schott M, Minich WB, Willenberg HS, et al. Relevance of TSH receptor stimulating and blocking autoantibody measurement for the prediction of relapse in Graves' disease. Horm Metab Res 2005;37:741–4.

[68] Hidaka Y, Tamaki H, Iwatani Y, et al. Prediction of post-partum Graves' thyrotoxicosis by measurement of thyroid stimulating antibody in early pregnancy. Clin Endocrinol (Oxf) 1994;41:15–20.

[69] Tamaki H, Amino N, Aozasa M, et al. Universal predictive criteria for neonatal overt thyrotoxicosis requiring treatment. Am J Perinatol 1988;5(2):152–8.

[70] Mortimer RH, Tyack SA, Galligan JP, et al. Graves' disease in pregnancy: TSH receptor binding inhibiting immunoglobulins and maternal and neonatal thyroid function. Clin Endocrinol (Oxf) 1990;32(2):141–52.

[71] Caplan RH, Pagliara AS, Wickis G. Thyroxine toxicosis: a common variant of hyperthyroidism. JAMA 1980;244:1934–8.

[72] Amino N, Yabu Y, Miyai K, et al. Serum ratio of triiodothyronine to thyroxine, and thyroxine-binding globulin and calcitonin concentrations in Graves' disease and destruction-induced thyrotoxicosis. J Clin Endocrinol Metab 1981;53:113–6.

[73] Yanagisawa T, Sato K, Takano K. Rapid differential diagnosis of Graves' disease and painless thyroiditis using T3/T4 ratio, TSH, and total alkaline phosphatase activity. Endocr J 2005;52(1):29–36.

[74] Burman KD, Monchik JM, Earll JM, et al. Ionized and total serum calcium and parathyroid hormone in hyperthyroidism. Ann Intern Med 1976;84:668–71.

[75] Sarlis NJ, Gourgiotis L. Thyroid emergencies. Rev Endocr Metab Disord 2003;4:129–36.

[76] Britto JM, Fenton AJ, Nicholson GC, et al. Osteoclasts mediate thyroid hormone stimulation of osteoclastic bone resorption. Endocrinology 1994;134:169–76.

[77] Intenzo CM, dePapp AE. Scintigraphic manifestations of thyrotoxicosis. Radiographics 2003;23(4):857–69.

[78] Meier DA, Kaplan MM. Radioactive iodine uptake and thyroid scintiscanning. Endocrinol Metab Clin North Am 2001;30(2):291–313.

[79] Cakir M. Marine-Lenhart syndrome. J Natl Med Assoc 2005;97(7):1036–8.

[80] Cavalieri RR. In vivo isotopic tests and imaging. In: Braverman LE, Utiger R, editors. Werner's and Ingbar's the thyroid. 6th edition. Philadelphia: Lipincott-Ranen; 1991. p. 437–45.

[81] Ryu UY, Vaidya PV, Schneider AB, et al. Thyroid imaging agents: a comparison of I-123 and Tc-99m pertechnetate. Radiology 1983;148:819–22.

[82] Kurita S, Sakurai M, Kita Y. Measurement of thyroid blood flow area is useful for diagnosing the cause of thyrotoxicosis. Thyroid 2005;15(11):1249–52.

[83] Bogazzi F, Bartalena L, Brogiani S. Color flow Doppler sonography rapidly differentiates type I and type II amiodarone-induced thyrotoxicosis. Thyroid 1997;7:541–5.

[84] Astwood E. Chemotherapy of hyperthyroidism. Harvey Lect 1945;40:195–235.

[85] Cooper D. Treatment of thyrotoxicosis. In: Braverman LE, Utiger RD, editors. Werner's and Ingbar's the thyroid. 9th edition. Philadelphia: Lipincott, Williams & Wilkins; 2005. p. 665–94.

[86] Sonnet E, Massart C, Gibassier J, et al. Longitudinal study of soluble intracellular adhesion molecule-1 (ICAM-1) in sera of patients with Graves' disease. J Endocrinol Invest 1999;22: 430–5.

[87] Tsatsoulis A, Vlachoyiannopoulos PG, Dalekos GN, et al. Increased serum interleukin-1 beta during treatment of hyperthyroidism with antithyroid drugs. Eur J Clin Invest 1995; 25:654–8.

[88] McGregor AM, Peterson MM, Mclachlan SM, et al. Carbimazole and the autoimmune response in Graves' disease. N Engl J Med 1980;303:302–7.

[89] Zantut-Wittman DE, Tambascia MA, da Silva Trevisan MA, et al. Antithyroid drugs inhibit in vivo HLA-DR expression in thyroid follicular cells in Graves' disease. Thyroid 2001;11:575–80.

[90] Tajiri J, Noguchi S. Antithyroid drug-induced agranulocytosis: special reference to normal white blood cell count agranulocytosis. Thyroid 2004;14:459–62.

[91] Romaldini JH, Bromberg N, Reis LC. Comparison of effects of high and low dosage regimens of antithyroid drugs in the management of Graves' hyperthyroidism. J Clin Endocrinol Metab 1983;57(3):563–70.

[92] Pujol P, Osman A, Jaffiol C, et al. TSH suppression combined with carbimazole for Graves' disease: effect on remission and relapse rate. Clin Endocrinol (Oxf) 1998;48(5): 635–40.

[93] Pfeilschifter J, Ziegler R. Suppression of serum thyrotropin with thyroxine in patients with Graves' disease: effects on recurrence of hyperthyroidism and thyroid volume. Eur J Endocrinol 1997;136(1):81–6.

[94] McIver B, Rae P, Toft A, et al. Lack of effect of thyroxine in patients with Graves' hyperthyroidism who are treated with an antithyroid drug. N Engl J of Med 1996;334(4):220–4.

[95] Shiroozu A, Okamura K, Yashizumi T, et al. Treatment of hyperthyroidism with a single daily dose of methimazole. J Clin Endocrinol Metab 1986;63(1):125–8.

[96] Nicholas WC, Fischer RG, Stevenson RA, et al. Single daily dose of methimazole compared to every 8 hours propylthiouracil in the treatment of hyperthyroidism. South Med J 1995;88(9):973–6.

[97] Bouma DJ, Kammer H. Single daily dose methimazole treatment of hyperthyroidism. West J Med 1980;132:13–5.

[98] He CT, Hsieh AT, Kuo SW, et al. Comparison of single daily dose methimazole and propylthiouracil in the treatment of Graves' hyperthyroidism. Clin Endocrinol (Oxf) 2004;60: 676–81.

[99] Nagasaka A, Hikada H. Effect of antithyroid agents 6-propyl-2-thiouracil and 1-methyl-2-mercaptoimidazole on human thyroid iodide peroxidase. J Clin Endocrinol Metab 1976;43: 152–8.

[100] Jansson R, Dahlberg PA, Lindstrom B, et al. Intrathyroidal concentrations of methimazole in patients with Graves' disease. J Clin Endocrinol Metab 1983;57:129–32.

[101] Okamura K, Ikenoue H, Shiroozu A, et al. Reevaluation of the effects of methylmercaptoimidazole and propylthiouracil in patients with Graves' hyperthyroidism. J Clin Endocrinol Metab 1987;65:719–23.

[102] Walter RM, Bartle WR. Rectal administration of propylthiouracil in the treatment of Graves' disease. Am J Med 1990;88:69–70.

[103] Nabil N, Miner DJ, Amatruda JM. Methimazole: an alternative route of administration. J Clin Endocrinol Metab 1982;54(1):180–1.

[104] Yeung S, Go R, Balasubramanyam A, et al. Rectal administration of iodide and propylthiouracil in the treatment of thyroid storm. Thyroid 1995;5(5):403–5.

[105] Jongjaroenprasert W, Akarawut W, Chantasart D, et al. Rectal administration of propylthiouracil in hyperthyroid patients: comparison of suspension enema and suppository form. Thyroid 2002;12(7):627–31.

[106] Okamura Y, Shigemusa C, Tatsuhara T. Pharmacokinetics of methimazole in normal subjects and hyperthyroid patients. Endocrinol Jpn 1986;33:605–15.

[107] Hodak SP, Huang C, Clarke D, et al. Intravenous methimazole in the treatment of refractory hyperthyroidism. Thyroid 2006;16(7):691–5.

[108] Werner MC, Romaldini JH, Farah CS, et al. Adverse effects related to thionamide drugs and their dose regimen. Am J Med Sci 1989;297:216–9.

[109] Pearce SH. Spontaneous reporting of adverse reactions to carbimazole and propylthiouracil in the UK. Clin Endocrinol (Oxf) 2004;61:589–94.

[110] Tajiri J, Noguchi S. Antithyroid drug-induced agranulocytosis: how has granulocyte colony-stimulating factor changed therapy? Thyroid 2005;15(3):292–7.

[111] Cooper DS, Goldminz D, Ridgway EC, et al. Agranulocytosis associated with antithyroid drugs. Effects of patient age and drug dose. Ann Intern Med 1983;98:26–9.

[112] Cooper DS. Antithyroid drugs for the treatment of hyperthyroidism caused by Graves' disease. Endocrinol Metab Clin North Am 1998;27:225–47.

[113] Sheng WH, Hung CC, Chen YC, et al. Antithyroid drug-induced agranulocytosis complicated by life-threatening infections. QJM 1999;92:455–61.

[114] Cooper D. Antithyroid drugs. N Engl J Med 2005;352:905–17.

[115] Hughes G. Management of thyrotoxicosis with a beta-adrenergic blocking agent. Br J Clin Pract 1966;20:579–81.

[116] Langley RW, Burch HB. Perioperative management of the thyrotoxic patient. Endocrinol Metab Clin North Am 2003;32:519–34.

[117] Taurog A. Hormone synthesis: thyroid iodine metabolism. In: Braverman LE, Utiger RD, editors. Werner's and Ingbar's the thyroid. 6th edition. Philadelphia: Lipincott, Williams, Wilkins; 1991. p. 51–97.

[118] Goldberg PA, Inzucchi SE. Critical issues in endocrinology. Clin Chest Med 2003;24: 583–606.

[119] Panzer C, Beazley R, Braverman L. Rapid preoperative preparation for severe hyperthyroid Graves' disease. J Clin Endocrinol Metab 2004;89:2142–4.

[120] Boehm TM, Burman KD, Barnes S, et al. Lithium and iodine combination therapy for thyrotoxicosis. Acta Endocrinol (Copenh) 1980;94:174–83.

[121] Spaulding SW, Burrow GN, Bermudez F, et al. The inhibitory effect of lithium on thyroid hormone release in both euthyroid and thyrotoxic patients. J Clin Endocrinol Metab 1972; 35(6):905–11.

[122] Solomon BL, Wartofsky L, Burman KD. Adjunctive cholestyramine therapy for thyrotoxicosis. Clin Endocrinol (Oxf) 1993;38:39–43.

[123] Mercado M, Mendoza-Zubieta V, Bautista-Osorio R, et al. Treatment of hyperthyroidism with a combination of methimazole and cholestyramine. J Clin Endocrinol Metab 1996; 81(9):3191–3.

[124] Tsai WC, Pei D, Wang T, et al. The effect of combination therapy with propylthiouracil and cholestyramine in the treatment of Graves' hyperthyroidism. Clin Endocrinol (Oxf) 2005; 62(5):521–4.

[125] Holm LE, Hall P, Lundell G, et al. Cancer risk after iodine-131 therapy for hyperthyroidism. J Natl Cancer Inst 1991;83(15):1072–6.

[126] Franklyn JA, Maissonneuve P, Sheppard M, et al. Cancer incidence and mortality after radioactive iodine treatment for hyperthyroidism: a population-based cohort study. Lancet 1999;353:2111–5.

[127] Sridama V, McCormick M, Kaplan EL, et al. Long-term follow-up study of compensated low-dose 131I therapy for Graves' disease. N Engl J Med 1984;311(7): 426–32.

[128] Nordyke RA, Gilbert FI Jr. Optimal iodine-131 dose for eliminating hyperthyroidism in Graves' disease. J Nucl Med 1991;32(3):411–6.

[129] Cevallos JL, Hagen GA, Maloof F, et al. Low-dosage 131-I therapy of thyrotoxicosis (diffuse goiters). A five-year follow-up study. N Engl J Med 1974;290(3):141–3.

[130] Burman K. Hyperthyroidism. In: Rakel R, Bope E, editors. Conn's current therapy. Philadelphia: Saunders; 2006. p. 806–11.

[131] McDermott MT, Kidd GS, Dodson LE, et al. Radioactive iodine-induced thyroid storm. Case report and literature review. Am J Med 1983;75(2):353–9.

[132] Bonnema SJ, Bennedbaek FN, Veje A, et al. Propylthiouracil before I-131 therapy of hyperthyroid diseases: effect on cure rate evaluated by a randomized clinical trial. J Clin Endocrinol Metab 2004;89(9):4439–44.

[133] Santos RB, Romaldini JH, Ward LS. Propylthiouracil reduces the effectiveness of radioactive iodine treatment in hyperthyroid patients with Graves' disease. Thyroid 2004;14: 525–30.

[134] Andrade VA, Gross JL, Maia AL. The effect of methimazole pretreatment on the efficacy of radioactive iodine therapy in Graves' hyperthyroidism: one-year follow-up of a prospective, randomized study. J Clin Endocrinol Metab 2001;86(8):3488–93.

[135] Bonnema SJ, Bennedbaek FN, Veje A, et al. Continuous methimazole therapy and its effect on the cure rate of hyperthyroidism using radioactive iodine: an evaluation by a randomized trial. J Clin Endocrinol Metab 2006;91(8):2946–51.

[136] Sabri O, Zimny M, Buell U, et al. Success rate of radioactive iodine therapy in Graves' disease: the influence of thyrostatic medication. J Clin Endocrinol Metab 1999;84(4):1229–33.

[137] Vitti P, Rago T, Chiovato L. Clinical features of patients with Graves' disease undergoing remission after antithyroid drug treatment. Thyroid 1997;7:369–75.

[138] Hedley AJ, Young RE, Jones SJ, et al. Antithyroid drugs in the treatment of hyperthyroidism of Graves' disease: long-term follow-up of 434 patients. Clin Endocrinol (Oxf) 1989;31: 209–18.

[139] Bartalena Luigi, Pinchera A, Marcocci C. Management of Graves' ophthalmopathy: reality and perspectives. Endocr Rev 2000;21(2):168–99.

[140] Kahaly GJ, Pitz S, Dittmar M, et al. Randomized, single blind trial of intravenous versus oral steroid monotherapy in Graves' orbitopathy. J Clin Endocrinol Metab 2005;90(9): 5234–40.

[141] Bartalena L, Marcocci C, Pincher A. Relation between therapy for hyperthyroidism and the course of Graves' ophthalmopathy. N Engl J Med 1998;338(2):73–8.

[142] Tallstedt L, Lundell G, Taube A. Occurrence of ophthalmopathy after treatment for Graves' hyperthyroidism. N Engl J Med 1992;326(26):1733–8.

[143] Hegedius L, Brix TH, Vestergaard P. Relationship between cigarette smoking and Graves' ophthalmopathy. J Endocrinol Invest 2004;27(3):265–71.

[144] Bartalena L, Marcocci C, Manetti L, et al. Cigarette smoking and treatment outcomes in Graves' ophthalmopathy. Ann Intern Med 1998;129:632–5.

[145] Siegel RD, Lee SL. Toxic nodular goiter: toxic adenoma and toxic multinodular goiter. Endocrinol Metab Clin North Am 1998;27(1):151–68.

[146] Bartalena L, Brogioni S, Grasso L, et al. Treatment of amiodarone-induced thyrotoxicosis, a difficult challenge: results of a prospective study. J Clin Endocrinol Metab 1996;81(8): 2930–3.

[147] Martino E, Aghini-Lombardi F, Mariotti S. Treatment of amiodarone associated thyrotoxicosis by simultaneous administration of potassium perchlorate and methimazole. J Endocrinol Invest 1986;9:201–7.

[148] Soldin OP, Braverman LE, Lamm SH. Perchlorate clinical pharmacology and human health: a review. Ther Drug Monit 2001;23:316–31.

[149] Erdogan MF, Gulec S, Tutar E, et al. A stepwise approach to the treatment of amiodarone-induced thyrotoxicosis. Thyroid 2003;13(2):205–9.

[150] Roti E, Minelli R, Braverman LE, et al. Thyrotoxicosis followed by hypothyroidism in patients treated with amiodarone: a possible consequence of a destructive process of the thyroid. Arch Intern Med 1993;153:886–92.

[151] Davis LE, Lucas MJ, Hankins GD, et al. Thyrotoxicosis complicating pregnancy. Am J Obstet Gynecol 1989;160:63–70.

[152] LeBeau SO, Mandel SJ. Thyroid disorders during pregnancy. Endocrinol Metab Clin North Am 2006;35:117–36.

[153] Davies TF, Ando T, Lin RY, et al. Thyrotropin receptor-associated diseases: from adeno-
      mata to Graves' disease. J Clin Invest 2005;115(8):1972–83.
[154] Rodien P, Bremont C, Duprez L, et al. Familial gestational hyperthyroidism caused by
      a mutant thyrotropin receptor hypersensitive to human chorionic gonadotropin. N Engl
      J Med 1998;339(25):1823–6.
[155] Goodwin TM, Montoro M, Hershman JM, et al. The role of chorionic gonadotropin in
      transient hyperthyroidism of hyperemesis gravidarum. J Clin Endocrinol Metab 1992;75:
      1333–7.
[156] Grossman M, Weintraub BD, Szudlinski MW. Novel insights into the molecular mecha-
      nisms of human thyrotropin action: structural, physiological, and therapeutic implications
      for the glycoprotein hormone family. Endocr Rev 1997;18:476–501.
[157] Bach-Huynh TG, Jonklaas J. Thyroid medications during pregnancy. Ther Drug Monit
      2006;28(3):431–41.
[158] Burrow GN. Thyroid function and hyperfunction during gestation. Endocr Rev 1993;14:
      194–202.
[159] Masiukiewicz US, Burrow GN. Hyperthyroidism in pregnancy: diagnosis and treatment.
      Thyroid 1999;9:647–52.
[160] Marchant B, Brownie BEW, Hart DM, et al. The placental transfer of propylthiouracil,
      methimazole, and carbimazole. J Clin Endocrinol Metab 1977;45:1187–93.
[161] Kalb RE, Grossman ME. The association of aplasia cutis congenita with therapy of mater-
      nal thyroid disease. Pediatr Dermatol 1986;3:327–30.
[162] Van Dijke CP, Heydendael RJ, de Kleine MJ. Methimazole, carbimazole, and congenital
      skin defects. Ann Intern Med 1987;106:60–1.
[163] Mortimer R, Connell G, Addison R, et al. Methimazole and propylthiouracil equally cross
      the perfused human term placental lobule. J Clin Endocrinol Metab 1997;82:3099–102.
[164] Momotani N, Noh J, Oyanagi H, et al. Antithyroid drug therapy for Graves' disease during
      pregnancy: optimal regimen for fetal thyroid status. N Engl J Med 1986;315:24–8.
[165] Mestman JH. Hyperthyroidism in pregnancy. Best Pract Res Clin Endocrinol Metab 2004;
      18(2):267–88.
[166] Brodsky JB, Cohen EN, Brown BW Jr, et al. Surgery during pregnancy and fetal outcome.
      Am J Obstet Gynecol 1980;138(8):1165–7.
[167] Fisher DA. Fetal thyroid function: diagnosis and management of fetal thyroid disorders.
      Clin Obstet Gynecol 1997;40:16–31.
[168] Davidson KM, Richards DS, Schatz DA, et al. Successful in utero treatment of fetal goiter
      and hypothyroidism. N Engl J Med 1991;324:543–6.
[169] Van Loon AJ, Derksen J, Bos AF, et al. In utero diagnosis and treatment of fetal goitrous
      hypothyroidism, caused by maternal use of propylthiouracil. Prenat Diagn 1995;15:
      599–604.

ELSEVIER
SAUNDERS

Endocrinol Metab Clin N Am
36 (2007) 657–672

ENDOCRINOLOGY
AND METABOLISM
CLINICS
OF NORTH AMERICA

The Nonthyroidal Illness Syndrome

Suzanne Myers Adler, MD[a,b,*],
Leonard Wartofsky, MD, MACP[a,b,c]

[a]*Department of Medicine, Washington Hospital Center, Room 2A-62,
110 Irving Street, NW, Washington, DC 20010, USA*
[b]*Georgetown University School of Medicine, Building D, Suite 232,
4000 Reservoir Road, Washington, DC 20007, USA*
[c]*Uniformed Services University of the Health Sciences, 4301 Jones Bridge Road,
Bethesda, MD 20814, USA*

The evaluation of altered thyroid function parameters in systemic illness and stress remains complex because changes occur at all levels of the hypothalamic-pituitary-thyroid axis. The so-called "nonthyroidal illness syndrome," also known as the low T3 syndrome or euthyroid sick syndrome, is not a true syndrome but rather reflects alterations in thyroid function tests in a variety of clinical situations that commonly include a low serum triiodothyronine (T3), normal to low thyroxine (T4), and a high reverse T3 (rT3). These typical changes may be observed in up to 75% of hospitalized patients [1]. We generally assess measurements of thyroid hormone levels and thyrotropin (TSH) to ascertain the systemic metabolic state of the patient. Despite accurate and precise techniques, these measurements may not be indicative of true thyroid hormone action at the cellular level because of alterations in intracellular thyroid hormone uptake, receptor binding, and hormone binding to their serum transport proteins in systemic illness [2–4]. Thyroid function abnormalities can occur within hours of acute illness, and the magnitude of these alterations correlates with severity of disease with the lowest T3 and T4 values associated with decreased survival. Although it has been concluded that the probability of death is 50% when serum T4 is less than 4 μg/dL and increases to 80% when serum T4 is less than 2 μg/dL, evidence suggests that low T3 is an independent predictor of survival [5–8], as are elevated rT3 and decreased T3/rT3 [9]. This article briefly summarizes thyroid function alterations generally seen in the euthyroid sick syndrome, provides an overview of specific thyroidal adaptations during several clinical conditions and secondary to specific pharmacologic

---
* Corresponding author. Department of Medicine, Washington Hospital Center, Room 2A-62, 110 Irving Street, NW, Washington, DC 20010, USA.
  E-mail address: adlers@georgetown.edu (S.M. Adler).

0889-8529/07/$ - see front matter © 2007 Elsevier Inc. All rights reserved.
doi:10.1016/j.ecl.2007.04.007

agents, and discusses the current controversy in thyroid hormone treatment of nonthyroidal illness.

Alterations of thyroid economy with nonthyroidal illness

Thyroid hormone parameters in nonthyroidal illness have been reviewed in detail elsewhere [10]. We provide a brief summary of the changes typically observed.

Triiodothyronine

Low serum T3 is the most common manifestation of altered thyroid economy in nonthyroidal illness. The enzyme 5'-deiodinase catalyzes the monodeiodination of approximately 35% to 40% of circulating T4 to produce the active hormone T3, thereby accounting for 80% to 90% of T3 in the circulation; the remaining 10% to 20% of T3 is directly secreted by the thyroid. Inhibition of 5'-deiodinase is believed to occur in nonthyroidal illness, resulting in a decrease in T4 to T3 conversion in a variety of tissues and hence low serum T3 concentrations [2].

Thyroxine

Generally, decreases of serum T4 are seen in nonthyroidal illness and can be due to hypothalamic-pituitary suppression, disordered iodine uptake, abnormal peripheral metabolism, or decreased binding to carrier proteins such as thyroid hormone binding globulin (TBG). Measurements of free T4 are commonly within the normal reference range but may be low or slightly increased depending upon the specific underlying disease process [10–12].

Serum reverse triiodothyronine

rT3 is usually elevated in nonthyroidal illness. T4 to rT3 conversion by 5-deiodinase is called the "inactivating pathway." With impairment of 5'-deiodinase activity reducing metabolism of T4 by the activating pathway, more T4 substrate is available for 5-deiodinase action via the inactivating pathway and hence conversion to rT3. In addition, 5'-deiodinase ordinarily converts rT3 to T2, and reduced activity of 5'-deiodinase slows clearance of rT3, further elevating rT3 levels. In the setting of low serum T3 and T4 in systemic illness, the differential diagnosis would include hypothyroidism. Previously, measurements of rT3 were said to be useful to differentiate non-thyroidal illness (with its high rT3) from hypothyroidism (which should be associated with low rT3), but subsequent studies have shown that rT3 does not accurately distinguish the two states [13].

Thyrotropin

TSH measurements most commonly within the normal reference range in nonthyroidal illness has been the strongest held evidence that these patients are "euthyroid" and is responsible for the continuing popularity of the designation "euthyroid sick syndrome." Depending upon the etiology of the underlying nonthyroid illness, TSH levels may be low, but only on rare occasions are TSH levels undetectable due to nonthyroidal illness alone. TSH may be transiently elevated even to greater than 20 mU/L during nonthyroidal illness recovery [2].

Altered thyroid economy in specific clinical conditions

Starvation and fasting

The fasting state causes a down-regulation in the hypothalamic-pituitary-thyroid axis and hence decreased thyroid hormone levels [14,15]. It may be difficult to distinguish between the effects on thyroid function of a given systemic illness versus those of the associated absolute or relative starvation because malnutrition is a component of many acute and chronic diseases. The decreased serum T3 in starvation is hypothesized to reflect an attempt by the organism to conserve energy by reducing metabolic expenditure. Investigative endeavors to restore serum T3 to the normal range during starvation have resulted in evidence of increased muscle catabolism [16,17]. Therefore, starvation-associated alterations in thyroid function different from those observed in the fed state may not be abnormal but rather may represent appropriate alterations reflecting maintenance of homeostasis.

In the fasting state, substantial decreases in serum total and free T3 are seen within 24 to 48 hours primarily due to the down-regulation of peripheral 5'-deiodination of T4 to T3. The increase in rT3 during fasting is mainly due to decreased metabolic clearance of rT3 by 5'-deiodinase rather than increased rT3 production from 5-deiodination of T4 to rT3 [10]. On the other hand, total T4 concentration may change little, and free T4 levels most commonly remain unchanged or may show slight increases due to fasting-induced elevations in plasma free fatty acids (known to occur during fasting), which inhibit hormone protein binding [18]. Free T4 returns to normal within 2 weeks of continued fasting [10], although total T4 may exhibit steady decreases corresponding to the fall in thyroid binding globulin seen with prolonged minimal caloric intake [19]. Long-term caloric restriction in humans (range, 3–15 years) with adequate protein intake is associated with a "chronic" low T3 syndrome [20].

Alterations in the regulation of thyroid hormone economy during starvation occur not only peripherally via effects on deiodination and hormone binding; changes also occur centrally. Reduced thyroidal secretion of thyroid hormones is thought to be due in part to suppression of TRH expression within the hypothalamic paraventricular nucleus leading to decreased stimulation of TSH production [21]. In addition, altered glycosylation of newly synthesized TSH reduces TSH bioactivity and hence decreases thyroid hormone secretion [21]. Not only are TSH and TRH levels decreased with prolonged fasting, but the TSH response to TRH is also blunted [22]. A key factor causing a fall in TRH expression is a rapid decrease in the hormone leptin, which is known to be a major signaling protein during the transition from the fed to the starved state [23]. Leptin is expressed mostly in adipose cells, and a decrease in leptin increases appetite, decreases energy expenditure, and modifies neuroendocrine function to favor survival during starvation [24]. The mechanisms by which leptin modifies TRH expression or TSH secretion are unclear: Leptin may act directly via leptin receptors on TRH neurons or indirectly via the hypothalamic melanocortin pathway [25]. Exogenous r-metHuLeptin administration has been shown to prevent the fasting-induced changes of TSH but has had no effect on the fasting-induced changes in T3 and rT3; this finding suggests that leptin has no direct effect on deiodinase activity [26], but more studies are needed to further elucidate these mechanisms.

Thyroid function is affected not only by caloric content but also by dietary composition. Reduced carbohydrate intake causes decreased T3, increased rT3, and decreased thyroid binding globulin levels [27]. Evidence suggests that in fasting subjects, refeeding with 50 g of carbohydrate (200 kcal) can reverse fasting-induced changes in T3 and rT3 [28], but refeeding with protein and fat cannot normalize T3 levels [29]. Because 5'-deiodinase contains selenium, a relationship between selenium deficiency and low T3 levels during fasting or nutritional deficiency had been surmised; however, several prospective, placebo-controlled trials have concluded that low T3 levels during starvation and other severe illnesses are not directly related to selenium deficiency [30].

Infectious disease

The development of the nonthyroidal illness syndrome during infection and sepsis involves central and peripheral mechanisms, including decreased TSH secretion from the pituitary, reduced thyroidal secretion of T4 and T3, and impaired peripheral T4 to T3 conversion. These changes contribute to low T4, free T4, T3, and TSH and occur early in the course of sepsis. Because increased cytokine release is predominantly observed in sepsis as compared with nonseptic diseases [31], attention has recently been focused on the role of cytokines in the development of nonthyroidal illness syndrome in the setting of sepsis and severe inflammatory states. Evidence suggests that the cytokines interleukin (IL)-1β, soluble IL-2 receptor, IL-6, tumor necrosis factor–α, and nuclear factor κB have roles in the direct suppression of TSH in sepsis [31–34]. Nutritional deprivation during sepsis and severe illness also contributes to altered thyroidal economy in these settings [35].

Although earlier reports hypothesized that endogenous glucocorticoids suppressed pituitary function, including TSH secretion in severe illness [36], more recently endogenous glucocorticoids were found to have little if any contribution to the development of nonthyroidal illness syndrome [31]. The degree of thyroid function test alterations directly relates to infection severity [37].

In most patients who have infections due to HIV, thyroid function parameters, including T3, free T4, and TSH, remain normal unless severe disease is present due to low CD4 cell counts [38–40]. One measurement that may be altered is the serum TBG. Increases in TBG have been observed in the HIV population for reasons that remain unclear but seem unrelated to hepatic dysfunction. The mechanism might relate to altered TBG sialylation, which is known to decrease TBG clearance as seen in pregnancy and other states of elevated serum estrogen levels [41]. In one study of patients who had *Pneumocystis carinii* pneumonia and AIDS, low serum T3 values were associated with increased mortality. In addition, serum rT3 levels were low in the outpatient setting and normalized after hospitalization for severe illness. Unlike other causes of nonthyroidal illness syndrome, rT3 levels were not markedly elevated in this group of patients who had AIDS [42]. In one study of HIV-infected patients receiving highly active antiretroviral therapy, 23 out of 182 patients (12.6%) demonstrated lower free T4 and higher TSH levels, which is suggestive of subclinical or mild hypothyroidism [43]. This could be due to immune reconstitution with the unmasking of underlying Hashimoto disease that was previously quiescent.

Cardiac disease

Thyroid hormone is a key modulator of cardiovascular functions, including heart rate, cardiac contractility, cardiac output, and peripheral vascular resistance [44,45]. Alterations in thyroid function tests in cardiac disorders are frequently observed with cardiac ischemia, congestive heart failure, and after coronary artery bypass grafting. Decreased T3, increased rT3, and decreased TSH and T4 have been found in acute myocardial infarction and unstable angina, with the degree of T3 decrease and rT3 increase proportional to the severity of disease. In these groups of patients, thyroid function test changes were not affected by β-blockers or thrombolytics [46]. One prospective study investigating thyroid function in cardiac arrest found total and free T3 to be significantly lower in patients after cardiac arrest induced by acute coronary syndrome as compared with patients who had acute uncomplicated myocardial infarction or healthy control subjects. There were no significant differences between total T4, free T4, and TSH levels among the groups. Much lower values of free and total T3, free and total T4, and TSH were found in those who sustained prolonged cardiac arrest than in those whose duration of cardiac arrest was shorter, and thyroid function tests normalized at 2 months in those who survived [47].

The prevalence of a nonthyroidal illness syndrome in congestive heart failure is approximately 18% according to a recent prospective trial [48] and may be as high as 23% [49]. Patients categorized as New York Heart Association (NYHA) class III-IV are more likely to have thyroid function test abnormalities consistent with nonthyroidal illness syndrome than are patients who have NYHA class I-II heart failure. Deaths in heart failure patients who have nonthyroidal illness syndrome are significantly more frequent than in heart failure patients who have normal thyroid function tests, and heart transplant normalizes thyroid function tests in patients who have heart failure and nonthyroidal illness syndrome [48]. In addition, so-called "subclinical" hypothyroidism (defined as a TSH level above the upper limit of normal but with a normal free T4) is even more prevalent than nonthyroidal illness syndrome in patients who have NYHA class II-III congestive heart failure [49]. Low T3 has been prospectively shown to be an independent predictor of mortality in hospitalized cardiac patients [50].

Renal disease

That impaired renal function can cause perturbations in thyroidal economy is not unexpected given the kidney's role in the metabolism and excretion of thyroid hormone. In the nephrotic syndrome characterized by proteinuria exceeding 3 g daily, hypoalbuminemia, hyperlipidemia, and edema, T3 levels are decreased. This was thought to be due to loss of TBG in the urine along with other proteins [51]; however, TBG levels are normal in many patients who have nephrotic syndrome and a preserved glomerular filtration rate (GFR) but are decreased if the degree of proteinuria is high secondary to a severely reduced GFR [52]. Serum rT3 levels are typically normal to low in nephrotic syndrome [52], in contrast to other forms of nonthyroidal illness syndrome typically characterized by elevated rT3. Glucocorticoids commonly given to treat nephrotic syndrome may complicate the interpretation of thyroid function tests because they may lower TSH secretion and decrease T4 to T3 conversion; in this setting, serum rT3 may be normal to elevated. Free T4 and free T3 are typically normal in nephrotic syndrome, and thyroid hormone supplementation should be reserved for patients who have at least mild TSH elevations as a consequence of large-scale proteinuria and excess thyroid hormone wasting in the urine or with low serum free T4 in the setting of glucocorticoid use.

End-stage renal disease (ESRD) alters the hypothalamic-pituitary-thyroid hormone axis in addition to peripheral thyroid hormone metabolism [53]. ESRD leads to decreased total and free T3 because of reduced T4 to T3 conversion. Enhanced clearance of T3 from plasma does not occur in renal failure and thus cannot account for the low serum T3 [10,54]. Chronic metabolic acidosis in ESRD may contribute to low free T3 levels [55], and low free T3 has been prospectively shown to be an independent predictor of mortality in hemodialysis patients [56]. Another striking difference from other nonrenal causes of nonthyroidal illness syndrome is the absence of a coexisting increase in the conversion of T4 to rT3 because rT3 levels are most commonly normal in ESRD [57–60]. Although the clearance rate of serum rT3 is impaired in ESRD, the apparent redistribution of rT3 from vascular to extravascular spaces and enhanced intracellular entry of rT3 may account for failure to observe a further increase in serum rT3 levels [37,60]. Total and free T4 are generally slightly decreased or normal, but free T4 may be increased in the setting of heparin used for anticoagulation during hemodialysis because heparin is known to inhibit T4 binding [61]. TSH levels are generally normal in ESRD, but TSH glycosylation is abnormal, which may affect the plasma half-life of TSH [53]. The TSH response to TRH is typically blunted, with a delayed peak and prolonged return to baseline, perhaps due to reduced renal clearance of TSH, TRH, or both [62–64]. Hemodialysis does not tend to normalize the abnormal thyroid function parameters observed in ESRD, but these alterations are largely reversed after renal transplant. Interpretation of thyroid function test in the renal transplant population is complicated by chronic posttransplant glucocorticoid use in many recipients, and persistent attenuation of the response of TSH to TRH may be attributable to steroids, especially if higher doses are used [10,53,54].

Hepatic disease

Normal liver function is important to thyroid metabolism because the liver is the principal site of T4 to T3 conversion via 5'-deiodination, thyroid hormone carrier protein (TBG and albumin) synthesis, T4 uptake, and secondary T4 and T3 release into the circulation. Abnormalities in thyroid function tests vary based on the type and severity of hepatic dysfunction. The abnormalities observed in cirrhosis, acute hepatitis, and chronic liver disease are described below.

The most common thyroid function test abnormalities in cirrhosis are low total T3, low free T3, and elevated rT3. The plasma T3:rT3 ratio is inversely related to the severity of cirrhosis [65,66]. Free T4 may increase and total T4 may decrease secondary to changes in TBG and albumin binding properties and concentrations. Although patients who have cirrhosis may have increased rather than normal TSH levels typically seen in nonthyroidal illness syndrome, they generally remain clinically euthyroid and have normal to delayed TSH and thyroid hormone responses to TRH injection [10,67].

The thyroid function test abnormalities that occur in acute hepatitis differ markedly from those seen with other forms of liver disease and severe illness. Increased TBG is released from the liver as an acute-phase reactant with concomitant elevations in serum total T3 and total T4 levels. Free T4 and TSH are most commonly normal, but minimal elevations in rT3 and reductions in free T3 may be observed [68]. Evidence suggests that the rT3:T3 ratio may have value in assessing the severity of hepatitis and the prognosis of patients who have fulminant hepatitis. For example, the rT3:T3 ratio quickly normalizes in survivors of fulminant hepatitis but does not improve in nonsurvivors [69].

Although diseases such as chronic autoimmune hepatitis and primary biliary cirrhosis are chronic diseases, their associated thyroid function test abnormalities more closely parallel those of acute hepatitis than those of cirrhosis. Similar to acute hepatitis, serum TBG levels are elevated, with an associated increase in total T4 and T3 concentrations. In contrast to cirrhosis and acute hepatitis, free T4 and free T3 levels are more likely to be low [67,70]. Because these forms of liver dysfunction have an autoimmune etiology, there is a higher incidence of coexisting autoimmune thyroid disease that must be distinguished from nonthyroidal illness syndrome. Up to 34% of patients who have primary biliary cirrhosis have antithyroid microsomal antibodies, and 20% have antithyroglobulin antibodies [71]. Such patients are likely to have Hashimoto thyroiditis and a propensity to develop subclinical or overt hypothyroidism with thyroid function test abnormalities superimposed upon those of the nonthyroidal illness syndrome. The degree of thyroid function abnormalities may not correlate with the severity of liver dysfunction in chronic autoimmune hepatitis and primary biliary cirrhosis in contrast to the stronger correlations in cirrhosis and acute hepatitis [10].

Effects of drugs on thyroid economy

Pharmacologic agents administered to patients who have systemic illness may confound the interpretation of thyroid function tests. A complete review of drug effects on the hypothalamic-pituitary-thyroid axis is beyond the scope of this article and has been reviewed previously [72,73]. The following section highlights the alterations in thyroid function parameters secondary to drugs commonly used in severe systemic illness.

Glucocorticoids

Often given in so-called stress doses in critical illness, glucocorticoids affect the hypothalamic-pituitary-thyroid axis at multiple levels, including the acute suppression of TSH secretion, down-regulation of T4 to T3 conversion by 5'-deiodinase, and decrease of TBG concentration and hormone-binding capacity [10]. Together, these alterations result in low TSH, low T3, low T4, and normal to slightly low free T4; these changes may be seen as soon as 24 to 36 hours after glucocorticoids are initiated [72,74–78].

Dopamine

Dopamine is administered intravenously in the intensive care setting for its high-dose pressor effects and, at some clinical centers, for its low-dose renal perfusion effects. Prolonged use of dopamine (ie, for several days) can result in precipitous TSH suppression and hence low T4, free T4, T3, and free T3, which may lead to secondary hypothyroidism with worsening prognosis until thyroid hormone replacement is given [10,79].

Amiodarone

Amiodarone, commonly administered for its antiarrhythmic effects, has a high iodine content reported to be 37% [10]. Amiodarone may increase or decrease thyroid hormone secretion and inhibits T4 to T3 conversion by 5'-deiodinase, resulting in decreased T3 and increased rT3 levels [80]. Amiodarone slows T4 metabolism, leading to T4 and free T4 elevations, and may cause short-term TSH increases [80]. Although the T4 effects may persist, T3 and TSH generally normalize after several months on amiodarone [37,81]. Most patients remain euthyroid on amiodarone, but the drug causes hypothyroidism in 5% to 25% of patients (more common in regions with adequate iodine intake) and hyperthyroidism in 2% to 10% of patients (especially in iodine-deficient regions) [45].

Furosemide

At common therapeutic doses, furosemide has little if any effect on thyroid parameters. At higher doses that may be used during hospitalization for aggressive diuresis (ie, >80 mg intravenously), furosemide causes a transient elevation in free T4 and a decrease in T4 due to the displacement of T4 from TBG. The magnitude of change depends on a number of factors including serum concentrations of albumin, which also bind furosemide [72,82–84].

Salicylates

Salicylates cause a transient increase in free T4 due to inhibition of T3 and T4 binding to TBG in a similar manner to furosemide. This effect is seen in high doses (ie, >2 g daily), and once a steady-state of the drug is achieved, free T4 normalizes with a 20% to 30% decrease in T4 [72,85–87].

Phenytoin

Phenytoin increases the rate of hepatic metabolism of T4 and T3 and may cause decreases in free T4 and rT3 but with generally normal TSH [2]. Free T4 measurements by equilibrium dialysis suggest that free T4 continues to be normal [72]. The effects of phenytoin on T3 and free T3 are variable, and these parameters may be depressed or remain normal in patients receiving this medication [88,89].

Beta-adrenergic-antagonists

Propranolol may cause minimal inhibition of 5'-deiodinase, thereby decreasing T3 and increasing rT3 [73], but propranolol does not cause increased thyroidal secretion [90].

Iodine

Iodine is a constituent of the intravenous contrast agents routinely used for CT studies and cardiac catheterization procedures. Iodine acutely reduces thyroid hormone secretion and exacerbate hypothyroidism. Conversely, large iodine loads can precipitate thyrotoxicosis in patients who have underlying autonomous thyroid function [2].

Thyroid hormone treatment during nonthyroidal illness

The commonly held notion that patients who have nonthyroidal illness are euthyroid continues to be debated [1,5,91–97]. The metabolic state in these patients has been deemed to be euthyroid based on generally normal TSH and free T4 measurements. Changes in thyroidal economy may play an adaptive role in times of stress, but consideration has also been given to the possibility that patients who have nonthyroidal illness and low thyroid hormone levels may not respond with elevated TSH due to central hypothyroidism from systemic illness. Because hypothyroidism exacerbates the condition of many underlying disease processes, thyroid hormone administration has been considered for treatment in patients who have nonthyroidal illness. Because thyroid hormone is not without adverse effects, including precipitating coronary ischemia, myocardial infarction, arrhythmia, or death at supraphysiologic thyroid hormone levels [98,99], the issue of thyroid hormone treatment continues to be controversial.

Work in models involving organ donors who had suffered brain death where thyroid hormone replacement was given in the organ transplant setting and benefits in cardiac inotropic function were observed [100,101] has led to investigations with thyroid hormone administration in systemic illness. During coronary artery bypass grafting and in the immediate postoperative period, total T3 decreases transiently. Several studies have investigated the use of intravenous T3 replacement during coronary artery bypass grafting, and although this normalizes decreases in total T3, no significant effect on perioperative morbidity and mortality has been found. Furthermore, although perioperative intravenous T3 administration resulted in lower systemic vascular resistance and improved cardiac output, there was no change in frequency of arrhythmia, hemodynamic stability, duration of stay in the intensive care unit, or inotropic drug requirements [102,103].

Evidence suggests that T3 administration may exert negative effects on protein and fat metabolism [16,104,105], adversely affect catecholamine levels found to increase as T3 and T4 levels decrease in critical illness [106], and cause deleterious cardiac effects. Thyroid hormone replacement during fasting [103], in patients who have ESRD who are on hemodialysis [107], and in burn victims [108] has shown no beneficial effects. In a recent study [109] involving patients who died in the intensive care unit, those who received a combination of T4 and T3 replacement therapy had higher serum

T3 levels and higher levels of T3 in liver and skeletal muscle, with a twofold greater increase in liver T3 than in serum T3. Patients who did not receive thyroid hormone replacement had decreased levels of T4 and T3 in the liver and skeletal muscle. Another study found that TRH infusion normalized peripheral thyroid hormone levels within 1 day in critically ill patients [110]; these investigators hypothesize that this may be a safer alternative to thyroid hormone administration with greater likelihood of avoiding supraphysiologic thyroid hormone levels.

If the clinician determines a trial of thyroid hormone replacement is warranted in a patient who has deteriorating clinical status and thyroid function test results suggestive of hypothyroidism, intravenous T3 administration is preferred over T4 due to reduced 5'-deiodinase activity and hence decreased conversion of T4 to metabolically active T3 in the sick patient. This was confirmed in one study in the intensive care unit that administered intravenous T4 sufficient to normalize T4 and free T4 and found that rT3 increased, whereas T3 did not; these investigators observed no survival benefit between those who did and did not receive thyroxine [111]. The answer to the question of whether or not thyroid hormone administration in nonthyroidal illness has a positive influence on outcome or prognosis in systemic illness is likely to remain unanswered until studies conclusively indicate morbidity and mortality benefits.

Summary

The evaluation of altered thyroid function parameters in systemic illness and stress remains complex because changes occur at all levels of the hypothalamic-pituitary-thyroid axis. Nonthyroidal illness syndrome is generally characterized by low serum T3, normal free T4 and TSH, and elevated rT3 values. Unique changes in thyroid function parameters are observed in various clinical states, including starvation and fasting, cardiac disease, renal disease, hepatic disease, and infection. Many pharmacologic agents cause changes in thyroidal economy that can complicate the interpretation of thyroid function parameters in systemic illness. Although alterations in thyroid parameters may represent adaptive changes to conserve energy expenditure by reducing metabolic activity, some argue that systemic illness may induce a central hypothyroidism. The issue of thyroid hormone replacement remains controversial in the nonthyroidal illness syndrome.

References

[1] Wartofsky L. The low T3 or "sick euthyroid syndrome": update 1994. Endocr Rev 1994;3: 248–51.
[2] Burman KD, Wartofsky L. Endocrine and metabolic dysfunction syndromes in the critically ill: thyroid function in the intensive care unit setting. Crit Care Clin 2001;17:43–57.

[3] Ekins R. Measurement of free hormones in blood. Endocr Rev 1990;5:5–46.

[4] Sarne DH, Refetoff S. Measurement of thyroxine uptake from serum by cultured human hepatocytes as an index of thyroid status: reduced thyroxine uptake from serum of patients with nonthyroidal illness. J Clin Endocrinol Metab 1985;61:1046–52.

[5] De Groot L. Dangerous dogmas in medicine: the nonthyroidal illness syndrome. J Clin Endocrinol Metab 1999;84:151–64.

[6] Maldonado LS, Murata GH, Hershman JM, et al. Do thyroid function tests independently predict survival in the critically ill? Thyroid 1992;2:119–23.

[7] Vaughan GM, Mason AD, McManus WF, et al. Alterations of mental status and thyroid hormones after thermal injury. J Clin Endocrinol Metab 1985;60:1221–5.

[8] De Marinis L, Mancini A, Masala R, et al. Evaluation of the pituitary-thyroid axis response to acute myocardial infarction. J Clin Invest 1985;8:507–11.

[9] Peeters RP, Wouters PR, van Toor H, et al. Serum rT3 and T3/rT3 are prognostic markers in critically ill patients and are associated with post-mortem tissue deiodinase activities. J Clin Endocrinol Metab 2005;90:4559–65.

[10] Wartofsky L, Burman KD. Alterations in thyroid function in patients with systemic illness: the "euthyroid sick syndrome". Endocr Rev 1982;3:164–217.

[11] Kaptein EM, Grieb DA, Spencer C, et al. Thyroxine metabolism in the low thyroxine state of critical nonthyroidal illnesses. J Clin Endocrinol Metab 1981;53:764–71.

[12] Chopra IJ. Simultaneous measurement of free thyroxine and free 3,5,3-triiodothyronine in undiluted serum by direct equilibrium dialysis/radioimmunoassay: evidence that free triio-dothyronine and free thyroxine are normal in many patients with the low triiodothyronine syndrome. Thyroid 1998;8:249–57.

[13] Burmeister LA. Reverse T3 does not reliably differentiate hypothyroid sick syndrome from euthyroid sick syndrome. Thyroid 1995;5:435–41.

[14] Suda AK, Pittman CS, Shimizu T, et al. The production and metabolism of 3,5,3-triiodo-thyronine and 3,3,5-triiodothyronine in normal and fasting subjects. J Clin Endocrinol Metab 1978;47:1311–9.

[15] Blake NG, Eckland DJ, Foster OJ, et al. Inhibition of hypothalamic thyrotropin-releasing hormone messenger ribonucleic acid during food deprivation. Endocrinology 1991;129: 2714–8.

[16] Gardner DF, Kaplan MM, Stanley CA, et al. Effect of triiodothyronine replacement n the metabolic and pituitary responses to starvation. N Engl J Med 1979;300:579–84.

[17] Burman KD, Wartofsky L, Dinterman RE, et al. The effect of T3 and reverse T3 adminis-tration on muscle protein catabolism during fasting as measured by 3-methylhistidine excretion. Metabolism 1979;28:805–13.

[18] Lim CF, Doctor R, Visser TJ, et al. Inhibition of thyroxine transport into cultured rat hepatocytes by serum of nonuremic critically ill patients: effects of bilirubin and non-esterified fatty acids. J Clin Endocrinol Metab 1993;76:1165–72.

[19] Stockholm KH. Decrease in serum free triiodothyronine, thyroxine-binding globulin and thyroxine-binding prealbumin whilst taking a very low-calorie diet. Int J Obes 1980;4: 133–8.

[20] Fontana L, Klein S, Holloszy JO, et al. Effect of long-term calorie restriction with adequate protein and micronutrients on thyroid hormones. J Clin Endocrinol Metab 2006;91: 3232–5.

[21] Weintraub BD, Gesundheit N, Taylor T, et al. Effect of TRH on TSH glycosylation and biological action. Ann NY Acad Sci 1989;553:205–13.

[22] Burman KD, Smallridge R, Osburne R, et al. Nature of suppressed TSH secretion during undernutrition: effect of fasting and refeeding on TSH responses to prolonged TRH infu-sions. Metabolism 1978;29:46–52.

[23] Ahima RS, Prabakaran D, Mantzoros C, et al. Role of leptin in the neuroendocrine response to fasting. Nature 1996;382:250–2.

[24] Flier JS, Harris M, Hollenberg AN. Leptin, nutrition, and the thyroid: the why, the where-fore, and the wiring. J Clin Invest 2000;105:859–61.

[25] Kim MS, Small CJ, Stanley SA, et al. The central melanocortin system affects the hypothal-amo-pituitary thyroid axis and may mediate the effect of leptin. J Clin Invest 2000;105:1005–11.

[26] Chan JL, Heist K, De Paoli AM, et al. The role of falling leptin levels in the neuroendocrine and metabolic adaptation to short-term starvation in healthy men. J Clin Invest 2003;111:1409–21.

[27] Danforth E Jr, Burger AG. The impact of nutrition on thyroid hormone physiology and action. Annu Rev Nutr 1989;9:201–27.

[28] Burman KD, Dimond RC, Harvey GS, et al. Glucose modulation of alterations in serum iodothyronine concentrations induced by fasting. Metabolism 1979;28:291–9.

[29] Azizi F. Effect of dietary composition on fasting-induced changes in serum thyroid hormones and thyrotropin. Metabolism 1978;27:935–42.

[30] Zimmerman MB, Kohrle J. The impact of iron and selenium deficiencies on iodine and thyroid metabolism: biochemistry and relevance to public health. Thyroid 2002;12:867–78.

[31] Monig H, Arendt T, Meyer M, et al. Activation of the hypothalamo-pituitary-adrenal axis in response to septic or non-septic disease: implications for the euthyroid sick syndrome. Intensive Care Med 1999;25:1402–6.

[32] Nagaya T, Miyuki F, Otsuka G, et al. A potential role of activated NF-kB in the pathogen-esis of euthyroid sick syndrome. J Clin Invest 2000;106:393–401.

[33] Reichlin S. Neuroendocrine-immune interactions. N Engl J Med 1993;329:1246–53.

[34] Lechan RM. Update on thyrotropin-releasing hormone. Thyroid Today 1993;16(1):1–11.

[35] Richmand DA, Molitch ME, O'Donnell TF. Altered thyroid hormone levels in bacterial sepsis: the role of nutritional adequacy. Metabolism 1980;29:936–42.

[36] Kallner G, Ljunggren JG. The role of endogenous cortisol in patients with non-thyroidal illness and decreased T3 levels. Acta Med Scand 1979;26:459–61.

[37] Cavalieri RR. The effects of disease and drugs on thyroid function tests. Med Clin North Am 1991;75:27–39.

[38] Grunfeld C, Pang M, Doerrier W, et al. Indices of thyroid function and weight loss in human immunodeficiency virus infection and the acquired immunodeficiency syndrome. Metabolism 1993;42:1270–6.

[39] Hommes MJT, Romijn JA, Endert R, et al. Hypothyroid-like regulation of the pituitary thyroid axis in stable human immunodeficiency virus infection. Metabolism 1993;42:556–61.

[40] Dobs AS, Dempsey MA, Ladenson PW, et al. Endocrine disorders in men infected with human immunodeficiency virus. Am J Med 1988;84:611–6.

[41] Sellmeyer DE, Grunfeld C. Endocrine and metabolic disturbances in human immunodefi-ciency virus infection and the acquired immune deficiency syndrome. Endocr Rev 1996;17:518–32.

[42] Lo Presti JS, Fried JC, Spencer CA, et al. Unique alterations of thyroid hormone indices in the acquired immunodeficiency syndrome (AIDS). Ann Intern Med 1989;110:970–5.

[43] Madeddu G, Spanu A, Chessa F, et al. 2006 Thyroid function in human immunodeficiency virus patients treated with highly active antiretroviral therapy (HAART): a longitudinal study. Clin Endocrinol (Oxf) 2006;64:375–83.

[44] Polikar R, Burger AG, Scherrer U, et al. The thyroid and the heart. Circulation 1993;87:1435–41.

[45] Klein I, Ojamaa K. Mechanisms of disease: thyroid hormone and the cardiovascular system. N Engl J Med 2001;334:501–9.

[46] Pavlou HN, Kliridis PA, Panagiotopoulos AA, et al. Euthyroid sick syndrome in acute ischemic syndromes. Angiology 2002;53:699–707.

[47] Iltumur K, Olmez G, Anturk Z, et al. Clinical investigation: thyroid function test abnormalities in cardiac arrest associated with acute coronary syndrome. Crit Care 2005;9:R416–24.

[48] Opasich C, Pacini F, Ambrosino N. Sick euthyroid syndrome in patients with moderate-to-severe chronic heart failure. Eur Heart J 1996;17:1860–6.

[49] Manowitz NR, Mayor GH, Klepper MJ, et al. Subclinical hypothyroidism and euthyroid sick syndrome in patients with moderate-to-sever congestive heart failure. Am J Ther 1996; 3:797–801.

[50] Iervasi G, Pingitore A, Landi P, et al. Low T3 syndrome: a strong prognostic predictor of death in patients with heart disease. Circulation 2003;107:708–13.

[51] Afrasiabi MA, Vaziri ND, Gwinup G, et al. Thyroid function studies in the nephrotic syndrome. Ann Intern Med 1979;90:335–8.

[52] Gavin LA, McMahon FA, Castle JN, et al. Alterations in serum thyroid hormones and thyroxine-binding globulin in patients with nephrosis: qualitative aspects. J Clin Invest 1978;46:125–30.

[53] Kaptein EM. Thyroid hormone metabolism and thyroid disease in chronic renal failure. Endocr Rev 1996;17:45–63.

[54] Lim VS, Fang VS, Katz AI, et al. Thyroid dysfunction in chronic renal failure: a study of the pituitary-thyroid axis and peripheral turnover kinetics of thyroxine and triiodothyronine. J Clin Invest 1977;60:522–34.

[55] Wiederkehr MR, Kalogiros J, Krapf R. Correction of metabolic acidosis improves thyroid and growth hormone axes in haemodialysis patients. Nephrol Dial Translpant 2004;19: 1190–7.

[56] Zoccali C, Mallamaci F, Tripepi G, et al. Low triiodothyronine and survival in end-stage renal disease. Kidney Int 2006;70:523–8.

[57] Chopra IJ. An assessment of daily production and significance of thyroidal secretion of 3,3,3',5'-triiodothyronine (reverse T3) in man. J Clin Invest 1976;58:32–40.

[58] Nicod P, Burger AG, Staheli V, et al. A radioimmunoassay for 3,3',5'-triiodo-L-thyronine in unextracted serum: method and clinical results. J Clin Endocrinol Metab 1976;48:823–9.

[59] Faber J, Heaf J, Kirkegaard C, et al. Simultaneous turnover studies of thyroxine, 3,3',5'- and 3,3'5'-triiodothyronine, 3,5-3,3'- and 3',5'-diodothyronine, and 3'-monoiodothyronine in chronic renal failure. J Clin Endocrinol Metab 1983;56:211–7.

[60] Kaptein EM, Feinstein E, Nicoloff JT, et al. Serum reverse triiodothyronine and thyroxine kinetics in patients with chronic renal failure. J Clin Endocrinol Metab 1983;57:181–9.

[61] Silverberg DS, Ulan RA, Fawcett DM, et al. Effects of chronic hemodialysis on thyroid function in chronic renal failure. Can Med Assoc J 1973;109:282–6.

[62] Ramirez G, O'Neill W, Jubiz W, et al. Thyroid dysfunction in uremia: evidence for thyroid and hypophyseal abnormalities. Ann Intern Med 1976;84:672–6.

[63] Czernichow P, Dauzet MC, Broyer M, et al. Abnormal TSH, PRL, and GH response to TSH releasing factor in chronic renal failure. J Clin Endocrinol Metab 1976;43: 630–7.

[64] Duntas L, Wolf CF, Keck FS, et al. Thyrotropin-releasing hormone: pharmacokinetic and pharmacodynamic properties in chronic renal failure. Clin Nephrol 1992;38:214–8.

[65] Guven K, Keletimur F, Yucesoy M. Thyroid function tests in non-alcoholic cirrhotic patients with hepatic encephalopathy. Eur J Med 1993;2:83–5.

[66] Malik R, Hodgson H. The relationship between the thyroid gland and the liver. Q J Med 2002;95:559–69.

[67] Borzio M, Caldara R, Borzio F, et al. Thyroid function tests in chronic liver disease: evidence for multiple abnormalities despite clinical euthyroidism. Gut 1983;24:631–6.

[68] Gardner DF, Carithers RL, Galen EA, et al. Thyroid function tests in patients with acute and resolved hepatitis B infection. Ann Intern Med 1982;96:450–2.

[69] Kano T, Kojima T, Takahashi T, et al. Serum thyroid hormone levels in patients with fulminant hepatitis: usefulness of rT3 and the rT3/T3 ratio as prognostic indices. Gastroenterol Jpn 1987;22:344–53.

[70] Schussler GC, Schaffner F, Korn F. Increased serum thyroid hormone binding and decreased free hormone in chronic active liver disease. N Engl J Med 1978;299:510–5.

[71] Elta GH, Sepersky RA, Goldberg MJ, et al. Increased incidence of hypothyroidism in primary biliary cirrhosis. Dig Dis Sci 1983;28:971–5.

[72] Surks MI, Sievert R. Drugs and thyroid function. NEJM 1995;333:1688–94.

[73] Cavalieri RR, Pitt-Rivers R. The effect of drugs on the distribution and metabolism of thyroid hormone. Pharmacol Rev 1981;33:55–80.

[74] Chopra IJ, Williams DE, Orgiazzi J, et al. Opposite effects of dexamethasone on serum concentrations of 3,3',5'-triiodothyronine (reverse T3) and 3,3'5-triiodothyronine (T3). J Clin Endocrinol Metab 1975;41:911–20.

[75] Duick DS, Warren DW, Nicoloff JT, et al. Effect of single dose dexamethasone on the concentration of serum triiodothyronine in man. J Clin Endocrinol Metab 1974;39:1151–4.

[76] Gamstedt A, Jarnerot G, Kagedal B. Dose related effects of betamethasone on iodothyro-nines and thyroid hormone-binding proteins in serum. Acta Endocrinol (Copenh) 1981;96: 484–90.

[77] De Groot LJ, Hoye K. Dexamethasone suppression of serum T3 and T4. J Clin Endocrinol Metab 1976;42:976–8.

[78] Lo Presti JS, Eigen A, Kaptein E, et al. Alterations in 3,3',5'-triiodothyronine metabolism in response to propylthiouracil, dexamethasone, and thyroxine administration in man. J Clin Invest 1989;84:1650–6.

[79] Heinen E, Herrmann J, Konigshausen T, et al. Secondary hypothyroidism in severe non-thyroidal illness? Horm Metab Res 1981;13:284–8.

[80] Melmed S, Nademance K, Reed AW, et al. Hyperthyroxinemia with bradycardia and normal thyrotropin secretion after chronic amiodarone administration. J Clin Endocrinol Metab 1981;53:997–1001.

[81] Borowski G, Garotano C, Rose L, et al. Effect of long-term amiodarone therapy on thyroid hormone levels and thyroid function. Am J Med 1985;78:443–50.

[82] Newnham HH, Hamblin PS, Long F, et al. Effect of oral furosemide on diagnostic indices of thyroid function. Clin Endocrinol (Oxf) 1987;26:423–31.

[83] Stockigt JR, Lim CF, Barlow JW, et al. Interaction of furosemide with serum thyroxine binding sites: in vivo and in vitro studies and comparison with other inhibitors. J Clin En-docrinol Metab 1985;60:1025–31.

[84] Stockigt JR, Topliss DJ. Assessment of thyroid function during high-dose furosemide ther-apy. Arch Intern Med 1989;149:973.

[85] Larsen PR. Salicylate-induced increases in free triiodothyronine in human serum: evidence of inhibition of triiodothyronine binding to thyroxine-binding-globulin and thyroxine-binding prealbumin. J Clin Invest 1972;51:1125–34.

[86] Faber J, Waetjen I, Siersbaek-Nielson K. Free thyroxine measured in undiluted serum by dialysis and ultrafiltration: effects of non-thyroidal illness and an acute load of salicylate of heparin. Clin Chim Acta 1993;223:159–67.

[87] Bishnoi A, Carlson HE, Gruber BL, et al. Effects of commonly prescribed nonsteroidal anti-inflammatory drugs on thyroid hormone measurements. Am J Med 1994;96:235–8.

[88] Smith PJ, Surks MI. Multiple effects of 5,5-diphenylhydantoin on the thyroid hormone system. Endocr Rev 1984;5:514–24.

[89] Cavalieri RR, Gavin LA, Wallace A, et al. Serum thyroxine, free T4, triiodothyronine and reverse-T3 in diphenylhydantoin-treated patients. Metabolism 1979;28:1161–5.

[90] Wartofsky L, Dimond RC, Noel GL, et al. Failure of propranolol to alter thyroid iodine release, thyroxine turnover, or the TSH and PRL response to TRH in patients with thyrotoxicosis. J Clin Endocrinol Metab 1975;41:485–90.

[91] Utiger RD. Altered thyroid function in nonthyroidal illness and surgery: to treat or not to treat? N Engl J Med 1995;333:1562–3.

[92] Chopra IJ. Euthyroid sick syndrome: is it a misnomer? J Clin Endocrinol Metab 1997;82: 329–34.

[93] Wartofsky L, Burman KD, Ringel MD. Trading one "dangerous dogma" for another? Thyroid hormone treatment of the "euthyroid sick syndrome". J Clin Endocrinol Metab 1999;84:1759.

[94] De Groot L. Dangerous dogmas in medicine: author's response. J Clin Endocrinol Metab 1999;84:1759–60.

[95] Van den Berghe G. Euthyroid sick syndrome. Curr Opin Anaesthesiol 2000;13:89–91.

[96] Stathatos N, Levetan C, Burman KD, et al. The controversy of the treatment of critically ill patients with thyroid hormone. Best Pract Res Clin Endocrinol Metab 2001;15:465–78.

[97] Stathatos N, Wartofsky L. The euthyroid sick syndrome: is there a physiologic rationale for thyroid hormone treatment? J Endocrinol Invest 2003;26:1174–9.

[98] Bergeron GA, Goldsmith R, Schiller NB. Myocardial infarction, severe reversible ischemia, and shock following excess thyroid administration in a woman with normal coronary arteries. Arch Intern Med 1988;148:1450–3.

[99] Bhasin N, Wallace W, Lawrence JB, et al. Sudden death associated with thyroid hormone abuse. Am J Med 1981;71:887–90.

[100] Novitzky D. Heart transplantation, euthyroid sick syndrome, and triiodothyronine replacement. J Heart Lung Transplant 1992;11:S196–8.

[101] Yokoyama Y, Novitzky D, Deal MT, et al. Facilitated recovery of cardiac performance by triiodothyronine following a transient ischemic insult. Cardiology 1992;81:34–45.

[102] Bennett-Guerrero E, Jimenez JL, White WD, et al. Cardiovascular effects of intravenous triiodothyronine in patients undergoing coronary artery bypass graft surgery: a random-ized, double-blind, placebo-controlled trial. JAMA 1996;275:687–92.

[103] Klemperer JD, Klein I, Gomez M, et al. Thyroid hormone treatment after coronary-artery bypass surgery. NEJM 1995;333:1522–7.

[104] Lim VS, Flanigan MJ, Zavala DC, et al. Protective adaptation of low serum triiodothyro-nine in patients with chronic renal failure. Kidney Int 1985;28:541–9.

[105] Axelrod L, Halter JB, Cooper DS, et al. Hormone levels and fuel flow in patients with weight loss and lung cancer: evidence for excessive metabolic expenditure and for an adap-tive response mediated by a reduced level of 3,5,3'-triiodothyronine. Metabolism 1983;32:924–37.

[106] Madsen M, Smeds S, Lennquist S. Relationship between thyroid hormone and catechol-amines in experimental trauma. Acta Chir Scand 1986;152:413–9.

[107] Lim VS, Tsalikian E, Flanigan MJ. Augmentation of protein degradation by L-triiodothy-ronine in uremia. Metabolism 1989;38:1210–5.

[108] Becker RA, Vaughan GM, Ziegler MG, et al. Hypermetabolic low triiodothyronine syndrome of burn injury. Crit Care Med 1982;10:870–5.

[109] Peeters RP, van der Geyten S, Wouters PJ, et al. Tissue thyroid hormone levels in critical illness. J Clin Endocrinol Metab 2005;90:6498–507.

[110] Van den Berghe G, Baxter RC, Weekers F, et al. The combined administration of GH-releasing peptide-2 (GHRP-2), TRH and GnRH to men with prolonged critical illness evokes superior endocrine and metabolic effects compared to treatment with GHRP-2 alone. Clin Endocrinol (Oxf) 2002;56:655–69.

[111] Brent GA, Hershman JM. Thyroxine therapy in patients with severe nonthyroidal illnesses and lower serum thyroxine concentration. J Clin Endocrinol Metab 1986;63:1–8.

ELSEVIER
SAUNDERS

Endocrinol Metab Clin N Am
36 (2007) 673–705

ENDOCRINOLOGY
AND METABOLISM
CLINICS
OF NORTH AMERICA

Thyroid and Bone

Jason A. Wexler, MD[a],*, John Sharretts, MD[b]

[a]*Division of Endocrinology, Washington Hospital Center, 110 Irving Street,
NW, Room 2A38A, Washington, DC 20010, USA*
[b]*MedStar Diabetes and Research Institute, Washington Hospital Center, 110 Irving Street,
NW, East Building, Suite 4114, Washington, DC 20010, USA*

Recent advances in bone research have sought to determine the molecular and hormonal mechanisms regulating bone function. Because the understanding of normal bone physiology has been so elusive, only in the past two decades have the actions of thyroid hormones on the bone begun to be understood. This article provides a summary of the numerous interactions between the thyroid gland and the skeleton, in the normal state, in disorders of thyroid function and as a result of thyroid malignancy. It recaps the current understanding of bone growth and development in the endochondral growth plate and the normal mechanisms of mature bone remodeling. The actions of thyroid hormones on these processes are described, and the clinical impact of thyroid disorders and their treatments on the bone are summarized. Finally, our current understanding of the physiology of bone metastases from thyroid cancer is covered.

Bone development and remodeling

Development of the fetal skeleton begins with the condensation of unspecialized mesenchymal cells. In the flat bones like the skull and scapula, these cells differentiate directly into osteoblasts by the process of intramembranous ossification. Mesenchymal cells clustered around blood vessels deposit aggregates of bone matrix, which are called bony spicules. The mesenchymal cells differentiate into osteoblasts that secrete osteoid and increase the size of the spicules. Adjacent bony spicules fuse to form trabeculae.

Endochondral bone formation is the major process that occurs in the long bones. A cartilage template is initially created that is subsequently replaced by ossified bone. The epiphysis and metaphysis originate from separate ossification centers, separated by the endochondral growth plate.

---

* Corresponding author.
E-mail address: jason.a.wexler@medstar.net (J.A. Wexler).

0889-8529/07/$ - see front matter © 2007 Elsevier Inc. All rights reserved.
doi:10.1016/j.ecl.2007.04.005

Chondroblasts are organized into discrete zones. The reserve zone, closest to the epiphysis, consists of undifferentiated progenitor cells in a matrix of type II collagen and proteoglycan. These chondroblasts undergo clonal expansion and become organized in columns in the proliferative zone. Proliferative chondrocytes secrete bone matrix and enlarge in size. The largest proliferative cells then undergo terminal differentiation into hypertrophic chondrocytes. Chondrocytes in the hypertrophic zone secrete Type X collagen, enlarge further, and undergo apoptosis, leaving a lacunae surrounding cartilaginous septae. Blood vessels from the primary spongiosum invade the primary spongiosum, and osteoblasts from the adjacent bone marrow penetrate to mineralize the newly formed bone [1,2].

Chondrocyte differentiation is mediated by a feedback loop involving parathyroid hormone-related peptide (PTHrP) and the Indian hedgehog factor (Ihh). Ihh is secreted by prehypertrophic chondrocytes and stimulates PTHrP. PTHrP stimulates proliferation and inhibits hypertrophic differentiation [3].

Mature bone is a dynamic system that continuously remodels itself. Bone is resorbed by osteoclasts and is replaced by osteoblasts. In the normal state, these actions are tightly coupled. Resorption begins with the activation of osteoclast precursors of the monocyte/macrophage lineage under the influence of macrophage colony-stimulating factor. Differentiated osteoclasts are induced to resorb bone via activation of receptor activator of nuclear factor κB (RANK) by RANK ligand (RANK-L), which is produced by osteoblasts and bone marrow stromal cells. These cells also produce the competitive inhibitor osteoprotegerin, a decoy binder of RANK-L, which helps regulate the process of resorption by inhibiting osteoclastogenesis and osteoclast maturation. Osteoblasts, which arise from mesenchymal lineage, invade the resorption cavity, lay down a new matrix, and remineralize the new bone [1,2]. Normally this sequence of events occurs over a 200-day cycle [4].

Thyroid receptors in the growth plate and bone

Thyroid hormone is synthesized as thyroxine (T4) in the thyroid gland. This pro-hormone is converted to the active hormone triiodothyronine (T3) in the gland and the peripheral tissues by the deiodinating enzymes D1 and D2. Some quantities of T4 and T3 are converted to inactive metabolites by the deiodinating enzyme D3 [5].

The thyroid hormone receptor (TR) is a nuclear receptor that acts as a transcription factor. T3 binds to TR as a heterodimer with the retinoid X receptor (RXR) to promote gene transcription. TR exists as several isoforms. TR β-2 is present primarily in the hypothalamus and is the major regulator of thyrotropin (thyroid-stimulating hormone [TSH]) synthesis. TR α-1, TR α-2, and TR β-1 are widely distributed throughout the body [6,7]. A number of inactive or negative acting isoforms, such as TR β-3, TR Δα-1, and TR Δα-2, are also present. The thyroid hormone receptors compete with the retinoic acid receptor, vitamin D receptor , and peroxi-some proliferator-activated receptor (PPAR) for heterodimeric partnership with RXR [5].

In the bone, TR α-2 and TR β-1 have been identified in reserve and pro-liferating chondrocytes, osteoblasts and bone marrow cultures and on osteo-blastoma and osteoclastoma cell lines. TR α-1 has also been identified, primarily in osteoblasts [6–12].

The TSH receptor (TSHr) is a membrane protein that regulates transcrip-tion via second messengers, such as cyclic adenosine monophosphate, and it has recently been demonstrated in osteoblast and osteoclast precursors, nor-mal human osteoblasts, and osteosarcoma cell lines [13,14].

In the growth plate, hypothyroidism leads to growth arrest, epiphyseal dysgenesis, delayed bone age, and short stature. Postmortem studies of hy-pothyroid rats reveal a disorganized growth plate with failure of hypertro-phic differentiation, abnormal matrix, and angiogenesis [7].

Juvenile hyperthyroidism causes accelerated growth, advanced bone ma-turity, and premature closure of the growth plate, leading to short stature. Resistance to thyroid hormone (RTH) is an autosomal dominant condition expressed by dysfunction of TR β and causes a variable phenotype, depend-ing on the specific mutation. Dysfunctional TR β causes impaired feedback to the hypothalamus, leading to elevated level of thyroid hormone and in-appropriately elevated TSH [15].

T3 has been demonstrated to regulate chondrocyte proliferation, pro-mote terminal differentiation, and induce mineralization and angiogenesis [16]. Thyroid hormone stimulates production of type II and X collagen and alkaline phosphatase (ALP), a marker of bone mineralization. There is evidence of peripheral deiodination in the growth plate, and it seems to be mainly by the thyroxine deiodinase D2 [17]. Hypothyroid rats have been demonstrated to have reduced collagen II and X in addition to the aforementioned structural abnormalities [7,18].

Thyroid hormones seem to have direct effects on growth plate chondro-cytes, mediated by TR, but also may have indirect influence mediated by growth factors and cytokines. Thyroid hormones stimulate the production of insulin-like growth factor (IGF)-1 and interleukin (IL)-6 and IL-8, which are thought to be important in regulating the cellular processes of bone for-mation and resorption [19,20].

An intermediate factor in the PTHrP/Ihh feedback loop, WSB-1 (a Hedgehog-inducible ubiquitin ligase subunit), seems to activate deiodinase D2, facilitating the formation of active thyroid hormone in the growth plate, which stimulates hypertrophic differentiation [21].

PPAR-γ seems to act as an inhibitor of T3-mediated differentiation, pos-sibly via competition for heterodimeric partnering with RXR. PPAR-γ activity inhibits T3-induced terminal differentiation, decreases TR α-1 transcription, reduces production of bone ALP and type X collagen, and promotes apoptosis [22,23].

Thyroid hormone action in the bone in genetically modified mice

A number of studies involving the genetic alteration of TR isoforms in mice have provided considerable insight into the activity of these receptors in the bone. These studies have been reviewed in detail previously [5,24], and the conclusions are summarized in the following section.

Deletion of all the TR α receptor isoforms (Thra[0/0]) produces mice that appear otherwise euthyroid, with normal fertility and growth hormone levels, but a hypothyroid skeletal phenotype characterized by growth retardation failed differentiation and impaired mineralization. Deletion of TR β isoforms (Thrb[−/−]) leads to a thyroid phenotype of RTH and goiter, but normal bone growth and mineralization, suggesting that TR α is the predominant isoform in bone [24,25].

Deletion of TR α and TR β isoforms (Thra[0/0]Thrb[−/−]) causes a worse skeletal phenotype than Thra(0/0). It has been speculated that TR β partially compensates for the absence of TR α in the bone or that decreased growth hormone and IGF-1 levels in this phenotype are the primary determinants of the skeletal abnormalities. A worse skeletal phenotype is seen in Pax8(−/−) mice, which have functional TR but agenesis of the thyroid gland and complete absence of T4. Further studies of these mice with concomitant mutations of TR have suggested that unliganded TR, specifically TR α isoforms, may exert an additional negative action on bone development [5].

Targeted mutation of TR β in mice with the PV mutation, a frameshift mutation of the carboxy-terminal 14 amino acids of TR β that causes impairment of T3 binding and transactivation and was derived from a human patient who had RTH and hypothyroid skeletal features, resulted in severe RTH in the mice, expressing a hyperthyroid phenotype in the developing bone manifested by increased ossification, growth retardation, and premature quiescence of the growth plate. This finding seems to be in concordance with the hypothesis that TR α and not TR β is the essential receptor regulating bone development [24,25].

Bone remodeling and thyroid hormones

The remodeling process is influenced by thyroid hormones. Thyroid hormone directly stimulates osteoblasts [26]. Osteoclast activity is increased by thyroid hormone but only in the presence of osteoblasts [27], indicating that the stimulation is mediated by cytokine signaling. Evidence suggests that the signaling may be independent of RANK-L [28]. Treatment with the β-selective thyroid agonist GC-1 (a synthetic analog that is selective for binding and activating functions of TR β1 over TR α1) does not seem to affect bone density in rats as compared with those treated with an equally potent dose of T3, suggesting a predominant effect by the TR α receptor in bone [29].

During bone remodeling, the bone structural unit, or osteon, is characterized by a certain structural thickness. In hyperthyroidism, the activation frequency is increased. The resorptive and formative phases are shortened in length. Resorption depth is normal, but completed wall thickness at the end of each cycle is reduced, leading to a loss of thickness with each cycle. In hypothyroidism, resorption depth is reduced, and completed wall thickness at the end of each cycle is increased [30].

Thyroid hormones may affect the bone turnover process indirectly. Numerous cytokines and growth factors have been implicated, including IL-6, IL-8, prostaglandin E2, IGF-1, and insulin-like growth factor binding protein (IGFBP)-2 and -4, osteocalcin, matrix metalloproteinase 13, matrix metalloproteinase 9, and ALP [19,20,31–35].

Disorders of thyroid function affect mineral metabolism. Hyperthyroid patients demonstrate increased dietary calcium intake but have reduced absorption and increased fecal and dermal calcium loss, leading to a negative calcium balance. Reduced 1,25-OH vitamin D levels in hyperthyroidism may contribute to decreased calcium absorption [30].

TSH seems to be an inhibitor of bone turnover. In cell culture, TSH inhibits osteoclast formation, resorption, and survival. It seems that the effect of TSH does not involve RANK-L or M-CSF, but rather inhibition of tumor necrosis factor (TNF)-α [36]. TSH also seems to suppress osteoblast activity, inhibiting vascular endothelial growth factor expression. Therefore, it seems that TSH regulates osteoclast and osteoblast function via completely independent mechanisms [13]. TSH also seems to stimulate production of D2 in osteoblast cultures, indicating that it may have a function in local activation of thyroid hormone [14].

In the mouse model, recent studies have been conducted using a genetically inactivated TSH. TSHR-null (tshr$[-/-]$) mice were hypothyroid, with reduced growth and bone mineralization. Heterozygote tshr($\pm$) mice, although otherwise clinically euthyroid, also displayed defective bone mineralization. Thyroid hormone replacement in the tshr($-/-$) mice improved growth defects but not mineralization. The investigators concluded that although TR predominantly influences bone maturation, TSHR is the primary regulator of bone remodeling [13,37].

Other data suggest that the interaction of TSH, T3, and the bone are more complex. Previous reviewers have speculated that the failure of mineralization in TSHR-null mice may be due to prenatal hypothyroidism occurring at a crucial stage in bone development or to insufficient duration of rescue with thyroid hormone in the postnatal period during the study [1]. The authors of the TSH receptor studies have speculated that the bone mineralization defect may be related to overexpression of TNF-α in the genetically modified mice. Supporting this hypothesis, tshr ($\pm$) mice also absent the TNF-α receptor demonstrated normal bone development and no osteoporosis [37].

A recent in vivo study has also called into question some of the conclusions drawn from the TSHR-null mice. Recombinant human TSH was

administered to women who had a history of differentiated thyroid carcinoma on suppressive thyroxine therapy. The transient increase in TSH resulted in a significant decrease in c-terminal telopeptides of CTX, an
increase in bone ALP, and no effect on serum osteoprotegerin levels [38].
This study confirmed the inhibitory effects of TSH on bone resorption but
did not reveal any evidence of inhibition of bone formation [1]. Alternatively, it may indicate that the inhibition of osteoclast function is more potent and that the effect on osteoblast activity was not measurable in the
study design.

If the TSH receptor does mediate bone turnover, it might be expected
that in patients who have Graves' disease and circulating TSH antibodies
the bone turnover would be mitigated compared with bone loss observed
in other hyperthyroid states; however, such an effect has not been seen
[1,39].

The apparent paradoxical findings in different forms of RTH may impli-
cate a complex interaction between TSH and thyroid hormones in bone
physiology. Hypothyroid bone phenotypes in mild thyroid resistance may
indicate TSH inhibition of bone remodeling due to elevated sensitivity to
TSH. The hyperthyroid skeletal changes in severe RTH phenotypes may
by contrast demonstrate a shift to dominance by thyroid hormone and perhaps up-regulation of the TR α receptors due to abnormal TR β function in
the presence of elevated thyroid hormone levels and despite marked elevations in TSH levels.

In summary, thyroid hormone and TSH play roles in bone growth and
development, mineralization, and remodeling. T3 seems to be essential to induce chondrocyte differentiation, hypertrophy, and angiogenesis, but TSH
may also play a complementary role in normal mineralization. T3 action
in mature and developing bone seems to be mediated primarily by TR α,
and local conversion by deiodinase D2 may play a role in local activation.
TSH seems to be an inhibitor of bone resorption and formation.

Thyroid disorders and fractures

Untreated hyperthyroidism causes severe osteoporosis and pathologic
fractures, but the long-term risk of fracture in patients previously treated
for hyperthyroidism and patients on replacement or suppressive therapy
for hypothyroidism is less understood. A number of studies in the medical
literature have attempted to investigate these issues.

A 1998 population-based study of 7209 previously hyperthyroid patients
treated with radioiodine demonstrated an increased risk in death due to
fracture, with the majority of the higher death risk attributable to fractures
of the femur [40].

A retrospective study of 864 hyperthyroid patients previously treated
with radioiodine showed an increased risk of self-reported fractures (relative risk [RR], 1.7), although there was not a statistically significant risk

of fracture in patients who had also been treated with methimazole or other antithyroid medications in addition to definitive therapy with radio-iodine [41].

Two smaller cohort studies of patients who had a history of thyroidec-tomy demonstrated no increase in overall fracture risk. Both studies re-vealed small but statistically significant increases in the risk of hip fracture in patients who had had thyroidectomy [42,43]. The Melton study, which evaluated 630 female patients, also demonstrated significant increases in rib, spine, and pelvis fractures among those who had previously under-gone surgery.

More recently, two large case-control studies by Vestergaard and Mose-kilde [44] have indicated that there is an increased risk of fractures among patients previously treated for hyperthyroidism. In 2002, researchers evalu-ated 11,776 hyperthyroid patients and found an increased risk of fracture around the time of diagnosis of hyperthyroidism (RR, 1.26–2.29), but no in-creased risk after the diagnosis of hyperthyroidism was made. Those pa-tients treated with thyroidectomy had a significantly lower risk of fracture after diagnosis. This study also evaluated 4473 hypothyroid patients and discovered an increased fracture risk in this group before and up to 2 years after the diagnosis (RR, 2.17–2.35).

In the 2005 study, 124,655 consecutive patients who had fractures were evaluated. The researchers found that there was an increased risk of fracture within 5 years of the diagnosis of hyperthyroidism and within 10 years of the diagnosis of hypothyroidism. Levothyroxine therapy was not associated with fractures, and the use of antithyroid medications was associated with a significantly reduced risk of fracture [45].

Subclinical hyperthyroidism is defined by normal serum free T4 and T3 values but thyrotropin (TSH) values below the normal reference range. Pa-tients who have subclinical hyperthyroidism may have few or no clinical symp-toms of hyperthyroidism. The risk of fracture due to subclinical hyperthyroidism is also not well defined, but one study attempted to address this issue.

A case-control study of 148 women over 65 years of age who had hip fracture and 149 women who had vertebral fracture demonstrated an in-crease risk of fractures at either site in those with TSH suppressed below 0.1 mIU/mL (RR, 4.5). When the fracture outcome was adjusted for TSH level, a history of hyperthyroidism remained an independent risk for frac-tures (RR, 2.2). Current use of levothyroxine conferred no risk for fracture in this study [46].

Four more studies have attempted to examine the risk of fracture on pa-tients treated with long-term levothyroxine. A case-control study of 116 post-menopausal women with hip fracture showed an increased risk of frac-ture among patients who had past or current hyperthyroidism (RR, 2.5) but no increased risk (RR, 0.67) among patients receiving levothyroxine replace-ment for hypothyroidism for 3 to 29 years [47].

An interview of 160 women who had a history of thyroid disease and 140 control subjects showed no increase of fractures in patients on thyroid replacement therapy. Although there was no significant increase in the overall rate of fractures in previously hyperthyroid patients in this study, fractures seemed to occur at a younger age in patients who had a history of hyperthyroidism compared with control subjects [48].

A questionnaire study of 408 patients receiving levothyroxine replacement and 408 control subjects demonstrated a temporary increase in fracture risk within 2 years of the diagnosis of primary idiopathic hypothyroidism. The risk was statistically significant in patients over 50 years of age [49].

Another study of 1180 patients on levothyroxine therapy compared fracture rates in patients on suppressive doses and those on normal replacement doses of levothyroxine. In this study, no difference in fracture rates was detected between the two groups [50].

In summary, it seems that a history of previously treated hyperthyroidism may impose a higher long-term risk for fractures, particularly fractures of the hip. In hyperthyroid patients, thyroidectomy and the use of antithyroid medication, specifically methimazole before definitive treatment, may decrease the risk of fractures in these patients.

Despite normal bone density, patients who have hypothyroidism may be at a higher risk of fractures. The greater risk does not seem to be related to a deleterious effect from the use of levothyroxine replacement because these patients seem to be at risk before and for 2 to 10 years after the diagnosis of hypothyroidism. Multiple studies have failed to link levothyroxine therapy with higher fracture rates. The mechanism for possible impaired bone strength in hypothyroid patients is unknown.

Bone density after hyperthyroidism

Because the risk of fractures is presumed to be related to the decreased bone mineral density (BMD) seen in patients who have hyperthyroidism, several small studies have been devised to assess the change in bone mass after treatment of hyperthyroidism. Although all of these studies have demonstrated improvement in bone density after restoration of the euthyroid state, the amount of improvement and the time frame evaluated has varied considerably.

In a study of 96 hyperthyroid patients treated with carbimizole, BMD in the calcaneus and forearm showed significant improvement within 3 to 6 months (12% and 1.5%, respectively) and normalization at both sites between 6 months and 3 years after therapy was initiated. Bone density in the calcaneus and the forearm increased 33% and 31%, respectively, at the endpoint of this study [51].

Two later studies showed improvement in bone density over baseline after 1 to 2 years of therapy, but bone density measurements remained significantly reduced compared with normal control subjects in both of these studies [52,53]. Three additional studies have demonstrated some improvement in

BMD with treatment of hyperthyroidism, although not necessarily a return to normal by the end of the study periods [54–56].

Several retrospective studies have compared bone density in previously treated hyperthyroid patients to matched control subjects. The largest of these studies involved 164 patients who had untreated or previously treated hyperthyroidism. Although bone density was significantly reduced in patients within the first 3 years after diagnosis, BMD was not significantly different from normal control subjects more than 3 years after treatment [57]. Three smaller studies have also found that bone density is normal in previously treated hyperthyroid patients [58–60].

A study of 106 postmenopausal women who had a history of treated hyperthyroidism demonstrated a decrease in bone density in all patients who received radioactive iodine. Patients who had previous hyperthyroidism treated with thyroidectomy who were receiving levothyroxine replacement were found to have reduced BMD. There was no significant decrease in bone density in patients who were euthyroid after thyroidectomy but not receiving levothyroxine replacement [61].

From the literature, a consensus has formed that treatment of hyperthyroidism improves BMD above baseline values. Although it is not certain that BMD can be restored to normal values in patients treated for hyperthyroidism, the data suggest that patients treated with thyroidectomy and antithyroid drugs may achieve greater improvement in bone density than those treated with radioactive iodine.

Therapy for reduced bone density in hyperthyroidism

Numerous agents have been studied to attempt to prevent the accelerated osteoporosis caused by hyperthyroidism. Studies have shown improvement in bone density with the use of the oral bisphosphonates risedronate, alendronate, and parenteral pamidronate [62–64]. Two additional studies of hyperthyroid rats treated with bisphosphonates have also demonstrated improvement in bone density in the laboratory setting [65,66]. One study has demonstrated an improvement in bone density with estrogen replacement in postmenopausal women [67]. Calcitonin has been shown to improve BMD in one study [68], but a previous investigation showed no improvement in bone density when calcitonin was added to antithyroid therapy with carbimazole [69]. Calcium and 1,25-$(OH)_2$ vitamin D3 supplementation may be beneficial in patients who have hyperthyroidism and concomitant hypoparathyroidism [70].

Endogenous subclinical hyperthyroidism and bone density

Although it is well established that overt hyperthyroidism has deleterious effects on bone density and the risk of fractures, the risk of untreated subclinical hyperthyroidism on the bone remains controversial. Two prospective cohort studies of women have found no decrease in bone density in women who have subclinical hyperthyroidism. The larger of these studies involved 458 women over 65 years of age divided into three groups (low, normal, or high TSH) who were followed over 4 to 6 years. No differences in bone density were observed among the three groups [71]. The smaller study followed 11 premenopausal women who had subclinical hyperthyroidism for 9 months to 2 years. No significant change was observed in bone density compared with control subjects. TSH levels were negatively correlated with plasma osteocalcin, serum alkaline phosphatase, and urine hydroxyproline measurements, but these markers of bone turnover were not significantly elevated when compared with control subjects [72].

In a cross-sectional study, 15 premenopausal women who had subclinical hyperthyroidism and suppressed TSH for 6 to 11 months before inclusion were evaluated. BMD in subclinical hyperthyroid subjects was not reduced compared with control subjects in this study [73]. Another cross-sectional study of premenopausal women compared bone density in 21 who had with Graves' disease and overt hyperthyroidism, 8 patients who had subclinical hyperthyroidism also due to Graves' disease, and 10 normal control subjects. Bone density was decreased only in the overt hyperthyroid group but not in those with subclinical disease [74].

Several studies have shown decreased bone density in patients who had untreated subclinical hyperthyroidism. A prospective study of 12 patients treated with radioiodine and 12 untreated patients followed over 2 years found that the untreated group experienced a 2% per year decline in bone density [75]. Two separate studies by one group compared patients who had previously untreated nodular goiter. In one study, subjects were divided into four groups: clinically hyperthyroid, subclinical hyperthyroidism, nontoxic nodular goiter, and matched control subjects. The investigators showed decreased bone density in postmenopausal subclinical hyperthyroid patients in the radius and femur but not the lumbar spine compared with control subjects. Overt hyperthyroid patients had reduced BMD at all sites tested. Bone density in the lumbar spine was significantly lower in postmenopausal hyperthyroid subjects than in premenopausal hyperthyroid subjects. Patients who had nontoxic goiter and premenopausal patients who had subclinical hyperthyroidism had no difference in BMD compared with control subjects [76]. In the other study, pre- and postmenopausal women who had overt or subclinical hyperthyroidism were compared with normal control subjects. Premenopausal hyperthyroid patients had reduced bone density in the spine but not in the femur. Postmenopausal patients who had overt and subclinical hyperthyroidism had reduced bone density in the spine and femoral neck. Premenopausal women who had subclinical hyperthyroidism did not demonstrate significant BMD reductions at either site compared with control subjects [77].

In a study of 60 patients who had subclinical hyperthyroidism due to multinodular goiter, bone density was decreased in the femoral neck and phalanges in pre- and postmenopausal subjects. Lumbar spine bone density was reduced only in the postmenopausal group [78].

A larger study of 413 subjects compared patients who had subclinical hyperthyroidism and subclinical hypothyroidism with euthyroid control subjects. Femoral neck bone density was reduced in the hypo- and hyperthyroid groups, whereas lumbar BMD did not differ among all three groups [79].

A prospective study of 16 postmenopausal women who had subclinical hyperthyroidism and multinodular goiter suggested that the deleterious effect of subclinical hyperthyroidism on bone density may be blunted with treatment. Eight subjects were treated with methimazole, and these patients had an increase in distal forearm BMD over 2 years as compared with the untreated group [80].

Although the effects of subclinical hyperthyroidism on bone remain in dispute, it would seem that postmenopausal women with this condition are at greatest risk of bone loss and that the axial skeleton is more likely to be affected than the lumbar spine.

Thyroid hormone therapy and bone density

The majority of clinical data involving thyroid conditions and bone density has been obtained from subjects receiving replacement doses of levothyroxine for hypothyroidism and those receiving TSH-suppressive doses for differentiated thyroid carcinoma, thyroid nodules, or nontoxic goiter. Studies have been difficult to compare because they have used different methodologies, patient selection criteria, treatment criteria, and endpoints. The following sections of this article briefly summarize key studies, reviews, and meta-analyses from the literature on this subject.

Suppressive doses of levothyroxine and bone density

At the time this article was written, we had found 22 studies demonstrating a reduction in bone density in at least some patients treated with doses of levothyroxine potent enough to suppress TSH [81–102]. In contrast, 18 studies have shown no decrease in bone density in patients treated with suppressive doses of levothyroxine [103–120]. Reductions in bone density have been demonstrated in pre- and postmenopausal women and in men. Significant decreases in BMD have been observed in patients who have a history of treated differentiated thyroid carcinoma and in those who have benign diseases such as nontoxic goiter. In these patients, reductions in bone density have been observed in the spine, pelvis, radius, femur, and calcaneus. Other studies have found that all patient types and skeletal sites have also been protected from bone loss despite suppressive doses of levothyroxine. Because these studies have used various methodologies of prospective and retrospective analysis, direct comparison of conflicting findings is difficult. Reviews and meta-analyses of these data are addressed in a subsequent section.

Replacement doses of levothyroxine and bone density

Three prospective trials involving hypothyroid patients on levothyroxine replacement therapy have demonstrated a reduction in bone density over the treatment period [121–123]. The longest of these followed patients for 1 year after their diagnosis. Considering that hypothyroid patients have increased bone density compared with normal subjects and that hypothyroidism causes an increase in the length of the bone remodeling cycle from a normal period of 200 days to over 700 days [30], these results are not surprising. It is expected that restoration of thyroid function ought to stimulate bone turn-over; however, it is not clear if this is a maladaptive process or a return to the normal state of bone resorption. One cross-sectional study has shown a reduction in bone density in cortical bone in 26 premenopausal women who had a history of Hashimoto's thyroiditis who were treated with levo-thyroxine for an average of 7.5 years [124].

One prospective study of postmenopausal women on thyroid-replace-ment therapy for 14 months demonstrated no reduction in bone density over the study period [125]. A case-control study of women receiving levo-thyroxine replacement demonstrated significant reductions in speed of sound and stiffness index ultrasound measurements at the heel but no signif-icant reduction in bone density scores compared with control subjects [126]. A cross-sectional study of women on thyroid hormone replacement for more than 5 years demonstrated no reduction in bone density in the treated group compared with normal control subjects [127]. In a cross-sectional study of men and women [128] and in a study of men only [129], investiga-tors found no significant deleterious effect on bone density in patients treated with levothyroxine compared with normal control subjects.

A longitudinal study of patients who had congenital hypothyroidism on thyroxine replacement and followed for 17 years demonstrated bone density scores within the normal range for age and gender [130].

Reviews and meta-analyses of levothyroxine therapy and bone density

Two groups of authors have attempted to clarify the conflicting results of prior studies of the effects of levothyroxine therapy on bone density through meta-analyses of available data. Faber and Galloe [131] compiled 13 cross-sectional studies of female patients on suppressive doses of levothyroxine. Fifty percent of the subjects were on treatment for differentiated thyroid carcinoma, the rest for benign thyroid disorders. Based on measurements of bone density at various skeletal sites, a theoretical skeleton composed of the distal forearm, femoral neck, and lumbar spine was created. No significant bone loss was detected in premenopausal women, but a 0.91% per year excess bone loss compared with normal individuals was observed in the postmeno-pausal group.

In a separate article, Uzzan and colleagues [132] compiled 41 cross-sectional studies and separately analyzed 25 subsets based on gender, menopausal status, skeletal site, and suppression versus replacement dose of levothyroxine. They concluded that suppressive levothyroxine therapy caused significant bone loss in postmenopausal women at the lumbar spine and hip but had no significant effect on premenopausal women or men. Paradoxically, thyroid replacement therapy was demonstrated to cause reduced bone density in premenopausal women at the spine and hip but did not have significant effects on bone in the other groups.

Several other authors have systematically reviewed the available studies in the publication databases involving thyroid hormone therapy and bone density. It has been suggested that methodologic differences among the many studies defy evaluation of the data by the technique of meta-analysis.

In a review article by Ross [133], the author concluded that suppressive therapy with levothyroxine had an adverse effect on bone density, that cortical bone was reduced more than trabecular bone, and that postmenopausal women were more likely to suffer bone loss than premenopausal women and men.

A review by Quan and colleagues [134], based on the evaluation of 11 studies of patients who had differentiated thyroid cancer, concluded that suppressive levothyroxine therapy had no significant effect on bone density in premenopausal women or men and that the effect on postmenopausal women was uncertain.

Heemstra and colleagues [135] more recently reviewed 21 studies of patients who had differentiated thyroid cancer on suppressive therapy and concluded that postmenopausal women were most at risk for reduction in bone density but that there was no evidence of significant risk to men or premenopausal women.

Schneider and Reiners [136] reviewed 63 studies, including those with prospective and cross-sectional data and those involving suppressive and replacement doses of levothyroxine. Thirty-one studies showed no significant effect on BMD, 23 showed partially beneficial or adverse effects, and nine studies showed an overall adverse effect on bone density with levothyroxine therapy. The authors concluded that evidence for the deleterious effects of levothyroxine on bone density in men and premenopausal women was the weakest and that the effects on postmenopausal women remained unclear.

Levothyroxine therapy at doses that suppress TSH may cause reductions in bone density, particularly in postmenopausal women. There is no evidence that the reduction in bone density confers an increased risk of fracture, but patients at high risk for osteoporosis for other reasons should be monitored closely. Osteoporosis prevention with bisphosphonates should be considered in these patients. There is no clear evidence that replacement therapy with levothyroxine causes osteoporosis, although a reduction in bone density may be seen early on after the initiation of therapy. Overt hyperthyroidism causes osteoporosis and fractures, but it is not clear if subclinical hyperthyroidism has any negative effects on bone density or increases the risk of fracture. Levothyroxine replacement therapy has not been definitively linked to osteoporosis or fractures, but a history of hypothyroidism may itself be a risk for reduced bone strength and an increased risk for fracture despite normal or even elevated BMD in those patients.

Markers of bone turnover in hyperthyroid states

Markers of bone turnover have been used to assess the changes in bone metabolism in hyperthyroid states and thyroid hormone therapy. Bone-specific ALP and serum osteocalcin are produced by osteoblasts and reflect bone formation. Numerous markers have been used to evaluate bone resorption, including tartrate-resistant acid phosphatase, urine hydroxyproline, urine deoxypyridinoline, serum levels of N-terminal and C-terminal telopeptides of type I collagen, urine N-terminal telopeptides of type I collagen crosslinks, and urine C-terminal telopeptides of CTX crosslinks.

Markers of bone turnover are elevated in overt hyperthyroidism but improve to normal with antithyroid therapy. The markers associated with formation, namely ALP, osteocalcin, and osteoprotegerin (OPG), stay elevated longer than markers associated with bone resorption [137–143]. Treatment with calcitonin or bisphosphonates, specifically alendronate and risedronate, hastens the normalization of markers of bone turnover [62,63,68].

Subclinical hyperthyroidism may increase markers of bone turnover [144,145], but studies have produced conflicting results [146,147]. Similarly, conflicting information has been obtained from studies of bone markers in patients on suppressive thyroxine therapy [146,148–152].

Overt and subclinical hypothyroidism may demonstrate a pattern of markers consistent with reduced bone turnover, evidenced by elevated OPG levels. OPG levels in these patients have been shown to return to normal levels with levothyroxine replacement therapy [153,154].

Although serum and urine markers of bone turnover are elevated in hyperthyroid states and improve with antithyroid therapy and antiresorptive therapy, it is not clear how these tests might be used to monitor bone metabolism in these patients or in patients receiving thyroxine therapy in TSH-suppressive doses.

Thyroid cancer and bone metastases

Skeletal metastases are an unusual complication for patients who have thyroid cancer. Although papillary thyroid cancer is the most common type of thyroid carcinoma, bone metastases occur in fewer than 2% of patients.

Because papillary thyroid cancer is so much more common than the other histologic types of thyroid cancer, it accounts for the vast majority of cases of skeletal metastases. Follicular thyroid cancer, on the other hand, metastasizes to bone in 7% to 20% of cases [155]. Because osseous metastases from thyroid cancer tend to be poorly differentiated, treatment options are limited and prognosis is poor, with mean survival estimated at 4 years [156].

Molecular aspects of bone metastases

For osseous metastases to occur, there must be several interactions between the malignant cell and the skeleton. First, the cancer cell must lose its cell–cell interactions and its cell-matrix cohesion. The adhesion of cells to their neighbors helps regulate major cellular processes including motility, growth, differentiation, and survival. Cell–cell adherens junctions (AJs), the most abundant type of intercellular adhesions, are important for maintaining tissue architecture and can limit cell movement and proliferation. AJs interact with calcium-dependent cadherin receptors on the surface of neighboring cells. The transmembrane assembly of cadherin receptors with the cytoskeleton stabilizes cell–cell adhesions and normal cell physiology.

The malignant potential of a cell is characterized by significant modifications in its cytoskeleton structure, decreased cellular adhesion, and aberrant adhesion-mediated signaling. The disruption of physiologic cell–cell adhesion in malignant cells may contribute to their improved ability to migrate and proliferate, leading to invasion and metastasis. This disruption can be achieved by inhibiting the expression of cadherin or catenin family members or by activating pathways that prevent the assembly of AJs.

The loss of E-cadherin (E-cadherin is the product of the *CDH1* gene) expression eliminates AJ formation and has been associated with the transition to carcinoma and acquisition of metastatic capacity in gastric cancer cell lines. Moreover, the reintroduction of AJs into cancer cell lines by restoration of cadherin expression has been shown to exert tumor-suppressive effects, including decreased proliferation and motility [157]. Although the specific role the cadherin–catenin system might play in the development of the metastatic potential of thyroid cancer is unknown, it is an important molecular pathway involved in the regulation of cell proliferation, invasion, and intracellular signaling during cancer progression.

After the loss of cell–cell interactions, the cancer cell must gain motility and take on the ability to invade other tissue. Eventually, the cell must navigate the vascular or lymphatic system and exit that environment so that it can take residence in a new, distant site. Once in its new site, the malignant cell must expand and multiply in number for it to become an established location for metastasis [158].

In recent years, investigators have begun to elucidate the mechanisms by which thyroid cancer metastasizes to bone. It is known, for example, that follicular thyroid cancer has decreased expression of caveolin-1 and caveolin-2, genes which are thought to function as tumor suppressors. Caveolin-1 and caveolin-2 are up-regulated in patients who have papillary and anaplastic thyroid cancer [159,160], so these genes may have pleiotropic effects depending on the thyroid cell type that is involved. Another molecule involved in the development of metastatic potential is focal adhesion kinase (FAK). FAK is expressed in high amounts in aggressive thyroid cancers and is thought to affect adhesion, motility, and distant site tumor growth [161]. In vitro data have shown that bone sialoprotein is up-regulated in thyroid cancer cells and may be important in determining the tissue invasiveness of a malignancy [162]. Other data have shown that follicular thyroid cancer cells express less fibronectin than normal cells and thus might lose their ability to suppress cellular adhesion and migration [163]. Finally, integrin $\alpha v\beta 3$ is expressed in high amounts in thyroid cancer cells and seems to enhance the ability of those cells to adhere to bone and form lytic lesions within the skeleton [164].

Development of skeletal metastases

Numerous studies have shown that thyroid cancer most often metastasizes to the vertebral bodies in those who have pre-existing or underlying osseous disease [165–167], although metastases to the long bones, pelvis, and skull can occur. Several features of bone physiology explain why the skeleton is a favorable site for metastasis. Because the bone is a highly vascular organ, it is a uniquely hospitable environment for hematogenous invasion. Moreover, the skeleton contains pockets lined by epithelial cells that do not possess a basement membrane, a characteristic that allows malignant cells to invade the bone more easily than other organs [168].

Once deposited into the skeleton, malignant cells up-regulate production of cell surface adhesion molecules, which enhance cellular attachment to the skeletal matrix. Malignant cells in the skeleton then release various cytokines that promote bone resorption and increase local angiogenesis [168]. Additionally, the malignant cells co-opt the skeletal matrix to ramp up production of fibroblast growth factors, transforming growth factors β, insulin-like growth factors I and II, platelet derived growth factors, and bone morphogenetic proteins that alter the normal bone remodeling process so that cellular division and survival are enhanced [169]. How these events occur is not known, but they likely involve direct tumor cell–bone interaction and humoral effects mediated through cytokines that regulate osteoclast and osteoblast activity.

Thyroid cancer most frequently causes lytic lesions when it metastasizes to bone [170]. The osteolytic process is ultimately driven by the receptor activator of the RANK/RANK-L/OPG pathway. RANK-L is present on the external membrane of stromal cells and is released by activated T cells. In this process, RANK-L binds to RANK and activates a sequence of signaling events (partly mediated through NF-κβ and Jun N-terminal kinase) that lead to recruitment and maturation of osteoclasts. Osteoclasts directly influence the resorption of bone and allow osteolytic lesions to take hold in the skeleton. This process is balanced by an opposing molecular mechanism. OPG, which is produced by osteoblasts, bone matrix, and some tumors, serves as an inhibitory check on osteoclast activity. OPG serves as a decoy receptor for RANK-L and prevents RANK-L from binding to RANK. In this way, OPG down-regulates osteoclast maturation and decreases osteoclastic resorption of bone [169,171].

Although the RANK/RANK-L/OPG pathway seems to be common to all osteolytic malignancies, how this process is regulated in thyroid cancer is unknown. In multiple myeloma, for example, not only is osteoclast activity enhanced, but osteoblast activity is diminished. This suggests that osteolytic tumors not only influence osteoclast activity through RANK/RANK-L/OPG but also affect osteoblast function [172]. The lytic lesions of multiple myeloma seem to release cytokine signals that influence Wnt. Wnts are a large family of growth factors that mediate fundamental biological processes like embryogenesis, organogenesis, and tumorigenesis. These proteins bind to a membrane receptor complex comprised of a frizzled G-protein–coupled receptor and a low-density lipoprotein receptor–related protein (LRP). The formation of this ligand-receptor complex initiates a number of intracellular signaling cascades that have been shown to play an important role in the regulation of bone formation. Mutations in LRP-5 have been linked to changes in BMD and fracture risk. Studies of knockout and transgenic mouse models for Wnt pathway components like Wnt-10b, LRP-5/6, secreted frizzled-related protein-1, dickkopf-2, Axin-2, and beta-catenin have demonstrated that these signaling components alter most aspects of osteoblast physiology, including proliferation, differentiation, bone matrix formation, mineralization, apoptosis, and coupling to osteoclastogenesis and bone resorption [173].

The Wnt pathway is not involved only in regulating osteoblast function; it is also involved in cell adhesion. A major route for signal transduction by AJs involves the regulation of β-catenin–T cell factor (TCF) signaling. β-catenin acts as a transcription factor in the nucleus by serving as a coactivator of the lymphoid enhancer factor/TCF family of DNA-binding proteins. β-catenin–mediated transcription is activated by the Wnt pathway, especially during embryonic development. Promotion of Wnt signaling involves the inhibition of β-catenin degradation by the proteasomes, resulting in its nuclear accumulation and eventually transcriptional activation of lymphoid enhancer factor/TCF target genes. Mutations in components that regulate β-catenin turnover and mutations in β-catenin that compromise the protein's degradation have been found in several human cancers. When the Wnt signaling pathway is inactive, free β-catenin is degraded by a protein complex so that it does not activate genes thought to be involved in cancer development. The binding of Wnt to Frizzled receptors activates Wnt signaling. Once the Wnt pathway is activated, other components, such as disheveled protein, a member of the Wnt signaling cascade, are activated and inhibit β-catenin phosphorylation by glycogen synthase kinase. This results in β-catenin accumulation in the nucleus, where it complexes with TCF and transactivates target genes such as *Cyclin D1* and *Myc*, which are thought to be crucial to the promotion of cell proliferation, invasion and cancer progression [157].

In one recent study, investigators analyzed the effects of a suppressive thyroid hormone therapy in men who had differentiated thyroid cancer on the RANK/RANK-L/OPG pathway and on bone metabolism. OPG was found to be significantly increased and RANK-L significantly decreased in patients who were on suppressive doses of levothyroxine compared with healthy control subjects. Additionally, CTX levels were significantly higher in patients than in control subjects. Therefore, suppressive levothyroxine therapy in men who have differentiated thyroid cancer seems to affect the RANK/RANK-L/OPG pathway and lead to more osteoclastic activity, but our understanding of how thyroid cancer metastasizes and proliferates in bone remains to be elucidated [174].

Screening for bone metastases

Although follicular thyroid cancer accounts for fewer than 15% of differentiated thyroid cancers, it has an incidence of bone metastases of 7% to 20%, so follicular thyroid cancer is the main focus of our discussion on bone metastases [156]. Any type of thyroid cancer can metastasize to osseous structures.

Detection of distant metastases may be difficult, and 131-I scanning has relatively poor sensitivity. Radiographs and bone scintigraphy are often used in the evaluation of skeletal metastases. These imaging techniques detect disease only after more than 50% of bone has been destroyed, and there are no prospective studies assessing their individual sensitivity and specificity in detecting osseous metastases from thyroid cancer [175]. Bone scintigraphy often detects skeletal metastases earlier than they appear on standard radiographs but only if there is a significant osteoblastic component. MRI is superb for imaging the medullary component of bone and detailing the intraosseous and extraskeletal extent of disease. CT is valuable in imaging for cortical erosion and subclinical fracture in osseous metastases. If a patient has pulmonary metastases or if there is a clinical suspicion for osseous metastases, it seems prudent to consider obtaining a metastatic skeletal survey or a bone scan and a chest CT without contrast. Once a bone lesion at a particular site is suspected, directed MRI or CT scan is most appropriate to better define the lesion(s). MRI or CT is particularly helpful in planning surgical approaches to destructive skeletal metastases [175].

In a recent study, PET, Technetium 99m sestamibi (Tc-MIBI) whole-body scan (WBS), and posttherapy 131-I imaging were compared under TSH stimulation for their ability to detect distant metastases. Three of the

19 patients had follicular thyroid cancer, and the rest had papillary thyroid carcinoma. PET was found to be superior to Tc-MIBI and 131-I scan in detecting distant spread. The 19 patients had 32 isolated lesions (10 lymph node, 15 lung, 6 bone, and 1 muscle) confirmed by histopathology or other imaging studies (radiograph, ultrasound, CT, MRI, and bone scan). PET detected 81.3%, MIBI detected 62.5%, and 131-I detected 68.8% of the total lesions. Lung metastases were detected in 73.3%, 46.7%, and 66.7% of cases, respectively. The three imaging modalities were comparable in detecting bone metastases, all detecting about 83% of lesions [176].

Role and efficacy of radioactive iodine for osseous metastases

Prospective, randomized studies of 131-I in the treatment of bone metastases from thyroid carcinoma are lacking. The best available data regarding this topic come from retrospective studies. A recent retrospective analysis of 2200 patients who had differentiated thyroid carcinoma identified 394 patients who had lung or bone metastases [177]. Twenty-eight patients had well differentiated follicular carcinoma, and 173 patients had less differentiated follicular carcinoma. Most patients underwent total thyroidectomy and received ablative therapy with 131-I. One third received postoperative external-beam radiation therapy (EBRT) after surgery to the neck. Patients who had detectable lung or bone disease on posttherapy scanning received an additional 100 mCi 131-I 3 months after a standard initial ablation dose of 100 mCi 131-I. The same occurred for patients who had a detectable thyroglobulin (Tg) level during levothyroxine therapy or Tg > 5 ng/mL off levothyroxine therapy. Patients who had radiographically proven bone metastases also received approximately 3000 rads of EBRT to the affected region in association with 131-I therapy. Patients who had less differentiated follicular cancer had lower survival rates than those who had well differentiated papillary or follicular carcinoma. Positive 131-I uptake was associated with improved prognosis. The risk of death was greatest in patients who had macronodular pulmonary metastases or multiple bone metastases. Ten-year survival was 96% in patients younger than 40 years of age who had normal chest radiographs but only 7% in patients over 40 years of age who had macronodular pulmonary or multiple bone metastases. Survival was 63% for all other patients. For patients who had a complete response, survival was 96% at 5 years, 93% at 10 years, and 89% at 15 years. Without a complete response, survival was 37%, 14%, and 8%, respectively. Response to 131-I therapy was improved the earlier disease was detected and treated. In addition to 131-I WBS, Tg measurement is an important and sensitive marker of detecting metastatic disease. Although prolonged survival was not proven to be linked to 131-I treatment alone, patients who survived more than 15 years after the detection of metastases had all been treated with 131-I alone or in combination with EBRT.

In the most recent report from this center, researchers were able to distinguish survival rates among 444 patients who had distant metastases from papillary and follicular thyroid carcinoma [178]. Among those who had radioiodine uptake, 20-year survival was 33% versus only 3% at 10 years for those without radioiodine uptake. Those who had lung metastases had 49% survival at 20 years, whereas those who had bone metastases had 20-year survival of only 8%. For patients who have lung and bone metastases, 20-year survival was 9%. Survival rates were not affected by the presence of neck recurrences. The discovery of metastases early versus late in the patient's course also did not affect survival.

Role and efficacy of intravenous bisphosphonates in treatment of bone metastases

Bone metastases from thyroid cancer, particularly those that are less differentiated, respond poorly if at all to traditional treatment regimens that include 131-I. Because bone metastases destroy bone architecture through a local osteolytic process, some investigators have proposed using inhibitors of osteoclast activity (eg, bisphosphonates) to slow or prevent the skeletal complications of osseous metastases. A small protocol enrolled 10 patients who had thyroid cancer and administered pamidronate 90 mg intravenously every month for 1 year [179]. Patients who received pamidronate reported significantly less bone pain by visual analog scale, improved performance status, and a beneficial impact on quality of life. Two of 10 patients demonstrated a partial radiographic response to therapy. The main side effects—fever, myalgias, and electrolyte abnormalities (mainly hypocalcemia)—were mild and short lived.

In a recent study, zoledronic acid (4 mg), a newer-generation bisphosphonate, was compared in a phase III randomized trial with pamidronate (90 mg) in patients who had breast cancer. Zoledronic acid significantly reduced the risk of developing a skeletal-related event (SRE), defined as a pathologic fracture, spinal cord compression, radiation therapy, or surgery to bone, by an additional 20% versus 9% for pamidronate [180]. Zoledronic acid was at least as effective as pamidronate in reducing the proportion of patients who had at least one SRE and in delaying the onset of SREs. Moreover, a retrospective subset analysis of patients who had at least one osteolytic lesion proved zoledronic acid more effective than pamidronate in reducing the risk and delaying the onset of SREs. Although there is no evidence to support improved survival rates, the widespread adoption of these agents (with the evidence favoring zoledronic acid) in the management of patients who have bone metastases from thyroid cancer should be considered because this therapy is easy to administer and well tolerated. In our center, we favor using zoledronic acid 4 mg intravenously on a monthly basis for 1 year followed by quarterly infusions indefinitely for patients who have thyroid cancer and bone metastases [181]. Prospective studies in thyroid cancer patients who have osseous metastases are required.

No discussion of bisphosphonates is complete without addressing the complication known as osteonecrosis of the jaw (ONJ). ONJ is characterized by areas of exposed bone in the mandible, maxilla, or palate that heal poorly or do not heal at all over a period of 2 months. The nonhealing lesions are often painful and typically associated with infection at the affected site [182].

A thorough review of this topic examined all case reports and case series of patients who had bisphosphonate-associated ONJ published in MEDLINE from 1966 to January 2006 [183]. Patients who had multiple myeloma and metastatic carcinoma to the skeleton who are receiving intravenous nitrogen-containing bisphosphonates (eg, pamidronate or zoledronic acid) are at greatest risk for ONJ (94% of published cases), but ONJ has been reported to occur with all of the available oral bisphosphonates (alendronate, risedronate, ibandronate). Eighty-five percent of affected patients have had multiple myeloma or metastatic breast cancer, and 4% have had osteoporosis. The estimated prevalence of ONJ in patients who have cancer is 6% to 10%, but the prevalence in those who have osteoporosis is unknown. The mandible is more commonly affected than the maxilla (2:1 ratio), 60% of cases are preceded by a dental surgical procedure, and the remaining 40% related to infection or trauma. Patients who have ONJ have typically been administered chemotherapy or glucocorticoids and have usually received intravenous bisphosphonates for 1.5 to 3 years [182].

Oversuppression of bone turnover is thought to represent the predominant mechanism for the development of this condition, but there may be other contributing factors, such as pre-existing dental infection, radiation exposure to the jaw, and a history of receiving chemotherapy. A recently issued recommendation calls for the eradication of all sites of potential jaw infection before bisphosphonate therapy is begun to lessen the need for subsequent dentoalveolar surgery. Conservative debridement of necrotic bone, pain control, infection management, use of antimicrobial oral rinses, and withdrawal of bisphosphonates are thought to be preferable to aggressive surgical measures for treating this condition [183].

Novel modalities for the treatment of bone metastases

Traditional therapy for differentiated thyroid cancer includes total thyroidectomy, removal of suspicious lymph nodes in the central compartment, and 131-I treatment. In cases of local or distant relapse, further surgery, 131-I therapy, or EBRT may be required. If none of those modalities is successful, novel treatments may be instituted to control the disease burden.

EBRT is a significant component of the therapeutic options available to patients who have skeletal metastases from thyroid cancer. The main objective of EBRT is to alleviate pain and the neurologic complications from osseous disease. Although data on this subject as it relates to thyroid cancer are lacking, it is thought that approximately 70% of patients experience pain relief with palliative EBRT [184]. Patients often report subjective improvement in their symptoms within 2 to 3 days, but some report improvement up to a month after therapy. EBRT must be tailored to the patient's life expectancy, the anatomic site of the skeletal metastasis, and the size of area to be treated. EBRT is often implemented after surgical treatment of pathologic fractures or impending fractures to improve the patient's functional status. EBRT is undergoing investigation as to whether its integration with newer therapeutic modalities, such as vertebroplasty and radiofrequency ablation, may provide additional benefit to patients.

Radiofrequency ablation (RFA) and ethanol injection (EtOH) are relatively new, minimally invasive techniques that have been used as adjuvant therapy in malignancies such as hepatocellular carcinoma or malignancies that have metastasized to the liver. RFA uses current to induce focal coagulative necrosis and eradicate small areas of tissue in a controlled fashion. Side effects of RFA include hoarseness (most likely caused by thermal injury to the recurrent laryngeal nerve) and skin burns (most likely caused by protrusion of the proximal portion of the electrode tip through the skin during the ablation procedure). Self-limited neck swelling and regional discomfort have been reported in almost all patients, but the symptoms typically resolved within 1 to 2 weeks. EtOH is thought to induce tissue necrosis as a result of cellular dehydration and protein denaturation. The role of these techniques in thyroid cancer is just beginning to be explored.

One study recently evaluated the RFA and EtOH experience in local and focal distant metastases [185]. In this study, 16 patients underwent RFA treatment of biopsy proven recurrent well differentiated thyroid cancer in the neck. Four patients underwent RFA for focal distant metastases. Three patients had solitary bone metastases, and one patient had a solitary pulmonary metastasis. Of the three patients treated with RFA for bone metastases, one presented at 1 year of follow-up with persistent disease. This individual was retreated with RFA and 131-I, and subsequent 131-I whole body scanning was negative. A second patient had persistent disease at the treated site and developed a new osseous metastasis. The third patient had biopsy proven absence of disease at the treated site, and subsequent 131-I WBS have been negative through 53 months of follow-up. The patient who had the pulmonary metastasis had no evidence of uptake in the lung fields on follow-up 131-I whole-body scanning despite persistent uptake in the neck after multiple rounds of 131-I treatment. Six patients underwent EtOH ablation, under local anesthesia and with ultrasound guidance, of biopsy proven recurrent thyroid cancer in the neck. RFA and EtOH were able to achieve resolution of solitary lymph node metastases from thyroid cancer in 18 of the 22 patients. The data for bone metastases were less robust, with only one of the three treated patients showing a response at the focal distant site.

RFA and EtOH have advantages and disadvantages. RFA has been found to reduce pain from thyroid cancer bone metastases, but data are lacking in terms of long-term resolution of disease at the treated sites. RFA produces a larger area of lesion destruction, but the energy it delivers can be finely modulated. Therefore, RFA can be used to treat a larger region of interest than EtOH, but RFA may be more likely to cause local tissue injury from its thermal effect. These techniques should be used carefully, especially when treating disease in the lateral aspect of the central compartment where the recurrent laryngeal nerve might be susceptible to the damaging treatment effect. This last comment in particular applies to ethanol injection because extravasation can be extremely toxic to local tissues, causing significant fibrosis. These techniques should be used only in selected patients by individuals experienced in these techniques.

The role of adjuvant EBRT in patients who have locally advanced follicular thyroid cancer has been studied only retrospectively [186]. The efficacy of EBRT to the thyroid bed or to the upper cervical and superior mediastinal lymph nodes is uncertain, with some studies showing no benefit or even worse outcomes compared with those who did not receive EBRT; survival seems to be unchanged with EBRT. It is possible that retrospective studies have failed to demonstrate an effect due to a selection bias favoring treatment of the more serious lesions. Some studies have shown improvements in local recurrence and disease-specific survival with EBRT in papillary thyroid cancer but not follicular thyroid cancer. Nonetheless, some centers offer EBRT to high-risk patients (age >45 years and resectable extrathyroidal disease) in conjunction with 131-I treatment. If EBRT is given, it is usually limited to the thyroid bed, but it can be tailored to the specific anatomic site of disease.

Newer techniques, such as conformal radiotherapy intensity modulated radiation therapy, can allow for more precise radiotherapy delivery to sites outside the thyroid bed where more normal tissue can be spared and acute and late toxicity may be mitigated [187]. In patients who have solitary bone metastases, for example, 50 Gy is usually given in several fractions over 4 weeks, but special caution must be taken to avoid delivering high doses (limited to 40 Gy) to the spinal cord. Side effects of EBRT include skin erythema, dry desquamation, and mucositis of the pharynx and esophagus. Long-term sequelae include skin hyperpigmentation and esophageal and tracheal stenosis. Patients receiving EBRT to the neck area almost invariably have some difficulty swallowing and neck pain during the last several weeks of therapy. We recommend EBRT to the neck for patients who have locally aggressive tumors, particularly for patients who have residual disease invading the trachea.

Another adjuvant therapeutic modality for treating skeletal metastases is cryotherapy. Cryotherapy used to be performed by introducing liquid nitrogen into the tumor bed. Although this technique was somewhat successful, side effects included the formation of nitrogen emboli, bone fractures secondary to local necrosis of skeletal tissue, and damage to local neurovascular structures. More recently, cryotherapy has been performed using an argon-based system that allows for the controlled formation of ice around a metallic probe. The technique is computer controlled and allows for the protection of surrounding structures. In one study, 27 patients underwent argon therapy (14 patients had metastatic bone disease). No patient suffered neurologic injury, and after 2 years only two of the surviving patients had a site recurrence (none from the metastatic group). There were no pathologic fractures [188]. In light of these data, cryotherapy seems to be a useful addition to the therapeutic armamentarium available for the treatment of osseous metastases of thyroid carcinoma with minimal risk to local surrounding structures. Definitive studies in this area are warranted.

Summary

Triiodothyronine and thyrotropin independently affect bone growth and development, mineralization, and remodeling. T3 effects seem to be mediated primarily by TR α. TSH is apparently an inhibitor of bone resorption and formation.

Previously treated hyperthyroidism is likely a long-term risk factor for fractures, particularly fractures of the hip. Thyroidectomy and methimazole may decrease the risk of fractures in these patients compared with treatment with radioactive iodine. Hypothyroidism may also be a risk factor for fractures, although the mechanism is not understood. Fracture risk does not seem to be related to levothyroxine replacement in hypothyroid patients.

Treatment of hyperthyroidism improves BMD but not necessarily to normal levels. Patients treated with thyroidectomy and antithyroid drugs may achieve greater improvement in bone density than those treated with radioactive iodine. The effects of subclinical hyperthyroidism on the bone are controversial.

TSH-suppressing doses of levothyroxine may cause reduced bone density, especially in postmenopausal women. Although it is not clear that this reduction in bone density creates an increased risk of fractures, high-risk patients need to be monitored for progression of osteoporosis. Replacement therapy with levothyroxine has not been shown to cause osteoporosis, although it may temporarily reduce bone density after the initiation of treatment.

We have learned much about the molecular biology and pathophysiology of bone metastases and how to treat them. Alterations of the RANK/RANK-L/OPG and Wnt pathways, along with changes in gene expression that affect cell adhesion, cell movement, and cell proliferation, have been studied and seem to be important to our understanding of how thyroid cancer metastasizes to bone. Total thyroidectomy and 131-I therapy remain the standard of care for patients who have osseous metastases from thyroid cancer, but newer additions to our treatment paradigm include intravenous bisphosphonates, EBRT, cryotherapy, alcohol ablation, and radiofrequency ablation. Although curing patients who have bone metastases is rare, using aggressive techniques against high-risk lesions can lead to palliation of symptoms and prolongation of survival, even in those who have persistent disease.

References

[1] Galliford TM, Murphy E, Williams AJ, et al. Effects of thyroid status on bone metabolism: a primary role for thyroid stimulating hormone or thyroid hormone? Minerva Endocrinol 2005;30:237.

[2] Kronenberg HM. Developmental regulation of the growth plate. Nature 2003;423:332.

[3] Bassett JH, Swinhoe R, Chassande O, et al. Thyroid hormone regulates heparin sulfate proteoglycan expression in the growth plate. Endocrinology 2006;147:295.

[4] Eriksen EF, Mosekilde L, Melsen F. Trabecular bone remodeling and bone balance in hyperthyroidism. Bone 1985;6:421.

[5] Bassett JH, Williams GR. The molecular actions of thyroid hormone in bone. Trends Endocrinol Metab 2003;14:356.

[6] Robson H, Siebler T, Stevens DA, et al. Thyroid hormone acts directly on growth plate chondrocytes to promote hypertrophic differentiation and inhibit clonal expansion and cell proliferation. Endocrinology 2000;141:3887.

[7] Stevens DA, Hasserjian RP, Robson H, et al. Thyroid hormones regulate hypertrophic chondrocyte differentiation and expression of parathyroid hormone-related peptide and its receptor during endochondral bone formation. J Bone Miner Res 2000;15:2431.

[8] Abu E, Bord S, Horner A, et al. The expression of thyroid hormone receptors in human bone. Bone 1997;21:137.

[9] Abu E, Horner A, Teti A, et al. The localization of thyroid hormone receptor mRNAs in human bone. Thyroid 2000;10:287.

[10] Allain TJ, Yen PM, Flanagan AM, et al. The isoform-specific expression of the tri-iodothyronine receptor in osteoblasts and osteoclasts. Eur J Clin Invest 1996;26:418.

[11] Siddiqi A, Parsons MP, Lewis JL, et al. TR expression and function in human bone marrow stromal and osteoblast-like cells. J Clin Endocrinol Metab 2002;87:906.

[12] Williams GR, Bland R, Sheppard MC. Characterization of thyroid hormone (T3) receptors in three osteosarcoma cell lines of distinct osteoblast phenotype: interactions among T3, vitamin D3, and retinoid signaling. Endocrinology 1994;135:2375.

[13] Abe E, Marians R, Yu W, et al. TSH is a negative regulator of skeletal remodeling. Cell 2003;115:151.

[14] Morimura T, Tsunekawa K, Kasahara T, et al. Expression of type 2 iodothyronine de-iodinase in human osteoblast is stimulated by thyrotropin. Endocrinology 2005;146:2077.

[15] Weiss RE, Refetoff S. Effect of thyroid hormone on growth: lessons from the syndrome of resistance to thyroid hormone. Endocrinol Metab Clin North Am 1996;25:719.

[16] Ishikawa Y, Genge BR, Wuthier RE, et al. Thyroid hormone inhibits growth and stimulates terminal differentiation of epiphyseal growth plate chondrocytes. J Bone Miner Res 1998;13:1398.

[17] Miura M, Tanaka K, Komatsu Y, et al. Thyroid hormones promote chondrocyte differentiation in mouse ATDC5 cells and stimulate endochondral ossification in fetal mouse tibias through iodothyronine deiodinases in the growth plate. J Bone Miner Res 2002;17:443.

[18] Okubo Y, Reddi AH. Thyroxine downregulates Sox9 and promotes chondrocyte hypertrophy. Biochem Biophys Res Commun 2003;306:186.

[19] Lakatos P, Foldes J, Horvath C, et al. Serum interleukin-6 and bone metabolism in patients with thyroid function disorders. J Clin Endocrinol Metab 1997;82:78.

[20] Lakatos P, Foldes J, Nagy Z, et al. Serum insulin-like growth factor-I, insulin-like growth factor binding proteins, and bone mineral content in hyperthyroidism. Thyroid 2000; 10:417.

[21] Dentice M, Bandyopadhyay A, Gereben B, et al. The Hedgehog-inducible ubiquitin ligase subunit WSB-1 modulates thyroid hormone activation and PTHrP secretion in the developing growth plate. Nat Cell Biol 2005;7:698.

[22] Shao YY, Wang L, Hicks DG, et al. Expression and activation of peroxisome proliferator-activated receptors in growth plate chondrocytes. J Orthop Res 2005; 23:1139.

[23] Wang L, Shao YY, Ballock RT. Peroxisome proliferator activated receptor-gamma (PPARgamma) represses thyroid hormone signaling in growth plate chondrocytes. Bone 2005;37:305.

[24] O'Shea PJ, Williams GR. Insight into the physiological actions of thyroid hormone receptors from genetically modified mice. J Endocrinol 2002;175:553.

[25] Gauthier K, Chassande O, Plateroti M, et al. Different functions for the thyroid hormone receptors TRalpha and TRbeta in the control of thyroid hormone production and post-natal development. EMBO J 1999;18:623.

[26] Mundy G, Shapiro J, Bandelin J, et al. Direct stimulation of bone resorption by thyroid hormones. J Clin Invest 1976;58:529.

[27] Allain TJ, McGregor AM. Thyroid hormones and bone. J Endocrinol 1993;139:9.

[28] Kanatani M, Sugimoto T, Sowa H, et al. Thyroid hormone stimulates osteoclast differentiation by a mechanism independent of RANKL-RANK interaction. J Cell Physiol 2004;201:17.

[29] Freitas FR, Moriscot AS, Jorgetti V, et al. Spared bone mass in rats treated with thyroid hormone receptor TR beta-selective compound GC-1. Am J Physiol Endocrinol Metab 2003;285:E1135.

[30] Mosekilde L, Eriksen E, Charles P. Effects of thyroid hormones on bone and mineral metabolism. Endocrinol Metab Clin North Am 1990;19:35.

[31] Harvey CB, O'Shea PJ, Scott AJ, et al. Molecular mechanisms of thyroid hormone effects on bone growth and function. Mol Genet Metab 2002;75:17.

[32] Milne M, Quail JM, Rosen CJ, et al. Insulin-like growth factor binding proteins in femoral and vertebral bone marrow stromal cells: expression and regulation by thyroid hormone and dexamethasone. J Cell Biochem 2001;81:229.

[33] Siddiqi A, Burrin JM, Wood DF, et al. Tri-iodothyronine regulates the production of interleukin-6 and interleukin-8 in human bone marrow stromal and osteoblast-like cells. J Endocrinol 1998;157:453.

[34] Simsek G, Karter Y, Aydin S, et al. Osteoporotic cytokines and bone metabolism on rats with induced hyperthyroidism; changes as a result of reversal to euthyroidism. Chin J Physiol 2003;46:181.

[35] Stevens DA, Harvey CB, Scott AJ, et al. Thyroid hormone activates fibroblast growth factor receptor-1 in bone. Mol Endocrinol 2003;17:1751.

[36] Hase H, Ando T, Eldeiry L, et al. TNFalpha mediates the skeletal effects of thyroid-stimulating hormone. Proc Natl Acad Sci U S A 2006;103:12849.

[37] Sun L, Davies T, Blair H, et al. TSH and bone loss. Ann N Y Acad Sci 2006;1068:309.

[38] Mazziotti G, Sorvillo F, Piscopo M, et al. Recombinant human TSH modulates in vivo C-telopeptides of type-1 collagen and bone alkaline phosphatase, but not osteoprotegerin production in postmenopausal women monitored for differentiated thyroid carcinoma. J Bone Miner Res 2005;20:480.

[39] Majima T, Komatsu Y, Doi K, et al. Negative correlation between bone mineral density and TSH receptor antibodies in male patients with untreated Graves' disease. Osteoporos Int 2006;17:1103.

[40] Franklyn J, Maisonneuve P, Sheppard M, et al. Mortality after the treatment of hyperthyroidism with radioactive iodine. N Engl J Med 1998;338:712.

[41] Vestergaard P, Rejnmark L, Weeke J, et al. Fracture risk in patients treated for hyperthyroidism. Thyroid 2000;10:341.

[42] Melton LJ 3rd, Ardila E, Crowson CS, et al. Fractures following thyroidectomy in women: a population-based cohort study. Bone 2000;27:695.

[43] Nguyen TT, Heath H 3rd, Bryant SC, et al. Fractures after thyroidectomy in men: a population-based cohort study. J Bone Miner Res 1997;12:1092.

[44] Vestergaard P, Mosekilde L. Fractures in patients with hyperthyroidism and hypothyroidism: a nationwide follow-up study in 16,249 patients. Thyroid 2002;12:411.

[45] Vestergaard P, Rejnmark L, Mosekilde L. Influence of hyper- and hypothyroidism, and the effects of treatment with antithyroid drugs and levothyroxine on fracture risk. Calcif Tissue Int 2005;77:139.

[46] Bauer D, Ettinger B, Nevitt M, et al. Risk for fracture in women with low serum levels of thyroid-stimulating hormone. Ann Intern Med 2001;134:561.

[47] Wejda B, Hintze G, Katschinski B, et al. Hip fractures and the thyroid: a case-control study. J Intern Med 1995;237:241.

[48] Solomon B, Wartofsky L, Burman K. Prevalence of fractures in postmenopausal women with thyroid disease. Thyroid 1993;3:17.

[49] Vestergaard P, Weeke J, Hoeck H, et al. Fractures in patients with primary idiopathic hypothyroidism. Thyroid 2000;10:335.

[50] Leese G, Jung R, Guthrie C, et al. Morbidity in patients on L-thyroxine: a comparison of those with a normal TSH to those with a suppressed TSH. Clin Endocrinol (Oxf) 1992; 37:500.

[51] Linde J, Friis T. Osteoporosis in hyperthyroidism estimated by photon absorptiometry. Acta Endocrinol (Copenh) 1979;91:437.

[52] Krolner B, Jorgensen J, Nielsen S. Spinal bone mineral content in myxoedema and thyrotoxicosis: effects of thyroid hormone(s) and antithyroid treatment. Clin Endocrinol (Oxf) 1983;18:439.

[53] Toh S, Claunch B, Brown P. Effect of hyperthyroidism and its treatment on bone mineral content. Arch Intern Med 1985;145:883.

[54] Acotto CG, Niepomniszcze H, Vega E, et al. Ultrasound parameters and markers of bone turnover in hyperthyroidism: a longitudinal study. J Clin Densitom 2004;7:201.

[55] Diamond T, Vine J, Smart R, et al. Thyrotoxic bone disease in women: a potentially reversible disorder. Ann Intern Med 1994;120:8.

[56] Rosen C, Adler R. Longitudinal changes in lumbar bone density among thyrotoxic patients after attainment of euthyroidism. J Clin Endocrinol Metab 1992;75:1531.

[57] Karga H, Papapetrou P, Korakovoni A, et al. Bone mineral density in hyperthyroidism. Clin Endocrinol (Oxf) 2004;61:466.

[58] Langdahl B, Loft A, Eriksen E, et al. Bone mass, bone turnover, body composition, and calcium homeostasis in former hyperthyroid patients treated by combined medical therapy. Thyroid 1996;6:161.

[59] Langdahl B, Loft A, Eriksen E, et al. Bone mass, bone turnover, calcium homeostasis, and body composition in surgically and radioiodine-treated former hyperthyroid patients. Thyroid 1996;6:169.

[60] Nielsen H, Mosekilde L, Charles P. Bone mineral content in hyperthyroid patients after combined medical and surgical treatment. Acta Radiol Oncol Radiat Phys Biol 1979;18:122.

[61] Grant D, McMurdo M, Mole P, et al. Is previous hyperthyroidism still a risk factor for osteoporosis in post-menopausal women? Clin Endocrinol (Oxf) 1995;43:339.

[62] Lupoli G, Nuzzo V, Di Carlo C, et al. Effects of alendronate on bone loss in pre- and postmenopausal hyperthyroid women treated with methimazole. Gynecol Endocrinol 1996;10:343.

[63] Majima T, LKomatsu Y, Doi K, et al. Clinical significance of risedronate for osteoporosis in the initial treatment of male patients with Graves' disease. J Bone Miner Metab 2006;24:105.

[64] Rosen H, Moses A, Gundberg C, et al. Therapy with parenteral pamidronate prevents thyroid hormone-induced bone turnover in humans. J Clin Endocrinol Metab 1993; 77:664.

[65] Kung A, Ng F. A rat model of thyroid hormone-induced bone loss: effect of antiresorptive agents on regional bone density and osteocalcin gene expression. Thyroid 1994;4:93.

[66] Rosen H, Sullivan E, Middlebrooks V, et al. Parenteral pamidronate prevents thyroid hormone-induced bone loss in rats. J Bone Miner Res 1993;8:1255.

[67] Franklyn J, Betteridge J, Holder R, et al. Effect of estrogen replacement therapy upon bone mineral density in thyroxine-treated postmenopausal women with a past history of thyrotoxicosis. Thyroid 1995;5:359.

[68] Akcay MN, Akcay G, Habib B. The effects of calcitonin on bone resorption in hyperthyroidism: a placebo-controlled clinical study. J Bone Miner Metab 2004;22:90.

[69] Jodar E, Munoz-Torres M, Escobar-Jimenez F, et al. Antiresorptive therapy in hyperthyroid patients: longitudinal changes in bone and mineral metabolism. J Clin Endocrinol Metab 1997;82:1989.

[70] Hawkins F, Escobar-Jimenez F, Jodar E, et al. Bone mineral density in hypoparathyroid women on LT4 suppressive therapy: effect of calcium and 1,25(OH)2 vitamin D3 treatment. J Musculoskelet Neuronal Interact 2003;3:71.

[71] Bauer D, Nevitt M, Ettinger B, et al. Low thyrotropin levels are not associated with bone loss in older women: a prospective study. J Clin Endocrinol Metab 1997;82:2931.

[72] Faber J, Overgaard K, Jarlov A, et al. Bone metabolism in premenopausal women with nontoxic goiter and reduced serum thyrotropin levels. Thyroidology 1994;6:27.

[73] Gurlek A, Gedik O. Effect of endogenous subclinical hyperthyroidism on bone metabolism and bone mineral density in premenopausal women. Thyroid 1999;9:539.

[74] Ugur-Altun B, Altun A, Arikan E, et al. Relationships existing between the serum cytokine levels and bone mineral density in women in the premenopausal period affected by Graves' disease with subclinical hyperthyroidism. Endocr Res 2003;29:389.

[75] Faber J, Jensen I, Petersen L, et al. Normalization of serum thyrotropin by means of radioiodine treatment in subclinical hyperthyroidism: effect on bone loss in postmenopausal women. Clin Endocrinol (Oxf) 1998;48:285.

[76] Foldes J, Tarjan G, Szathmari M, et al. Bone mineral density in patients with endogenous subclinical hyperthyroidism: is this thyroid status a risk factor for osteoporosis? Clin Endocrinol (Oxf) 1993;39:521.

[77] Foldes J, Lakatos P, Zsadanyi J, et al. Decreased serum IGF-I and dehydroepiandrosterone sulphate may be risk factors for the development of reduced bone mass in postmenopausal women with endogenous subclinical hyperthyroidism. Eur J Endocrinol 1997;136:277.

[78] Tauchmanova L, Nuzzo V, Del Puente A, et al. Reduced bone mass detected by bone quantitative ultrasonometry and DEXA in pre- and postmenopausal women with endogenous subclinical hyperthyroidism. Maturitas 2004;48:299.

[79] Lee WY, Oh KW, Rhee EJ, et al. Relationship between subclinical thyroid dysfunction and femoral neck bone mineral density in women. Arch Med Res 2006;37:511.

[80] Mudde A, Houben A, Nieuwenhuijzen Kruseman A. Bone metabolism during anti-thyroid drug treatment of endogenous subclinical hyperthyroidism. Clin Endocrinol (Oxf) 1994;41: 421.

[81] Chen CH, Chen JF, Yang BY, et al. Bone mineral density in women receiving thyroxine suppressive therapy for differentiated thyroid carcinoma. J Formos Med Assoc 2004;103: 442.

[82] De Rosa G, Testa A, Giacomini D, et al. Prospective study of bone loss in pre- and postmenopausal women on L-thyroxine therapy for non-toxic goiter. Clin Endocrinol (Oxf) 1997;47:529.

[83] Diamond T, Nery L, Hales I. A therapeutic dilemma: suppressive doses of thyroxine significantly reduce bone mineral measurements in both premenopausal and postmenopausal women with thyroid carcinoma. J Clin Endocrinol Metab 1991;72:1184.

[84] Franklyn J, Betteridge J, Holder R, et al. Bone mineral density in thyroxine treated females with or without a previous history of thyrotoxicosis. Clin Endocrinol (Oxf) 1994;41:425.

[85] Garton M, Reid I, Loveridge N, et al. Bone mineral density and metabolism in premeno-pausal women taking L-thyroxine replacement therapy. Clin Endocrinol (Oxf) 1994;41:747.

[86] Giannini S, Nobile M, Sartori L, et al. Bone density and mineral metabolism in thyroidec-tomized patients treated with long-term L-thyroxine. Clin Sci (Lond) 1994;87:593.

[87] Gonzalez D, Marutalen C, Correa P, et al. Bone mass in totally thyroidectomized patients: role of calcitonin deficiency and exogenous thyroid treatment. Acta Endocrinol (Copenh) 1991;124:521.

[88] Jodar E, Begona Lopez M, Garcia L, et al. Bone changes in pre- and postmenopausal women with thyroid cancer on levothyroxine therapy: evolution of axial and appendicular bone mass. Osteoporos Int 1998;8:311.

[89] Karner I, Hrgovic Z, Sijanovic S, et al. Bone mineral density changes and bone turnover in thyroid carcinoma patients treated with supraphysiologic doses of thyroxine. Eur J Med Res 2005;10:480.

[90] Khmara IM, Tolkachev Iu V. [Bone tissue mineral density in patients with thyroid gland cancer on levothyroxine natrium therapy]. Klin Med (Mosk) 2005;83:61 [in Russian].

[91] Kung A, Yeung S. Prevention of bone loss induced by thyroxine suppressive therapy in postmenopausal women: the effect of calcium and calcitonin. J Clin Endocrinol Metab 1996;81:1232.

[92] Kung AW, Lorentz T, Tam SC. Thyroxine suppressive therapy decreases bone mineral den-sity in post-menopausal women. Clin Endocrinol (Oxf) 1993;39:535.

[93] Lehmke J, Bogner U, Felsenberg D, et al. Determination of bone mineral density by quan-titative computed tomography and single photon absorptiometry in subclinical hyperthy-roidism: a risk of early osteopaenia in post-menopausal women. Clin Endocrinol (Oxf) 1992;36:511.

[94] Mazokopakis EE, Starakis IK, Papadomanolaki MG, et al. Changes of bone mineral den-sity in pre-menopausal women with differentiated thyroid cancer receiving L-thyroxine sup-pressive therapy. Curr Med Res Opin 2006;22:1369.

[95] McDermott MT, Perloff JJ, Kidd GS. A longitudinal assessment of bone loss in women with levothyroxine-suppressed benign thyroid disease and thyroid cancer. Calcif Tissue Int 1995;56:521.

[96] Muller C, Bayley T, Harrison J, et al. Possible limited bone loss with suppressive thyroxine therapy is unlikely to have clinical relevance. Thyroid 1995;5:81.

[97] Paul T, Kerrigan J, Kelly A, et al. Long-term L-thyroxine therapy is associated with de-creased hip bone density in premenopausal women. JAMA 1988;259:3137.

[98] Piolo G, Pedrazzoni M, Palummeri E, et al. Longitudinal study of bone loss after thyroid-ectomy and suppressive thyroxine therapy in premenopausal women. Acta Endocrinol (Co-penh) 1992;126:238.

[99] Ross D, Neer R, Ridgway E, et al. Subclinical hyperthyroidism and reduced bone density as a possible result of prolonged suppression of the pituitary-thyroid axis with L-thyroxine. Am J Med 1987;82:1167.

[100] Schneider D, Barrett-Connor E, Morton D. Thyroid hormone use and bone mineral den-sity in elderly women: effects of estrogen. JAMA 1994;271:1245.

[101] Stall G, Harris S, Sokoll L, et al. Accelerated bone loss in hypothyroid patients overtreated with L-thyroxine. Ann Intern Med 1990;113:265.

[102] Stepan J, Limanova Z. Biochemical assessment of bone loss in patients on long-term thy-roid hormone treatment. Bone Miner 1992;17:377.

[103] Appetecchia M. Effects on bone mineral density by treatment of benign nodular goiter with mildly suppressive doses of L-thyroxine in a cohort women study. Horm Res 2005;64:293.

[104] Baldini M, Gallazzi M, Orsatti A, et al. Treatment of benign nodular goitre with mildly sup-pressive doses of L-thyroxine: effects on bone mineral density and on nodule size. J Intern Med 2002;251:407.

[105] Bauer M, Fairbanks L, Berghofer A, et al. Bone mineral density during maintenance treatment with supraphysiological doses of levothyroxine in affective disorders: a longitudinal study. J Affect Disord 2004;83:183.

[106] De Rosa G, Testa A, Maussier M, et al. A slightly suppressive dose of L-thyroxine does not affect bone turnover and bone mineral density in pre- and postmenopausal women with nontoxic goitre. Horm Metab Res 1995;27:503.

[107] Florkowski CM, Brownlie BE, Elliot JR, et al. Bone mineral density in patients receiving suppressive doses of thyroxine for thyroid carcinoma. N Z Med J 1993;106:443.

[108] Franklyn J, Betteridge J, Daykin J, et al. Long-term thyroxine treatment and bone mineral density. Lancet 1992;340:9.

[109] Gorres G, Kaim A, Otte A, et al. Bone mineral density in patients receiving suppressive doses of thyroxine for differentiated thyroid carcinoma. Eur J Nucl Med 1996;23:690.

[110] Grant DJ, McMurdo ME, Mole PA, et al. Suppressed TSH levels secondary to thyroxine replacement therapy are not associated with osteoporosis. Clin Endocrinol (Oxf) 1993;39: 529.

[111] Guo C, Weetman A, Eastell R. Longitudinal changes of bone mineral density and bone turnover in postmenopausal women on thyroxine. Clin Endocrinol (Oxf) 1997;46:301.

[112] Hawkins F, Rigopoulou D, Papapietro K, et al. Spinal bone mass after long-term treatment with L-thyroxine in postmenopausal women with thyroid cancer and chronic lymphocytic thyroiditis. Calcif Tissue Int 1994;54:16.

[113] Heijckmann AC, Huijberts MS, Geusens P, et al. Hip bone mineral density, bone turnover and risk of fracture in patients on long-term suppressive L-thyroxine therapy for differentiated thyroid carcinoma. Eur J Endocrinol 2005;153:23.

[114] Larijani B, Gharibdoost F, Pajouhi M, et al. Effects of levothyroxine suppressive therapy on bone mineral density in premenopausal women. J Clin Pharm Ther 2004;29:1.

[115] Marcocci C, Golia F, Bruno-Bossio G, et al. Carefully monitored levothyroxine suppressive therapy is not associated with bone loss in premenopausal women. J Clin Endocrinol Metab 1994;78:818.

[116] Marcocci C, Golia F, Vignali E, et al. Skeletal integrity in men chronically treated with suppressive doses of L-thyroxine. J Bone Miner Metab 1997;12:72.

[117] Nuzzo V, Lupoli G, Esposito Del Puente A, et al. Bone mineral density in premenopausal women receiving levothyroxine suppressive therapy. Gynecol Endocrinol 1998;12:333.

[118] Rosen H, Moses A, Garber J, et al. Randomized trial of pamidronate in patients with thyroid cancer: bone density is not reduced by suppressive doses of thyroxine, but is increased by cyclic intravenous pamidronate. J Clin Endocrinol Metab 1998;83:2324.

[119] Sajjinanont T, Rajchadara S, Sriassawaamorn N, et al. The comparative study of bone mineral density between premenopausal women receiving long term suppressive doses of levothyroxine for well-differentiated thyroid cancer with healthy premenopausal women. J Med Assoc Thai 2005;88(Suppl 3):S71.

[120] Toh S, Brown P. Bone mineral content in hypothyroid male patients with hormone replacement: a 3-year study. J Bone Miner Res 1990;5:463.

[121] Coindre J, David J, Riviere L, et al. Bone loss in hypothyroidism with hormone replacement: a histomorphometric study. Arch Intern Med 1986;146:48.

[122] Meier C, Beat M, Guglielmetti M, et al. Restoration of euthyroidism accelerates bone turnover in patients with subclinical hypothyroidism: a randomized controlled trial. Osteoporos Int 2004;15:209.

[123] Ribot C, Tremollieres F, Pouilles J, et al. Bone mineral density and thyroid hormone therapy. Clin Endocrinol (Oxf) 1990;33:143.

[124] Kung A, Pun K. Bone mineral density in premenopausal women receiving long-term physiological doses of levothyroxine. JAMA 1991;265:2688.

[125] Ross D. Bone density is not reduced during the short-term administration of levothyroxine to postmenopausal women with subclinical hypothyroidism: a randomized, prospective study. Am J Med 1993;95:385.

[126] Hadji P, Hars O, Sturm G, et al. The effect of long-term, non-suppressive levothyroxine treatment on quantitative ultrasonometry of bone in women. Eur J Endocrinol 2000;142: 445.

[127] Hanna F, Pettit R, Ammari F, et al. Effect of replacement doses of thyroxine on bone mineral density. Clin Endocrinol (Oxf) 1998;48:229.

[128] Langdahl B, Loft A, Eriksen E, et al. Bone mass, bone turnover and body composition in former hypothyroid patients receiving replacement therapy. Eur J Endocrinol 1996;134: 702.

[129] Schneider D, Barrett-Connor E, Morton D. Thyroid hormone use and bone mineral density in elderly men. Arch Intern Med 2005;155:1995.

[130] Salerno M, Lettiero T, Esposito-del Puente A, et al. Effect of long-term L-thyroxine treatment on bone mineral density in young adults with congenital hypothyroidism. Eur J Endocrinol 2004;151:689.

[131] Faber J, Galloe A. Changes in bone mass during prolonged subclinical hyperthyroidism due to L-thyroxine treatment: a meta-analysis. Eur J Endocrinol 1994;130:350.

[132] Uzzan B, Campos J, Cucherat M, et al. Effects on bone mass of long term treatment with thyroid hormones: a meta-analysis. J Clin Endocrinol Metab 1996;81:4278.

[133] Ross D. Hyperthyroidism, thyroid hormone therapy, and bone. Thyroid 1994;4:319.

[134] Quan ML, Pasieka JL, Rorstad O. Bone mineral density in well-differentiated thyroid cancer patients treated with suppressive thyroxine: a systematic overview of the literature. J Surg Oncol 2002;79:62.

[135] Heemstra KA, Hamdy NA, Romijn JA, et al. The effects of thyrotropin-suppressive therapy on bone metabolism in patients with well-differentiated thyroid carcinoma. Thyroid 2006;16:583.

[136] Schneider R, Reiners C. The effect of levothyroxine therapy on bone mineral density: a systematic review of the literature. Exp Clin Endocrinol Diabetes 2003;111:455.

[137] Amato G, Mazziotti G, Sorvillo F, et al. High serum osteoprotegerin levels in patients with hyperthyroidism: effect of medical treatment. Bone 2004;35:785.

[138] Cooper D, Kaplan M, Ridgway E, et al. Alkaline phosphatase isoenzyme patterns in hyperthyroidism. Ann Intern Med 1979;90:164.

[139] MacLeod J, McHardy K, Harvey R, et al. The early effects of radioiodine therapy for hyperthyroidism on biochemical indices of bone turnover. Clin Endocrinol (Oxf) 1993; 38:49.

[140] Mochizuki Y, Banba N, Hattori Y, et al. Correlation between serum osteoprotegerin and biomarkers of bone metabolism during anti-thyroid treatment in patients with Graves' disease. Horm Res 2006;66:236.

[141] Mosekilde L, Christensen M, Melsen F, et al. Effect of antithyroid treatment on calcium-phosphorus metabolism in hyperthyroidism. I: chemical quantities in serum and urine. Acta Endocrinol (Copenh) 1978;87:743.

[142] Mosekilde L, Melsen F, Bagger J, et al. Bone changes in hyperthyroidism: interrelationships between bone morphometry, thyroid function and calcium-phosphorus metabolism. Acta Endocrinol (Copenh) 1977;85:515.

[143] Nagasaka S, Sugimoto H, Nakamura T, et al. Antithyroid therapy improves bony manifestations and bone metabolic markers in patients with Graves' thyrotoxicosis. Clin Endocrinol (Oxf) 1997;47:215.

[144] Kumeda Y, Inaba M, Tahara H, et al. Persistent increase in bone turnover in Graves' patients with subclinical hyperthyroidism. J Clin Endocrinol Metab 2000;85:4157.

[145] Loviselli A, Rizzolo E, Mastinu R, et al. High serum circulating telopeptide type I in multinodular goiter. Horm Metab Res 2003;35:377.

[146] Kisakol G, Kaya A, Gonen S, et al. Bone and calcium metabolism in subclinical autoimmune hyperthyroidism and hypothyroidism. Endocr J 2003;50:657.

[147] Sekeroglu MR, Altun ZB, Algun E, et al. Serum cytokines and bone metabolism in patients with thyroid dysfunction. Adv Ther 2006;23:475.

[148] Harvey R, McHardy K, Reid D, et al. Measurement of bone collagen degradation in hyperthyroidism and during thyroxine replacement therapy using pyridinium cross-links as specific urinary markers. J Clin Endocrinol Metab 1991;72:1189.
[149] Mikosch P, Jauk B, Gallowitsch H, et al. Suppressive levothyroxine therapy has no significant influence on bone degradation in women with thyroid carcinoma: a comparison with other disorders affecting bone metabolism. Thyroid 2001;11:257.
[150] Mikosch P, Obermayer-Pietsch B, Jost R, et al. Bone metabolism in patients with differentiated thyroid carcinoma receiving suppressive levothyroxine treatment. Thyroid 2003;13:347.
[151] Ross D, Ardisson L, Nussbaum S, et al. Serum osteocalcin in patients taking L-thyroxine who have subclinical hyperthyroidism. J Clin Endocrinol Metab 1991;72:507.
[152] Schneider P, Berger P, Kruse K, et al. Effect of calcitonin deficiency on bone density and bone turnover in totally thyroidectomized patients. J Endocrinol Invest 1991;14:935.
[153] Guang-Da X, Hui-Ling S, Zhi-Song C, et al. Alteration of plasma concentrations of OPG before and after levothyroxine replacement therapy in hypothyroid patients. J Endocrinol Invest 2005;28:965.
[154] Guang-da X, Hui-ling S, Zhi-song C, et al. Changes in plasma concentrations of osteoprotegerin before and after levothyroxine replacement therapy in hypothyroid patients. J Clin Endocrinol Metab 2005;90:5765.
[155] Hundahl SA, Fleming ID, Fremgen AM, et al. A National Cancer Data Base report on 53,856 cases of thyroid carcinoma treated in the U.S., 1985–1995 [see comments]. Cancer 1998;83:2638.
[156] Pacini F, Schlumberger M, Dralle H, et al. European consensus for the management of patients with differentiated thyroid carcinoma of the follicular epithelium. Eur J Endocrinol 2006;154:787.
[157] Conacci-Sorrell M, Zhurinsky J, Ben-Ze'ev A. The cadherin-catenin adhesion system in signaling and cancer. J Clin Invest 2002;109:987.
[158] Lipton A. Pathophysiology of bone metastases: how this knowledge may lead to therapeutic intervention. J Support Oncol 2004;2:205.
[159] Aldred MA, Ginn-Pease ME, Morrison CD, et al. Caveolin-1 and caveolin-2,together with three bone morphogenetic protein-related genes, may encode novel tumor suppressors down-regulated in sporadic follicular thyroid carcinogenesis. Cancer Res 2003;63:2864.
[160] Aldred MA, Huang Y, Liyanarachchi S, et al. Papillary and follicular thyroid carcinomas show distinctly different microarray expression profiles and can be distinguished by a minimum of five genes. J Clin Oncol 2004;22:3531.
[161] Owens LV, Xu L, Dent GA, et al. Focal adhesion kinase as a marker of invasive potential in differentiated human thyroid cancer. Ann Surg Oncol 1996;3:100.
[162] Bellahcene A, Albert V, Pollina L, et al. Ectopic expression of bone sialoprotein in human thyroid cancer. Thyroid 1998;8:637.
[163] Chen KT, Lin JD, Chao TC, et al. Identifying differentially expressed genes associated with metastasis of follicular thyroid cancer by cDNA expression array. Thyroid 2001;11:41.
[164] Pecheur I, Peyruchaud O, Serre CM, et al. Integrin alpha(v)beta3 expression confers on tumor cells a greater propensity to metastasize to bone. FASEB J 2002;16:1266.
[165] Bernier MO, Leenhardt L, Hoang C, et al. Survival and therapeutic modalities in patients with bone metastases of differentiated thyroid carcinomas. J Clin Endocrinol Metab 2001;86:1568.
[166] Marcocci C, Pacini F, Elisei R, et al. Clinical and biologic behavior of bone metastases from differentiated thyroid carcinoma. Surgery 1989;106:960.
[167] Zettinig G, Fueger BJ, Passler C, et al. Long-term follow-up of patients with bone metastases from differentiated thyroid carcinoma: surgery or conventional therapy? Clin Endocrinol (Oxf) 2002;56:377.
[168] Orr FW, Lee J, Duivenvoorden WC, et al. Pathophysiologic interactions in skeletal metastasis. Cancer 2000;88:2912.

[169] Roodman GD. Mechanisms of bone metastasis. N Engl J Med 2004;350:1655.
[170] Castillo LA, Yeh SD, Leeper RD, et al. Bone scans in bone metastases from functioning thyroid carcinoma. Clin Nucl Med 1980;5:200.
[171] Guise TA, Mundy GR. Cancer and bone. Endocr Rev 1998;19:18.
[172] Matsumoto T, Abe M. Bone destruction in multiple myeloma. Ann N Y Acad Sci 2006; 1068:319.
[173] Bodine PV, Komm BS. Wnt signaling and osteoblastogenesis. Rev Endocr Metab Disord 2006;7:33–9.
[174] Mikosch P, Igerc I, Kudlacek S, et al. Receptor activator of nuclear factor kappaB ligand and osteoprotegerin in men with thyroid cancer. Eur J Clin Invest 2006;36:566.
[175] Brage ME, Simon MA. Evaluation, prognosis, and medical treatment considerations of metastatic bone tumors. Orthopedics 1992;15:589.
[176] Iwata M, Kasagi K, Misaki T, et al. Comparison of whole-body 18F-FDG PET, 99mTc-MIBI SPET, and post-therapeutic 131I-Na scintigraphy in the detection of metastatic thyroid cancer. Eur J Nucl Med Mol Imaging 2004;31:491.
[177] Schlumberger M, Challeton C, De Vathaire F, et al. Radioactive iodine treatment and external radiotherapy for lung and bone metastases from thyroid carcinoma. J Nucl Med 1996;37:598.
[178] Durante C, Haddy N, Baudin E, et al. Long-term outcome of 444 patients with distant metastases from papillary and follicular thyroid carcinoma: benefits and limits of radioiodine therapy. J Clin Endocrinol Metab 2006;91:2892.
[179] Vitale G, Fonderico F, Martignetti A, et al. Pamidronate improves the quality of life and induces clinical remission of bone metastases in patients with thyroid cancer. Br J Cancer 2001;84:1586.
[180] Rosen LS, Gordon DH, Dugan W Jr, et al. Zoledronic acid is superior to pamidronate for the treatment of bone metastases in breast carcinoma patients with at least one osteolytic lesion. Cancer 2004;100:36.
[181] Wartofsky L, Van Norstrand D, editors. Thyroid cancer: a comprehensive guide to clinical management. 2nd edition. Totowa (NJ): Humana Press; 2006.
[182] Bilezikian JP. Osteonecrosis of the jaw: do bisphosphonates pose a risk? N Engl J Med 2006;355:2278.
[183] Woo SB, Hellstein JW, Kalmar JR. Narrative [corrected] review: bisphosphonates and osteonecrosis of the jaws. Ann Intern Med 2006;144:753.
[184] Frassica DA. General principles of external beam radiation therapy for skeletal metastases. Clinical Orthopaedics & Related Research 2003;415:S158–64.
[185] Monchik JM, Donatini G, Iannuccilli J, et al. Radiofrequency ablation and percutaneous ethanol injection treatment for recurrent local and distant well-differentiated thyroid carcinoma. Ann Surg 2006;244:296.
[186] Tsang RW, Brierley JD, Simpson WJ, et al. The effects of surgery, radioiodine, and external radiation therapy on the clinical outcome of patients with differentiated thyroid carcinoma. Cancer 1998;82:375.
[187] Brierley JD, Tsang RW. External-beam radiation therapy in the treatment of differentiated thyroid cancer. Semin Surg Oncol 1999;16:42.
[188] Robinson D, Yassin M, Nevo Z. Cryotherapy of musculoskeletal tumors: from basic science to clinical results. Technol Cancer Res Treat 2004;3:371.

ENDOCRINOLOGY
AND METABOLISM
CLINICS
OF NORTH AMERICA

ELSEVIER
SAUNDERS

Endocrinol Metab Clin N Am
36 (2007) 707–735

Thyroid Nodules: Clinical Importance, Assessment, and Treatment

Hossein Gharib, MD, MACP, MACE[a,b,*],
Enrico Papini, MD, FACE[c]

[a]Mayo Clinic College of Medicine, Rochester, MN 55905, USA
[b]Division of Endocrinology, Diabetes, Metabolism, and Nutrition, Mayo Clinic,
200 First Street SW, Rochester, MN 55905, USA
[c]Department of Endocrine & Metabolic Diseases, Regina Apostolorum Hospital,
Albano Laziale, Italy 00041

Since the previous publication on thyroid nodule diagnosis and treatment in Endocrinology and Metabolism Clinics of North America a decade ago [1], many advances have occurred in the diagnosis and management of thyroid nodular disease. The introduction of new thyroid-stimulating hormone (TSH) assays, widespread application of fine-needle aspiration (FNA) biopsy, and the increasing availability and use of high-resolution ultrasonography (US) have facilitated, modified, and improved the management of thyroid nodules.

Although these new techniques have vastly improved patient care, controversy continues in some areas, including the evaluation of thyroid micronodules discovered incidentally on US, the use of US-guided FNA, management of nodules with cytologically suspicious FNA results, thyroxine (T4) therapy for benign nodules, and routine serum calcitonin measurement in patients presenting with a nodular thyroid. This article reviews many of these issues, focusing on advances and controversies. Recent practice management guidelines published by the American Association of Clinical Endocrinologists in collaboration with Associazione Medici Endocrinologi [2] and by the American Thyroid Association [3] are the main sources of the evidence-based recommendations. Published data are categorized using recent criteria suggested for grading, and the level of evidence is noted for all references in the bibliography [4].

* Corresponding author. Division of Endocrinology, Diabetes, Metabolism, and Nutrition, Mayo Clinic, 200 First Street SW, Rochester, MN 55905, USA.
E-mail address: hossein.gharib@mayo.edu (H. Gharib).

Clinical importance

Thyroid nodules are common. They are discovered by palpation in 3% to 7% [5,6], by US in 20% to 76% in the general population [7,8], and by autopsy in approximately 50% [9,10]. Prevalence increases linearly with age, exposure to ionizing radiation, and iodine deficiency. Thyroid nodules are more common in women than in men. In the Framingham population study, follow-up indicated new nodules in 1.3% in 15 years, calculated as an annual incidence of 100 cases per 100,000 persons per year [6]. With an incidence of 0.1% per year, an estimated 300,000 new nodules will be identified in the United States in 2007, with a 10% lifetime probability of a nodule developing [7,10,11]. The clinical significance of these data cannot be overstated.

The clinical importance of thyroid nodules, besides the infrequent local compressive symptoms or thyroid dysfunction, is primarily the possibility of thyroid cancer, which occurs in about 5% of all thyroid nodules regardless of their size [7,11,12]. Because of the high prevalence of nodular thyroid disease, it is not economically feasible or clinically necessary to perform a complete structural and functional assessment for all or even most thyroid nodules. Therefore, it is essential to develop and follow a systematic, cost-effective strategy for diagnosis and treatment of thyroid nodules and to avoid unnecessary, potentially harmful surgery.

Diagnosis

History and physical examination

Clinical evaluation begins with a detailed patient history and careful thyroid palpation. Most patients present with an asymptomatic mass discovered by a physician on routine neck palpation or by the patient during self-examination. Many disorders, benign and malignant, can cause thyroid nodules (Box 1) [5,10]. Newly diagnosed thyroid nodules should be evaluated primarily to rule out thyroid malignancy [5,7,10]. An inquiry should be made about family history of benign or malignant thyroid disease. Thyroid cancer (medullary thyroid carcinoma [MTC] or papillary thyroid carcinoma [PTC]), multiple endocrine neoplasia type 2, familial polyposis coli, Cowden disease, and Gardner syndrome are rare disorders but should be considered [13]. Presentation of nodules during childhood and adolescence should induce caution; the malignancy rate for nodules in young persons is 2-fold higher than in adult patients. Previous disease or treatments concerning the neck (history of childhood head/neck radiation), rapidity of onset, and rate of growth of the neck swelling should be documented. Appearance of a new mass, slow but progressive nodule growth, a firm or hard solitary or dominant nodule, or the presence of adjacent cervical adenopathy is suspicious for malignancy and should prompt further evaluation

---

Box 1. Common causes of thyroid nodules

Benign
    Colloid nodule
    Hashimoto thyroiditis
    Simple or hemorrhagic cyst
    Follicular adenoma
    Subacute thyroiditis
Malignant
    Primary
        Follicular cell-derived carcinoma:
            PTC, follicular thyroid carcinoma, anaplastic thyroid
                carcinoma
        C-cell–derived carcinoma:
            MTC
        Thyroid lymphoma
    Secondary
        Metastatic carcinoma

[5,10,11]. Box 2 highlights features associated with increased risk of cancer in thyroid nodules.

Ultrasonography

Brightness-mode US is the most sensitive test to detect lesions in the thyroid. It accurately measures the dimensions, identifies the structure, and evaluates diffuse changes in the thyroid parenchyma. US is noninvasive, relatively inexpensive, and can identify nodules not apparent on physical examination, isotope scanning, or other imaging techniques (Fig. 1) [14]. US

Box 2. Increased risk of malignancy in thyroid nodule

- History of childhood head/neck irradiation
- Family history of PTC, MTC, or multiple endocrine neoplasia type 2 (MEN2)
- Age <20 or >70 years
- Male sex
- Enlarging nodule
- Abnormal cervical adenopathy
- Fixed nodule
- Vocal cord paralysis

should not be a substitute for a physical examination or be performed on an otherwise normal thyroid gland or as a screening test in the general population. Because of the high prevalence of small, clinically inapparent thyroid nodules and the minimal aggressiveness of most thyroid cancers, US should be used as a screening test only if well-known risk factors are present (Box 3).

Sonographic examination should be ordered for all patients who have a history of familial thyroid cancer, multiple endocrine neoplasia type 2, or childhood head/neck irradiation, even if the thyroid appears normal by palpation [2,14]. The finding of adenopathy suspicious for malignancy in the anterior or lateral neck compartments warrants US examination of the lymph nodes and thyroid because of the risk of nodal metastasis from an otherwise unrecognized papillary microcarcinoma.

It is recommended that all patients who have a nodular thyroid, with a palpable solitary nodule or a multinodular goiter (MNG), be evaluated by US [2,3]. US examination should search for additional, unsuspected nodules; measure nodule number and size; record sonographic appearances to assess risk of malignancy; and select lesions that require US-guided FNA (US-FNA) biopsy [7,14]. A recent report showed that using thyroid US can result in an improved and important management change for many patients who have "presumed" thyroid nodules: 44% of patients had no nodule or had unsuspected but clinically important nodules that warranted further evaluation [15].

Ultrasound-guided fine-needle aspiration

In recent years, US-FNA has become increasingly popular because of increased precision and the ability to guide the biopsy needle to the desired location in real time (Fig. 2) [14]. The cardinal indications for US-FNA, listed in Box 4, include nondiagnostic results by palpation-guided FNA, impalpable or small (<1.5 cm) nodules, a nodule with solid and cystic

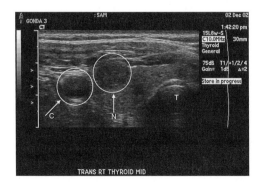

Fig. 1. Transverse ultrasonographic view of the right thyroid lobe showing a 1.2-cm hypoechoic nodule (N), which was benign by fine-needle aspiration biopsy. C, carotid artery; T, trachea.

Box 3. Thyroid ultrasonographic examination

Not indicated
- As screening test in general population
- In patient who has low risk for thyroid cancer and normal thyroid on palpation

Indicated
- In a patient who has a palpable nodule
- In a patient who has history of neck irradiation
- In a patient who has family history of MTC, MEN2, or PTC
- If unexplained cervical adenopathy is present

---

components, and abnormal cervical adenopathy. Recent studies show that US-FNA decreases nondiagnostic rates from 15% to between 3.5% and 7% [16,17].

Thyroid micronodules that are not clinically apparent (14%–24% of those with a diameter >10 mm) are detected by US in about half (27%–72%) of the women evaluated [5,7,10,11]. The prevalence of cancer ranges from 5.4% to 7.7% in studies regarding the cytologic evaluation of nonpalpable thyroid lesions and seems to be similar to that reported for palpable lesions (5.0%–6.5%) [18,19]. Few clinical criteria for malignancy exist for most nonpalpable lesions, and patients who have palpable thyroid nodules seldom present with history or physical examination findings suggestive of thyroid carcinoma [20]. Therefore, to avoid the inappropriate use of US-FNA, it is essential to determine which thyroid lesions are at risk of malignancy on the basis of US characteristics.

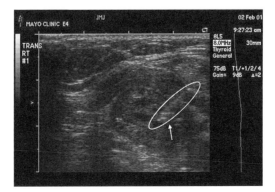

Fig. 2. A 50-year-old woman had multiple small thyroid nodules. US showed the largest nodule to be a complex, predominantly cystic mass in the right lobe measuring 2.6 × 1.7 cm. The nodule was benign by US-FNA. Arrow illustrates needle tip (*circled*) accurately placed in the nodule.

Box 4. Indications for ultrasonography fine-needle aspiration

- Palpation-guided FNA nondiagnostic
- Complex (solid/cystic) nodule
- Palpable small nodule (<1.5 cm)
- Impalpable incidentaloma
- Abnormal cervical nodes
- Nodule with suspicious US features

Ultrasound prediction of malignancy

Although no single US characteristic can unequivocally distinguish benign and malignant nodules, several US features and, more importantly, a combination of features, have been evaluated as predictors of malignancy [18,21].

Solitary versus multiple nodules. The risk of cancer is not significantly higher for solitary nodules than for glands with several nodules, whether the nodules are palpable or impalpable [18–25]. In glands with multiple nodules, selection for FNA should be based on US features rather than on size or clinically "dominant" nodules [18,23,25]. Although criteria for selection of 1 or more nodules for US-FNA is a matter of debate, Table 1 summarizes recent recommendations from three different professional societies (Fig. 3) [2,3,25].

Size. Nodule size is not predictive of malignancy. Cancer is not less frequent in small nodules (diameter <10 mm); thus, an arbitrary diameter cutoff of 10 or 15 mm for cancer risk should be discouraged in clinical practice [2,18]. The lower size limit of a micronodule that should be chosen for biopsy is also controversial. US-FNA should be considered for nodules smaller

Table 1
Biopsy recommendations for multiple nodules

Guidelines	Recommendation
ACE [2]	In multinodular thyroid glands, the cytologic sampling should be focused on lesions characterized by suspicious US features rather than on larger nodules.
ATA [3]	If two or more thyroid nodules >1–1.5 cm are present, those who have a suspicious US appearance should be aspirated preferentially.
SRU [25]	In patients who have multiple discreet nodules, the selection should be based primarily on US characteristics rather than nodule size.

Abbreviations: AACE, American Association of Clinical Endocrinologists; ATA, American Thyroid Association; SRU, Society of Radiologists in Ultrasound; US, ultrasonographic.

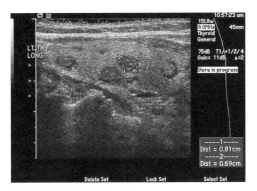

Fig. 3. Sagittal ultrasonographic view of the left thyroid lobe in a 71-year-old woman with a small, nontender, irregular thyroid on palpation. US showed multiple benign-appearing, subcentimeter nodules (1 and 2) bilaterally.

than 10 mm if associated with punctate microcalcifications, if a history of neck irradiation is present, or in a young patient (see Box 2). Because some microcarcinomas can have aggressive clinical behavior, early diagnosis by FNA of a small (<10 mm) PTC followed by immediate thyroidectomy may not only decrease morbidity but also be curative [18,26].

Ultrasound features and color Doppler findings. The specificity of US features for diagnosing cancer varies from 85% to 95% for microcalcifications (small intranodular punctate hyperechoic spots, with scanty or no posterior acoustic shadowing) (Fig. 4), from 83% to 85% for irregular or indistinct nodule margins, and about 81% for chaotic appearance of intranodular vascular images [18,21,25]. The predictive value of these US features for cancer is in part diminished by their low sensitivity (29.0%–59.2%, 55.1%–77.5%, and 74.2%, respectively), and no US sign by itself can reliably predict malignancy. The association of hypoechoic appearance of the nodule with at least one or more US features suggestive of malignancy effectively indicates a subset of nonpalpable thyroid nodules at high risk for malignancy [18,21]. The presence of at least two suspicious sonographic criteria reliably identifies 85% to 93% of thyroid gland neoplastic lesions, thus decreasing the number of US-FNA procedures to about one third of the nonpalpable nodules (Table 2) [18,23,27].

Color Doppler US evaluates nodule vascularity. The assumption is that hypervascularity with chaotic arrangement of blood vessels favors malignancy, whereas peripheral flow indicates a benign nodule. Reports have failed to consistently identify cancer on color Doppler alone (Fig. 5) [25].

Extracapsular growth. Hypoechoic nodules with irregular borders, extension beyond the thyroid capsule, invasion into perithyroid muscles, and

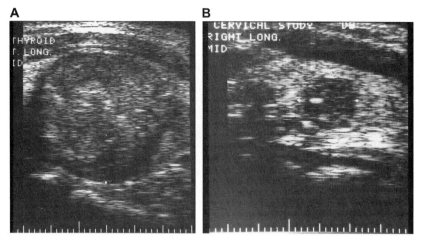

Fig. 4. Calcifications in thyroid nodules in two patients. (*A*) Nodule with a hypoechoic pattern and multiple fine calcifications. FNA biopsy showed papillary thyroid carcinoma, which was confirmed at surgery. (*B*) Transverse view of the right thyroid lobe showing a solid nodule with scattered calcifications suggestive of cancer. FNA biopsy results suggested medullary thyroid carcinoma, which was confirmed at thyroidectomy.

infiltration of the recurrent laryngeal nerve are sonographic features that warrant cytologic evaluation [23,27,28].

Complex or cystic lesions. Complex thyroid nodules have solid and cystic components, often with a dominant cystic part, and are frequently benign. These lesions are common, frequently smaller than 3 or 4 cm in diameter, and asymptomatic. US-FNA is necessary to document the morphology because some PTCs may be cystic (Fig. 6) [25,28].

Table 2
Value of ultrasonography features predicting thyroid malignancy

US feature	Sensitivity, %	Specificity, %	Positive predictive value, %	Negative predictive value, %	Relative risk
Microcalcifications	26.1–59.1	85.8–95.0	24.3–70.7	41.8–94.2	4.97
Hypoechogenicity	26.5–87.1	43.4–94.3	11.4–68.4	73.5–93.8	1.92
Irregular margins or no halo	17.4–77.5	38.9–85.0	9.3–60.0	38.9–97.8	16.83
Solid	69.0–75.0	52.5–55.9	15.6–27.0	88.0–92.1	4.2[a]
Intranodule vascularity	54.3–74.2	78.6–80.8	24.0–41.9	85.7–97.4	14.29
More tall than wide	32.7	92.5	66.7	74.8	10.5[a]

Abbreviation: US, ultrasonography.
[a] Unpublished data from a series of 400 patients undergoing surgery for thyroid nodular disease. Regina Apostolorum Hospital, Albano, Rome. *Courtesy of* Papini E and Guglielmi R.
Modified from Frates MC, Benson CB, Charboneau JW, et al. Society of Radiologists in Ultrasound. Management of thyroid nodules detected at US: Society of Radiologists in Ultrasound consensus conference statement. Radiology 2005;237:795; with permission.

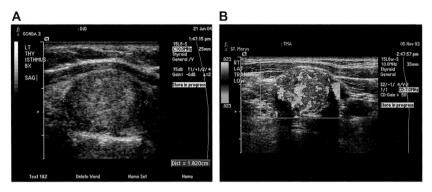

Fig. 5. US images of a left lobe thyroid nodule. (*A*) The 1.7 × 1.4-cm solid left lobe thyroid nodule was hypoechoic. (*B*) Color Doppler flow imaging shows hypervascularity. FNA biopsy showed papillary thyroid carcinoma, which was confirmed at surgery.

Nodule shape. A rounded appearance or a "more tall (anteroposterior) than wide (transverse)" shape of the nodule and a "marked hypoechogenicity" of a solid lesion (hypoechoic even compared with the cervical muscles) are newly described US patterns suggestive of malignancy [29].

Suspicious cervical adenopathy. Enlarged cervical lymph nodes that have a rounded appearance by US, no hilus, cystic changes, microcalcifications, or chaotic hypervascularity have a high probability for malignancy. These nodes and any coexistent, especially ipsilateral, thyroid nodules, whatever their size, always warrant US-FNA biopsy [25,26,28].

Other imaging techniques

MRI and CT are not recommended for routine use because they are costly and rarely diagnostic for malignancy in nodular thyroid disease.

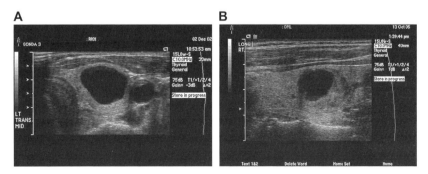

Fig. 6. Transverse US images of two mostly cystic thyroid nodules. The similarity between the cysts mandates US-FNA biopsy to accurately distinguish a benign (*A*) from a malignant (*B*) nodule.

MRI and CT are of value to assess size, substernal extension, and positional relationship of the goiter to surrounding structures (Fig. 7). Caution should be used with CT contrast medium that contains iodine because it decreases subsequent iodine 131 (^{131}I) uptake. Positron emission tomography with [^{18}F] fluorodeoxyglucose may add functional information to anatomic visualization provided by US [30]. The high cost of these procedures makes them impractical for routine clinical assessment of thyroid nodules.

Fine-needle aspiration biopsy

Thyroid FNA biopsy is the most accurate test for determining malignancy and is an integral part of thyroid nodule evaluation [2,31–42].

Palpation-guided fine-needle aspiration
Detailed descriptions of the palpation-guided FNA procedure, its problems, and progress to date have been published elsewhere [31–33,36–40,42].

Ultrasound-guided fine-needle aspiration
Commercially available US machines equipped with 7.5- to 10.0-MHz transducers give a clear, concise, and continuous visualization of the thyroid gland and permit real-time visualization of the needle tip during the FNA procedure to ensure accurate sampling of the desired area (see Fig. 2). The small-sized transducers currently in use are especially convenient for US-FNA. After the biopsy sites are identified, the needle is inserted through a steering device (US-guided FNA) or just above the center of the

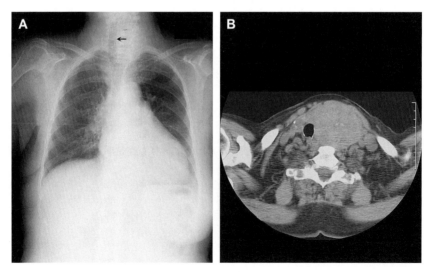

Fig. 7. Images of a large, asymmetric multinodular goiter. (*A*) Chest radiography shows marked tracheal deviation to the right (*arrow*). (*B*) Chest CT confirmed the presence of a large substernal goiter on the left to the level of tracheal bifurcation.

transducer (US-assisted FNA). Because of the direct visualization of the needle, accidental damage to vital neck structures, such as the trachea, carotid artery, jugular vein, or laryngeal nerve, is easily avoided [43]. The needle should be directed to the peripheral rather than the central part of the nodule to avoid cystic degenerative areas in the nodule center, whereas in pure cysts, the center of the lesion should be reached first to completely drain the fluid.

Cystic fluid should be submitted to the laboratory for cytologic analysis. Most colloid fluids are clear-yellow; watery, clear-colorless fluid is likely of parathyroid origin and should have parathyroid hormone measurement. Hemorrhagic fluid carries a higher risk of malignancy. In mixed or mostly fluid complex lesions, the needle should be directed to the root of hubs or pedicles growing into the cystic lumen (the inner area of the pedicle facing the lumen usually contains necrotic debris and cells with degenerative changes). After complete drainage of the fluid, the solid areas and the peripheral borders of the lesion should be carefully sampled.

Cytologic diagnosis

FNA results are categorized as diagnostic (satisfactory) or nondiagnostic (unsatisfactory). The specimen is "diagnostic," "adequate," or "satisfactory" if it contains no less than six groups of well-preserved thyroid epithelial cells consisting of at least 10 cells in each group. Nondiagnostic or unsatisfactory smears with an inadequate number of cells result from acellular cystic fluid, bloody smears, or poor techniques in preparing slides [32,34]. Benign (negative) cytology, the most common finding, is indicative of a colloid nodule, macrofollicular adenoma, lymphocytic thyroiditis, granulomatous thyroiditis, or benign cyst [32]. The most common benign diagnosis is "colloid nodule," which may come from a normal thyroid gland, a benign nodule, an MNG, or a macrofollicular adenoma (Fig. 8).

Malignant (positive) results are reliably identified by an experienced cytopathologist; the cytopathologist's expertise in thyroid cytology is crucial in ensuring proper interpretation of smears [31,33,37]. PTC is the most common malignancy; aspirates are characterized by increased cellularity, tumor cells arranged in sheets and papillary cell groups, and typical nuclear abnormalities, which include intranuclear holes and grooves. Other malignant lesions include MTC, anaplastic carcinoma, and high-grade metastatic cancers [33]. Suspicious (indeterminate) specimens are those for which a clear cytologic diagnosis cannot be made [31,33,35] and include follicular neoplasms, Hürthle cell neoplasms, atypical PTC, or lymphoma. Follicular neoplasms are the most common and are hypercellular with microfollicular arrangement and decreased or absent colloid. Hürthle cell neoplasm is diagnosed if the aspirate contains almost exclusively Hürthle cells, usually with absent or scanty colloid lacking a lymphoid cell population, similar to what is usually found in Hashimoto thyroiditis. Nondiagnostic (unsatisfactory)

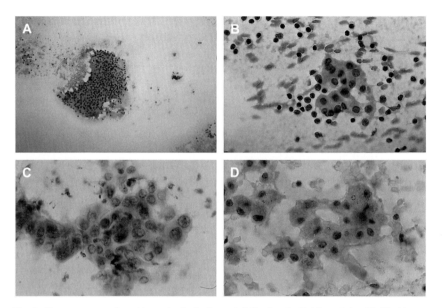

Fig. 8. Four common thyroid cytologic findings. (*A*) Benign (colloid) nodule. (*B*) Hashimoto thyroiditis. (*C*) Papillary thyroid carcinoma. (*D*) Unsatisfactory (nondiagnostic) smear.

aspirates have few or no epithelial cells for proper cytodiagnosis and account for up to 20% of all specimens [36,44,45]. The criteria for judging aspirates as inadequate are somewhat arbitrary and are influenced by the standards of a given laboratory, the nature of the cystic nodule, and the expertise of the cytopathologist.

Overall, 70% of FNA specimens are benign, 5% malignant, 10% suspicious, and 15% unsatisfactory [2,31–33,37]. The final FNA report is critical in dictating whether the patient's management should be medical or surgical. According to recent reviews and reports, FNA has improved patient selection for thyroidectomy, such that cancer yield at surgery has increased from 15% before the use of FNA to 50% with FNA use [39,46]. The sensitivity and specificity of FNA in experienced hands are excellent (Table 3).

A major concern with FNA is the possibility of a false-negative result (ie, a missed malignancy) [37,39]. Although the false-negative rate ranges from 1% to 11%, it is less than 2% in most clinics with adequate FNA experience. Box 5 illustrates some suggestions for minimizing false-negative results.

Biopsy often causes mild temporary pain and is occasionally associated with a minor hematoma. No serious adverse effects and no seeding of tumor cells in the needle track have been reported [37,42]. The consensus is that FNA is a safe, useful, and cost-effective procedure [2,3,37,39].

Some clinicians have debated whether routine rebiopsy is necessary after benign cytologic results [2,47]. For physicians or clinics just beginning to perform FNA, routine rebiopsy may provide reassurance with the procedure

Table 3
Summary characteristics for thyroid fine-needle aspiration: results of literature survey

Feature	Mean	Range	Definition
Sensitivity, %	83	65–98	Likelihood that patient who has disease has positive test results
Specificity, %	92	72–100	Likelihood that patient without disease has negative test results
Positive predictive value, %	75	50–96	Fraction of patients who have positive test who have disease
False-negative rate, %	5	1–11	FNA negative; histology positive for cancer
False-positive rate, %	5	0–7	FNA positive; histology negative for cancer

Abbreviation: FNA, fine-needle aspiration.

From AACE/AME Task Force on Thyroid Nodules. American Association of Clinical Endocrinologists and Associazione Medici Endocrinologi medical guidelines for clinical practice for the diagnosis and management of thyroid nodules. Endocr Pract 2006;12(1):63102; with permission.

and decrease false-negative rates; however, we believe that successive FNA biopsies do not change nodule management and suggest rebiopsy only of an enlarging nodule, a recurrent cyst, a large (>4–5 cm) nodule, or demonstrated lack of shrinkage on T4 therapy (Box 6) [2,39].

Thyroglobulin in fine-needle aspiration of cervical lymph nodes

An important recent advance in thyroid cancer practice is the demonstration that thyroglobulin (Tg) can be measured in lymph node or nodule aspirates (FNA-Tg) [48]. The appearance of cervical adenopathy in patients who have thyroid cancer requires diagnostic US-FNA for confirmation of metastasis and appropriate management.

Cytologic examination and measurement of Tg can be performed on the same specimen. To measure Tg, the needle is rinsed with 1 mL of normal saline solution immediately after FNA biopsy, and Tg levels are measured on the needle washout by immunoradiometric or chemiluminescence assays. The procedure does not require an additional puncture (washout is

---

Box 5. Ways to minimize false-negative results

- Follow-up cytologically benign nodules
- Aspirate multiple nodule sites
- Aspirate multiple nodules in MNG
- Submit cyst fluid for examination
- Review slides with experienced cytopathologist

From AACE/AME Task Force on Thyroid Nodules. American Association of Clinical Endocrinologists and Associazione Medici Endocrinologi medical guidelines for clinical practice for the diagnosis and management of thyroid nodules. Endocr Pract 2006;12(1):63–102; with permission.

Box 6. Indications for repeat biopsy

- Follow-up of benign nodule
- Enlarging nodule
- Recurrent cyst
- Nodule >4 cm
- Initial FNA nondiagnostic
- No nodule shrinkage after T4 therapy

From AACE/AME Task Force on Thyroid Nodules. American Association of Clinical Endocrinologists and Associazione Medici Endocrinologi medical guidelines for clinical practice for the diagnosis and management of thyroid nodules. Endocr Pract 2006;12:63–102; with permission.

---

performed after smear preparation), requires little extra time, and is easy to do. In one report [48], FNA-Tg levels were markedly elevated in metastatic lymph nodes in patients awaiting thyroidectomy and in patients postthyroidectomy. FNA-Tg sensitivity, evaluated through histologic examination, was 84.0%, and the combination of cytology plus FNA-Tg increased FNA sensitivity from 76% to 92.0% [48]. This test is attractive because the clinical performance of FNA-Tg is unaffected by the presence of Tg antibodies in the serum [49].

Immunohistochemical markers

Several molecular markers and assays have shown promise in clarifying suspicious FNA results. For example, HBME-1 is a monoclonal antibody that reportedly stains papillary cancer positively but does not stain benign follicular tumors [46,50]. In addition, galectin-3, which acts as a cell-death suppressor, is reported to distinguish benign from malignant thyroid follicular tumors [51]. Other markers, such as thyroid peroxidase and telomerase, have been reported to identify or exclude malignancy with variable success [52]. Despite most studies showing markers to have high sensitivity or specificity, no markers have high sensitivity and specificity for correctly diagnosing thyroid cancer. Therefore, no single specific tumor marker is available to regularly and reliably distinguish benign from malignant thyroid cellular tumors [2,46].

Laboratory evaluation

Measurement of serum TSH is the most useful test in the initial evaluation of thyroid nodules because of the high sensitivity of the TSH assay in detecting early or subtle thyroid dysfunction [53,54]. The measurement of serum free thyroid hormones and thyroid peroxidase antibody (TPOAb) levels should be the second diagnostic step, which is needed for confirmation and definition of thyroid dysfunction if TSH levels are outside the normal range [55].

Third-generation TSH assays, with detection limits of about 0.01 mIU/mL, should be used in clinical practice. These assays detect TSH levels even in cases of mild hypo- or hyperthyroidism and make possible a reliable diagnosis of subclinical disease [55–57]. If serum TSH is within the normal range, determination of free thyroid hormones adds no further relevant information. If TSH levels are low, measurement of free T4 and free triiodothyronine is required to confirm hyperthyroidism. To limit unnecessary laboratory testing, the following practical strategy is suggested by the American Association of Clinical Endocrinologists guidelines for most patients with thyroid nodules [2]: normal serum TSH—no further testing; high serum TSH—measure free T4 and TPOAb to evaluate hypothyroidism; low serum TSH—measure free T4 and free triiodothyronine to evaluate hyperthyroidism.

TPOAb should be measured in patients who have increased levels of serum TSH [57]. High levels of serum TPOAb associated with a firm, diffusely enlarged thyroid is highly suggestive of autoimmune disease (Hashimoto thyroiditis). Occasionally, a nodular goiter may represent Hashimoto thyroiditis [57]. Anti-Tg antibody assays are not routinely used and should be reserved for the few patients who have sonographic and clinical findings suggestive of chronic lymphocytic thyroiditis with normal or negative serum TPOAb titers [58].

Serum Tg concentration correlates with iodine intake and the size of the thyroid gland rather than with the nature or function of the nodule. Because Tg concentration does not influence management, measurement of Tg is seldom used in nodule diagnosis [2,59].

Serum calcitonin is a good marker for C-cell disease and correlates well with tumor burden [60]. Although MTC accounts for only 5% of thyroid cancers, several prospective studies show a prevalence of MTC ranging from 0.4% to 1.4% in patients who have nodular thyroid disease [61,62]. Therefore, to detect and treat early unsuspected C-cell disease, routine calcitonin measurement in all patients who have a nodular thyroid has been recommended by European studies [63–65]. There is no consensus on this issue because of the unproven clinical significance of C-cell hyperplasia or medullary microcarcinoma in studied patients, the possibility of false-positive results that necessitate further unnecessary work-up, and lack of data that this practice is cost-effective [46,61,62,66,67].

Two recent thyroid practice guidelines have not endorsed routine calcitonin determination [2,3]. Calcitonin should be measured in patients who have a family history of MTC, multiple endocrine neoplasia type 2, or pheochromocytoma, or when FNA results suggest MTC. A baseline serum calcitonin value of 10 to 100 pg/mL is considered abnormal (normal, <10 pg/mL) and should be followed by pentagastrin stimulation. If a patient has a marked response to pentagastrin, thyroidectomy frequently reveals microscopic

MTC [61,62,65]. Pentagastrin is no longer available for clinical use in the United States.

Radioisotope scanning

Thyroid scanning is the only technique that allows for assessment of thyroid nodular function and detects areas of autonomy within the thyroid gland. Based on the pattern of radioisotope uptake, nodules may be classified as hyperfunctioning ("hot") or hypofunctioning ("cold") (Fig. 9). Hot nodules are seldom, if ever, malignant, whereas cold ones have a reported cancer risk between 5% and 15%. Because the vast majority (80%–90%) of thyroid lesions are cold and only a small minority of these are malignant, the predictive value of hypofunctioning nodules for malignancy is low. The diagnostic specificity is further decreased in small lesions (<1 cm), which may not be identified by scanning [68–70].

Thyroid scintigraphy can be performed with $^{99m}TcO_4^-$ or ^{123}I, although the latter is preferred. The role of scintigraphy in the diagnostic work-up of thyroid nodules is generally limited to (1) a single nodule with suppressed TSH, in which case no FNA is necessary; (2) a large toxic or nontoxic MNG, especially with substernal extension; and (3) when searching for ectopic thyroid tissue, such as struma ovarii or sublingual thyroid.

Management

Clinical management of thyroid nodules is influenced by the combined results of TSH measurement, FNA biopsy, and US and depends primarily on cytologic diagnosis.

Fine-needle aspiration–positive nodule

If cytologic results are positive for primary thyroid malignancy, surgery is almost always needed [2,3,71,72]. Cancer due to metastasis requires further investigations aimed at finding the primary lesion, which often precludes thyroid surgery. If preoperative FNA results suggest PTC, a near-total or total thyroidectomy is preferred [2,3,73,74]. With the exception of intrathyroidal microcarcinomas with no evidence of nodal involvement, lymph nodes within the central compartment of the neck (level 6) should be removed [2,3,71].

It is recommended that all patients undergoing thyroid surgery be evaluated by US preoperatively [2]. Abnormal lymph nodes identified by US should be removed and sent for pathologic examination at cervical exploration. If central compartment (level 6) nodes are positive for cancer, ipsilateral modified neck dissection should follow [71–74]. In patients who have a solitary, small (<1 cm) nodule (without lymph node involvement) proved to be PTC by preoperative FNA or by frozen section at surgery, lobectomy plus isthmectomy may be sufficient treatment. This issue continues to be debated [3,71,72,74].

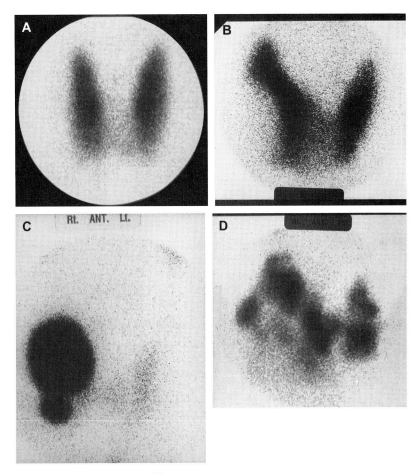

Fig. 9. Four different iodine 123 (^{123}I) thyroid scintigraphy patterns. (*A*) Normal thyroid show-ing homogeneous function in both lobes. (*B*) Nonfunctioning "cold" nodule in the right thyroid lobe. (*C*) Hyperfunctioning "hot" right thyroid nodule, with suppressed serum thyroid-stimu-lating hormone level and suppressed uptake of ^{123}I in the rest of the thyroid gland. (*D*) Typical pattern of a multinodular goiter with irregular, patchy uptake of an enlarged thyroid gland, including areas of normal, decreased, and increased ^{123}I uptake.

Fine-needle aspiration–negative nodule

Administration of T4 with TSH suppression is aimed at shrinking nodule size, arresting further nodule growth, and preventing the appearance of new nodules [2,3,46,75–80]. Although some reports show that nodule shrinkage is more frequent in patients who have long-term TSH suppression than in untreated patients [76–78], a clinically significant (>50%) decrease in nod-ule volume is obtained with T4 only in a minority of patients (ie, 20% of those who have palpable thyroid nodules) [46,75,79]. The growth of most thyroid nodules seems to be minimally dependent on TSH levels, and the observed beneficial effect of T4 may be explained by a decrease in volume of the still-TSH–dependent perinodular thyroid tissue. Nodule volume reduction is more likely in small, recently diagnosed nodules, in lesions with colloid features at FNA evaluation, and in geographic regions with borderline iodine deficiency [76,80].

T4 treatment is not free of adverse effects, and therapy should be targeted toward partial TSH suppression. Sustained subclinical hyperthyroidism is associated with a substantial decrease in bone density in postmenopausal women [81–83] and a 3-fold increase in atrial fibrillation, with increased morbidity and mortality from cardiovascular diseases [84–86].

Routine use of T4 suppressive therapy in nodular thyroid disease is not recommended [2,3,5,75]. The use of T4 may be considered in patients from iodine-deficient areas, in younger patients who have small nodules and colloid features on cytology, and in small MNGs with no evidence of functional autonomy [2]. The use of T4 should be avoided for large thyroid nodules or long-standing goiters, particularly if the TSH value is less than 0.5 mIU/mL; in postmenopausal women or persons older than 60 years; and in patients who have osteoporosis, cardiovascular disease, or systemic illnesses (Box 7). T4 treatment induces a clinically significant volume reduction only in a minority of patients, and the parameters of such a response are not known. Often, commitment to chronic therapy seems inevitable, but therapy should never be fully TSH suppressive because of the adverse effects of prolonged subclinical hyperthyroidism. If the nodule does not shrink or grows during the course of T4 therapy, US-FNA and possible surgery may be necessary.

Most thyroid nodules do not need specific treatment if malignancy and abnormal thyroid function have been excluded [2,3,5]. Unless the nodule (or nodules) is causing local symptoms or the patient's concerns are excessive, treatment aimed at volume debulking or growth prevention is unnecessary on the basis of the usually slow growth rate of benign thyroid lesions [87,88]. Clinical and US follow-up should be performed every 1 to 2 years.

Fine-needle aspiration–suspicious nodule

Indeterminate FNA results occur because the morphologic criteria used to distinguish benign from malignant lesions are poorly defined. No clear-cut

---

Box 7. Thyroxine-suppressive therapy for benign nodules

Not recommended:
- As routine treatment
- If TSH <0.5 mIU/mL
- In large nodule or MNG
- For postmenopausal women
- In patients with cardiac disease

cytologic criteria are available to help the clinician with the diagnosis. Overall, about 20% of indeterminate specimens are malignant, but cancer risk varies from 15% for "follicular neoplasm" to 60% for "atypical PTC" specimens [31,33,39]. It has been suggested that patients who have follicular neoplasm nodules undergo radioisotope scanning to rule out a hyperfunctioning, and therefore benign, process that may not require surgery. Because most follicular neoplasms are nonfunctional on these scans, this suggestion may not be cost-effective [31]. Reaspiration is not helpful; it typically creates confusion and does not provide useful information for management [35]. Clinical criteria such as sex, age, nodule size (<4 cm), and nodule consistency have been reported to favor [89] and not favor malignancy [46]. It is generally agreed that cytologically suspicious lesions are best surgically excised [2,3,39]. Current immunohistochemical or molecular markers do not reliably or regularly separate benign from malignant follicular neoplams [46], and their application in clinical practice is not endorsed [2,3].

Fine-needle aspiration–nondiagnostic nodule

An unsatisfactory specimen usually results from a cystic nodule that yields few or no follicular cells; reaspiration yields satisfactory smears in about 50% of cases [36]. US-FNA improves FNA accuracy and decreases the rates of nondiagnostic specimens. Two recent European studies showed that rates of nondiagnostic specimens (8.7% and 16%) decreased (to 3.5% and 7%, respectively) with the use of US-FNA [16,17]. Despite experienced centers, repeat biopsy, and US-FNA, a residual 5% of nodules remain nondiagnostic, which creates a management dilemma for the clinician [44,45,90]. Nondiagnostic, large (>3–4 cm), recurrent cysts or solid nodules should be treated surgically.

Therapeutic techniques

Surgery

Surgical options include lobectomy plus isthmectomy for a benign nodule, less-than-total thyroidectomy for MNG, and near-total or total thyroidectomy for malignant disease [3,71,72]. When established to be caused by thyroid enlargement, the presence or persistence of dysphagia, choking, shortness of breath (especially when supine), hoarseness, and neck pressure or pain are indications for thyroidectomy. A single toxic nodule or a toxic MNG may be treated surgically [2]. Patients who have cytologically suspicious nodules can be treated with thyroid lobectomy plus isthmectomy or total thyroidectomy; the latter is preferred if the patient is hyperthyroid, has a history of radiation, or has bilateral nodules. Frozen section should be performed at the time of surgery to help guide surgical decision making but may be of limited use in distinguishing benign from malignant follicular lesions [91].

Radioiodine

The aim of radioiodine (^{131}I) treatment is the ablation of thyroid autonomy, restoration of normal thyroid function, and reduction of thyroid mass (Box 8) [92,93]. Toxic nodular goiters are usually more radioresistant than toxic diffuse goiters, and higher ^{131}I doses (30–100 mCi) may be needed for successful treatment [94]. ^{131}I therapy is successful in more than 85% of patients who have hyperfunctioning nodules or toxic MNGs [95]. After treatment with ablative doses of ^{131}I, thyroid volume can decrease considerably (median decrease, 35% at 3 months and 45% at 24 months); 80% to 90% of patients become euthyroid. Hypothyroidism may develop after radioiodine treatment if the mass of normal thyroid tissue is too small, if its function is decreased because of concomitant autoimmune thyroiditis, or if there is damage to the thyroid consequent to contiguous cross-radiation from hot nodules [96]. Although rare (occurring in <1% of patients), immunogenic hyperthyroidism may occur due to induction of TSH receptor autoantibodies after ^{131}I treatment of toxic nodular goiter [97]. ^{131}I therapy can be repeated after 6 months if thyrotoxicosis is not cured, as documented by persistent low TSH levels.

^{131}I is preferred over thyroidectomy for small, nontoxic goiters (volume <100 mL) without suspected thyroid malignancy, in patients previously treated with surgery, or in those at risk for surgical intervention. ^{131}I is not the treatment of choice if compressive symptoms are present, in larger nodules requiring high doses of ^{131}I (which may be resistant to treatment), or if an immediate resolution of hyperthyroidism is medically indicated [92,93]. High doses of ^{131}I may increase cancer risk in the residual goiter, a consideration that disfavors its use in younger patients [92]. The only absolute contraindications to ^{131}I treatment are pregnancy (which should be excluded by a pregnancy test) and breast feeding [98]; treatment should be avoided for an arbitrary period of 3 to 6 months.

Recombinant human thyroid-stimulating hormone

The use of ^{131}I for nontoxic nodular goiter has been more successful in areas with mild iodine deficiency, in which 24-hour ^{131}I uptake is greater than in patients in the United States who have higher iodine intake [99–102]. In areas of high iodine intake, many patients who have MNG have low or low-normal ^{131}I uptake, which is often accompanied by partial or

---

Box 8. ^{131}I therapy for nodular thyroid

- An effective alternative to surgery for patients with high-risk or previous thyroidectomy
- Can be effective in toxic and nontoxic MNG
- Risk of malignancy in residual thyroid tissue unknown
- Contraindicated in pregnancy and lactation

complete suppression of serum TSH levels, thus rendering ^{131}I likely ineffective as a treatment option. The administration of small doses (0.1–0.3 mg) of recombinant human TSH (rhTSH) to patients who have low-uptake MNG increases ^{131}I uptake by more than 4-fold in 24 to 72 hours [103,104]. This allows for delivery of sufficient radiation to the thyroid to cause a decrease in size and amelioration of compressive symptoms within 2 months. As in patients who have high-uptake MNG, the average decrease in goiter size is 40% and 60% by the end of the first and second years, respectively [105,106].

rhTSH may cause a transient but clinically significant and symptomatic goiter enlargement of up to 24% and increased posttherapy hypothyroidism [107]. All patients should undergo US-FNA to rule out malignancy before ^{131}I treatment. rhTSH is approved only for scanning and Tg stimulation in patients who have thyroid cancer; its use to augment ^{131}I treatment is considered "off-label."

Nonsurgical minimally invasive procedures

Percutaneous ethanol injection

Percutaneous ethanol injection (PEI) is a US-guided, mini-invasive procedure that has been used for the nonsurgical management of some thyroid nodules [108–116].

Thyroid cysts. PEI is an effective alternative to surgery in the treatment of complex nodules with a dominant fluid component. Aspiration of thyroid cysts decreases the volume, but recurrences are common, and surgery is often required to remove large, relapsing lesions. Prospective randomized studies have shown that PEI is significantly superior to aspiration alone in reducing nodule volume [113,114]. A reduction of greater than 50% of the baseline size is obtained in nearly 90% of cases treated with PEI [111,114].

The recurrence rate of cysts after PEI is low, with the best results reported in large or symptomatic cystic lesions [11]. In one report, fluid reaccumulation was noted in only 5% of the treated nodules, and in two thirds of patients, one injection was curative [112]. In another randomized study comparing T4 suppression with PEI, the investigators found greater nodule shrinkage with PEI, and only 1 of 38 complex (predominantly cystic) nodules recurred after a 12-month follow-up [114]. Moreover, PEI reduced symptoms in 75% of treated patients, whereas simple fluid aspiration reduced symptoms in only 24% of treated patients. PEI seems to be safe in experienced hands; adverse effects of pain and dysphonia are reportedly transient and mild. Frequently, a single injection results in complete disappearance or significant size reduction of the treated cyst [2]. Only occasionally does a large or multilobulated cystic nodule require several injections.

Autonomously functioning thyroid nodules. Short-term successful results of PEI for toxic autonomously functioning thyroid nodules range from 64%

to more than 95% [115,117], but after 5 years, serum TSH is detectable in only 35% of those treated [113]. PEI reportedly induces a decrease in volume of 60% to 75%, but a small residual amount of tissue persists, which accounts for the high rate of relapse [113]. PEI is not recommended for treatment of toxic solitary or multinodular goiters, in part because of a high recurrence rate and in part because ^{131}I and surgery are effective and safe.

Cold solid nodules. A clinically significant decrease in nodule size after PEI has been reported in patients who have benign, solitary, solid nodules that are cold on scintigraphy [116,118]. The procedure seems to be more effective than T4 therapy in decreasing nodule volume and in relieving local pressure symptoms. The response is much less impressive and adverse effects are more common than in treatment of cysts [113].

In summary, PEI is an appropriate treatment for recurrent thyroid cysts if FNA has excluded the possibility of malignancy. PEI may be considered for autonomously functioning thyroid nodules with a large fluid component for preliminary drainage and debulking before radioiodine treatment [119]. PEI is not suitable for cold thyroid nodules because it requires repeated treatments, induces unpleasant adverse effects (eg, transient cervical pain), and can be complicated by recurrent laryngeal nerve damage.

Laser thermal ablation

Although percutaneous laser thermal ablation (PLA) has been used for many years to treat advanced cancer, it has been applied to the thyroid only recently. PLA is a minimally invasive procedure that is proposed as an alternative to surgery for thyroid nodules causing local symptoms or cosmetic concerns [120–123]. With US guidance and after local anesthesia, a 21-gauge needle is carefully inserted into the thyroid mass, and a thin optical fiber is advanced into the needle sheath. The fiber tips are seen as hyperechoic spots, and the area to be treated appears as an echogenic area enlarging over time on US [122]. The echogenic zone on US correlates poorly with the actual extent of thermal necrosis. US and color Doppler studies offer a precise definition of the laser-induced damage only a few hours after the procedure.

Adverse effects of PLA include burning cervical pain, which decreases rapidly as the energy is turned off. Localized pain can be treated with oral analgesics. Other problems, such as permanent dysphonia, skin burning, or damage to neck structures, have not been observed [120,121]. PLA is an outpatient procedure that lasts about 30 minutes, and patients can be dismissed shortly after the treatment.

In patients who have large nodules, one to three sessions of PLA or a single treatment with multiple fibers induces a nearly 50% decrease in nodule volume and alleviation of local symptoms [122–124]. Despite its apparent efficacy and because of the potential for major complications, PLA use should be restricted to specialized centers and is considered an experimental procedure.

Radiofrequency ablation

Radiofrequency (RF) ablation is a relatively novel procedure that is used widely for inoperable liver tumors [125]. On the basis of experience in animal models [126], RF is under evaluation as a nonsurgical therapeutic modality for the ablation of benign and malignant thyroid lesions [127].

Treatment is performed with an RF generator and an internally cooled electrode. After local anesthesia, a small skin incision is made, and a 17-gauge straight needle with a 1-cm active tip is inserted into the lesion along its longest axis. The RF energy is applied for at least 12 minutes with progressive increase of power output. Pain can be controlled during the procedure with conscious sedation and after treatment with oral analgesics. RF ablation induces substantial volume reduction, but a few relevant complications have been reported: cervical hematoma, burn at the puncture site, and vocal cord palsy due to recurrent laryngeal nerve damage. RF ablation is considered an experimental procedure.

Summary

Thyroid nodules are common and carry a 5% risk of malignancy. The challenge of management is to identify benign nodules and to accurately diagnose and treat malignant thyroid disease early. The current treatment plan—using TSH measurement, US, and FNA as initial tests, followed by US-FNA whenever necessary—seems to be practical, efficient, and cost-effective. US-FNA is gaining popularity because of its increased diagnostic accuracy and because new US machines are easy to operate and less costly. An ever-increasing number of practicing endocrinologists are using US in the office. The smallest size of a micronodule and the number of nodules in the thyroid gland that should undergo US-FNA are matters of debate. Routine T4 therapy for cytologically benign nodules and routine measurement of serum calcitonin are not recommended. New treatment options include the use of ^{131}I for large symptomatic MNGs; rhTSH to increase the efficacy of ^{131}I therapy; and PEI for benign, large, or recurrent cysts.

Acknowledgment

Editing, proofreading, and reference verification were provided by the Section of Scientific Publications, Mayo Clinic.

References

[1] Gharib H. Changing concepts in the diagnosis and management of thyroid nodules. Endocrinol Metab Clin North Am 1997;26(4):777–800.
[2] AACE/AME Task Force on Thyroid Nodules. American Association of Clinical Endocrinologists and Associazione Medici Endocrinologi medical guidelines for clinical practice for the diagnosis and management of thyroid nodules. Endocr Pract 2006;12(1):63–102.

[3] Cooper DS, Doherty GM, Haugen BR, et al, The American Thyroid Association Guidelines Taskforce. Management guidelines for patients with thyroid nodules and differentiated thyroid cancer. Thyroid 2006;16:109–42.

[4] American Association of Clinical Endocrinologists Ad Hoc Task Force for Standardized Production of Clinical Practice Guidelines. American Association of Clinical Endocrinologists protocol for standardized production of clinical practice guidelines. Endocr Pract 2004;10(4):353–61.

[5] Hegedus L. Clinical practice: the thyroid nodule. N Engl J Med 2004;351(17):1764–71.

[6] Vander JB, Gaston EA, Dawber TR. The significance of nontoxic thyroid nodules: final report of a 15-year study of the incidence of thyroid malignancy. Ann Intern Med 1968;69(3): 537–40.

[7] Tan GH, Gharib H. Thyroid incidentalomas: management approaches to nonpalpable nodules discovered incidentally on thyroid imaging. Ann Intern Med 1997;126(3): 226–31.

[8] Ezzat S, Sarti DA, Cain DR, et al. Thyroid incidentalomas: prevalence by palpation and ultrasonography. Arch Intern Med 1994;154(16):1838–40.

[9] Mortensen JD, Woolner LB, Bennett WA. Gross and microscopic findings in clinically normal thyroid glands. J Clin Endocrinol Metab 1955;15(10):1270–80.

[10] Ross DM. Diagnostic approach to and treatment of thyroid nodules. I. In: Rose BD, editor. Wellesley (MA): UpToDate; 2005.

[11] Filetti S, Durante C, Torlontano M. Nonsurgical approaches to the management of thyroid nodules. Nat Clin Pract Endocrinol Metab 2006;2(7):384–94.

[12] Belfiore A, Giuffrida D, La Rosa GL, et al. High frequency of cancer in cold thyroid nodules occurring at young age. Acta Endocrinol (Copenh) 1989;121(2):197–202.

[13] Loh KC. Familial nonmedullary thyroid carcinoma: a meta-review of case series. Thyroid 1997;7(1):107–13.

[14] Baskin HJ. Ultrasound of thyroid nodules. In: Baskin HJ, editor. Thyroid ultrasound and ultrasound-guided FNA biopsy. Boston: Kluwer Academic Publishers; 2000. p. 71–86.

[15] Marqusee E, Benson CB, Frates MC, et al. Usefulness of ultrasonography in the management of nodular thyroid disease. Ann Intern Med 2000;133(9):696–700.

[16] Danese D, Sciacchitano S, Farsetti A, et al. Diagnostic accuracy of conventional versus sonography-guided fine-needle aspiration biopsy of thyroid nodules. Thyroid 1998;8(1): 15–21.

[17] Carmeci C, Jeffrey RB, McDougall IR, et al. Ultrasound-guided fine-needle aspiration biopsy of thyroid masses. Thyroid 1998;8(4):283–9.

[18] Papini E, Guglielmi R, Bianchini A, et al. Risk of malignancy in nonpalpable thyroid nodules: predictive value of ultrasound and color-Doppler features. J Clin Endocrinol Metab 2002;87(5):1941–6.

[19] Hagag P, Strauss S, Weiss M. Role of ultrasound-guided fine-needle aspiration biopsy in evaluation of nonpalpable thyroid nodules. Thyroid 1998;8(11):989–95.

[20] Belfiore A, La Rosa GL, La Porta GA, et al. Cancer risk in patients with cold thyroid nodules: relevance of iodine intake, sex, age, and multinodularity. Am J Med 1992; 93(4):363–9.

[21] Mandel SJ. Diagnostic use of ultrasonography in patients with nodular thyroid disease. Endocr Pract 2004;10(3):246–52.

[22] Cochand-Priollet B, Guillausseau PJ, Chagnon S, et al. The diagnostic value of fine-needle aspiration biopsy under ultrasonography in nonfunctional thyroid nodules: a prospective study comparing cytologic and histologic findings. Am J Med 1994;97(2):152–7. Erratum in: Am J Med 1994;97(3):311.

[23] Papini E. The dilemma of non-palpable thyroid nodules. J Endocrinol Invest 2003;26(1): 3–4.

[24] Tan GH, Gharib H, Reading CC. Solitary thyroid nodule: comparison between palpation and ultrasonography. Arch Intern Med 1995;155(22):2418–23.

[25] Frates MC, Benson CB, Charboneau JW, et al, Society of Radiologists in Ultrasound. Management of thyroid nodules detected at US: Society of Radiologists in Ultrasound consensus conference statement. Radiology 2005;237(3):794–800.

[26] Pacini F, Schlumberger M, Dralle H, et al, European Thyroid Cancer Taskforce. European consensus for the management of patients with differentiated thyroid carcinoma of the follicular epithelium. Eur J Endocrinol 2006;154(6):787–803.

[27] Frasoldati A, Valcavi R. Challenges in neck ultrasonography: lymphadenopathy and·parathyroid glands. Endocr Pract 2004;10(3):261–8.

[28] Solbiati L, Osti V, Cova L, et al. Ultrasound of thyroid, parathyroid glands and neck lymph nodes. Eur Radiol 2001;11(12):2411–24. Epub 2001 Oct 25.

[29] Kim EK, Park CS, Chung WY, et al. New sonographic criteria for recommending fine-needle aspiration biopsy of nonpalpable solid nodules of the thyroid. AJR Am J Roentgenol 2002;178(3):687–91.

[30] Kim TY, Kim WB, Ryu JS, et al. 18F-fluorodeoxyglucose uptake in thyroid from positron emission tomogram (PET) for evaluation in cancer patients: high prevalence of malignancy in thyroid PET incidentaloma. Laryngoscope 2005;115(6):1074–8.

[31] Gharib H. Fine-needle aspiration biopsy of thyroid nodules: advantages, limitations, and effect. Mayo Clin Proc 1994;69(1):44–9.

[32] Goellner JR, Gharib H, Grant CS, et al. Fine needle aspiration cytology of the thyroid, 1980 to 1986. Acta Cytol 1987;31(5):587–90.

[33] Gharib H, Goellner JR. Fine-needle aspiration biopsy of thyroid nodules. Endocr Pract 1995;1(6):410–7.

[34] Gharib H, Goellner JR, Zinsmeister AR, et al. Fine-needle aspiration biopsy of the thyroid: the problem of suspicious cytologic findings. Ann Intern Med 1984;101(1):25–8.

[35] Cersosimo E, Gharib H, Suman VJ, et al. "Suspicious" thyroid cytologic findings: outcome in patients without immediate surgical treatment. Mayo Clin Proc 1993;68(4): 343–8.

[36] Chow LS, Gharib H, Goellner JR, et al. Nondiagnostic thyroid fine-needle aspiration cytology: management dilemmas. Thyroid 2001;11(12):1147–51.

[37] Gharib H, Goellner JR. Fine-needle aspiration biopsy of the thyroid: an appraisal. Ann Intern Med 1993;118(4):282–9.

[38] Caruso D, Mazzaferri EL. Fine needle aspiration biopsy in the management of thyroid nodules. Endocrinologist 1991;1:1194–202.

[39] Castro MR, Gharib H. Thyroid fine-needle aspiration biopsy: progress, practice, and pitfalls. Endocr Pract 2003;9(2):128–36.

[40] Jeffrey PB, Miller TR. Fine-needle aspiration cytology of the thyroid. Pathology (Phila) 1996;4(2):319–35.

[41] Hamberger B, Gharib H, Melton LJ III, et al. Fine-needle aspiration biopsy of thyroid nodules: impact on thyroid practice and cost of care. Am J Med 1982;73(3):381–4.

[42] Hamburger JI, Hamburger SW. Fine needle biopsy of thyroid nodules: avoiding the pitfalls. NY State J Med 1986;86(5):241–9.

[43] Haber RS. Ultrasound-guided fine needle aspiration biopsy of thyroid nodules. In: Baskin HJ, editor. Thyroid ultrasound and ultrasound-guided FNA biopsy. Boston: Kluwer Academic Publishers; 2000. p. 125–36.

[44] Schmidt T, Riggs MW, Speights VO Jr. Significance of nondiagnostic fine-needle aspiration of the thyroid. South Med J 1997;90(12):1183–6.

[45] McHenry CR, Walfish PG, Rosen IB. Non-diagnostic fine needle aspiration biopsy: a dilemma in management of nodular thyroid disease. Am Surg 1993;59(7):415–9.

[46] Castro MR, Gharib H. Continuing controversies in the management of thyroid nodules. Ann Intern Med 2005;142(11):926–31.

[47] Flanagan MB, Ohori NP, Carty SE, et al. Repeat thyroid nodule fine-needle aspiration in patients with initial benign cytologic results. Am J Clin Pathol 2006;125(5): 698–702.

[48] Frasoldati A, Toschi E, Zini M, et al. Role of thyroglobulin measurement in fine-needle aspiration biopsies of cervical lymph nodes in patients with differentiated thyroid cancer. Thyroid 1999;9(2):105–11.

[49] Boi F, Baghino G, Atzeni F, et al. The diagnostic value for differentiated thyroid carcinoma metastases of thyroglobulin (Tg) measurement in washout fluid from fine-needle aspiration biopsy of neck lymph nodes is maintained in the presence of circulating anti-Tg antibodies. J Clin Endocrinol Metab 2006;91(4):1364–9. Epub 2006 Jan 24.

[50] Miettinen M, Karkkainen P. Differential reactivity of HBME-1 and CD15 antibodies in benign and malignant thyroid tumors: preferential reactivity with malignant tumours. Virchows Arch 1996;429(4–5):213–9.

[51] Bartolazzi A, Gasbarri A, Papotti M, et al, Thyroid Cancer Study Group. Application of an immunodiagnostic method for improving preoperative diagnosis of nodular thyroid lesions. Lancet 2001;357(9269):1644–50.

[52] Segev DL, Clark DP, Zieger MA, et al. Beyond the suspicious thyroid fine needle aspirate: a review. Acta Cytol 2003;47(5):709–22.

[53] Spencer CA, LoPresti JS, Patel A, et al. Applications of a new chemiluminometric thyrotropin assay to subnormal measurement. J Clin Endocrinol Metab 1990;70(2):453–60.

[54] Spencer CA, Takeuchi M, Kazarosyan M. Current status and performance goals for serum thyrotropin (TSH) assays. Clin Chem 1996;42(1):140–5.

[55] Baloch Z, Carayon P, Conte-Devolx B, et al, Guidelines Committee, National Academy of Clinical Biochemistry. Laboratory medicine practice guidelines: laboratory support for the diagnosis and monitoring of thyroid disease. Thyroid 2003;13(1):3–126.

[56] Nicoloff JT, Spencer CA. Clinical review 12: the use and misuse of the sensitive thyrotropin assays. J Clin Endocrinol Metab 1990;71(3):553–8.

[57] Ross DS. Laboratory assessment of thyroid disfunction. In: Rose BD, editor. UpToDate. Waltham (MA): UpToDate; 2005.

[58] Hegedus L, Bonnema SJ, Bennedbaek FN. Management of simple nodular goiter: current status and future perspectives. Endocr Rev 2003;24(1):102–32.

[59] Aghini-Lombardi F, Antonangeli L, Martino E, et al. The spectrum of thyroid disorders in an iodine-deficient community: the Pescopagano survey. J Clin Endocrinol Metab 1999;84(2):561–6.

[60] Cohen R, Campos JM, Salaun C, et al, Groupe d'Etudes des Tumeurs a Calcitonine (GETC). Preoperative calcitonin levels are predictive of tumor size and postoperative calcitonin normalization in medullary thyroid carcinoma. J Clin Endocrinol Metab 2000;85(2):919–22.

[61] Kotzmann H, Schmidt A, Scheuba C, et al. Basal calcitonin levels and the response to pentagastrin stimulation in patients after kidney transplantation or on chronic hemodialysis as indicators of medullary carcinoma. Thyroid 1999;9(9):943–7.

[62] Erdogan MF, Gullu S, Baskal N, et al. Omeprazole: calcitonin stimulation test for the diagnosis follow-up and family screening in medullary thyroid carcinoma. J Clin Endocrinol Metab 1997;82(3):897–9.

[63] Pacini F, Fontanelli M, Fugazzola L, et al. Routine measurement of serum calcitonin in nodular thyroid diseases allows the preoperative diagnosis of unsuspected sporadic medullary thyroid carcinoma. J Clin Endocrinol Metab 1994;78(4):826–9.

[64] Niccoli P, Wion-Barbot N, Caron P, et al, The French Medullary Study Group. Interest of routine measurement of serum calcitonin: study in a large series of thyroidectomized patients. J Clin Endocrinol Metab 1997;82(2):338–41.

[65] Elisei R, Bottici V, Luchetti F, et al. Impact of routine measurement of serum calcitonin on the diagnosis and outcome of medullary thyroid cancer: experience in 10,864 patients with nodular thyroid disorders. J Clin Endocrinol Metab 2004;89(1):163–8.

[66] Bennedbaek FN, Perrild H, Hegedus L. Diagnosis and treatment of the solitary thyroid nodule: results of a European survey. Clin Endocrinol (Oxf) 1999;50(3):357–63.

[67] Bennedbaek FN, Hegedus L. Management of the solitary thyroid nodule: results of a North American survey. J Clin Endocrinol Metab 2000;85(7):2493–8.

[68] McHenry CR, Slusarczyk SJ, Askari AT, et al. Refined use of scintigraphy in the evaluation of nodular thyroid disease. Surgery 1998;124(4):656–61.

[69] Meier DA, Kaplan MM. Radioiodine uptake and thyroid scintiscanning. Endocrinol Metab Clin North Am 2001;30(2):291–313.

[70] Tollin SR, Fallon EF, Mikhail M, et al. The utility of thyroid nuclear imaging and other studies in the detection and treatment of underlying thyroid abnormalities in patients with endogenous subclinical thyrotoxicosis. Clin Nucl Med 2000;25(5):341–7.

[71] Thyroid Carcinoma Task Force, American Association of Clinical Endocrinologists, American College of Endocrinology. AACE/AAES medical/surgical guidelines for clinical practice: management of thyroid carcinoma. Endocr Pract 2001;7(3):202–20.

[72] British Thyroid Association. Guidelines for the management of thyroid cancer in adults. London: Royal College of Physicians of London and the British Thyroid Association; 2001. [cited 2005 Aug 2]. Available at: http://www.british-thyroid-association.org/complete%20guidelines.pdf.

[73] Mazzaferri E. Thyroid cancer: impact of therapeutic modalities on prognosis. In: Fagin JA, editor. Thyroid cancer. Boston: Kluwer Academic; 1998. p. 255–84.

[74] Schlumberger MJ. Papillary and follicular thyroid carcinoma. N Engl J Med 1998;338(5):297–306.

[75] Gharib H, Mazzaferri EL. Thyroxine suppressive therapy in patients with nodular thyroid disease. Ann Intern Med 1998;128(5):386–94.

[76] Papini E, Petrucci L, Guglielmi R, et al. Long-term changes in nodular goiter: a 5-year prospective randomized trial of levothyroxine suppressive therapy for benign cold thyroid nodules. J Clin Endocrinol Metab 1998;83(3):780–3.

[77] Wemeau JL, Caron P, Schvartz C, et al. Effects of thyroid-stimulating hormone suppression with levothyroxine in reducing the volume of solitary thyroid nodules and improving extranodular nonpalpable changes: a randomized, double-blind, placebo-controlled trial by the French Thyroid Research Group. J Clin Endocrinol Metab 2002;87(11):4928–34.

[78] Papini E, Bacci V, Panunzi C, et al. A prospective randomized trial of levothyroxine suppressive therapy for solitary thyroid nodules. Clin Endocrinol (Oxf) 1993;38(5):507–13.

[79] Castro MR, Caraballo PJ, Morris JC. Effectiveness of thyroid hormone suppressive therapy in benign solitary thyroid nodules: a meta-analysis. J Clin Endocrinol Metab 2002;87(9):4154–9.

[80] La Rosa GL, Ippolito AM, Lupo L, et al. Cold thyroid nodule reduction with L-thyroxine can be predicted by initial nodule volume and cytological characteristics. J Clin Endocrinol Metab 1996;81(12):4385–7.

[81] Faber J, Galloe AM. Changes in bone mass during prolonged subclinical hyperthyroidism due to L-thyroxine treatment: a meta-analysis. Eur J Endocrinol 1994;130(4):350–6.

[82] Uzzan B, Campos J, Cucherat M, et al. Effects on bone mass of long term treatment with thyroid hormones: a meta-analysis. J Clin Endocrinol Metab 1996;81(12):4278–89.

[83] Schneider R, Reiners C. The effect of levothyroxine therapy on bone mineral density: a systematic review of the literature. Exp Clin Endocrinol Diabetes 2003;111(8):455–70.

[84] Biondi B, Palmieri EA, Filetti S, et al. Mortality in elderly patients with subclinical hyperthyroidism. Lancet 2002;359(9308):799–800.

[85] Sawin CT, Geller A, Wolf PA, et al. Low serum thyrotropin concentrations as a risk factor for atrial fibrillation in older persons. N Engl J Med 1994;331(19):1249–52.

[86] Parle JV, Maisonneuve P, Sheppard MC, et al. Prediction of all-cause and cardiovascular mortality in elderly people from one low serum thyrotropin result: a 10-year cohort study. Lancet 2001;358(9285):861–5.

[87] Costante G, Crocetti U, Schifino E, et al. Slow growth of benign thyroid nodules after menopause: no need for long-term thyroxine suppressive therapy in post-menopausal women. J Endocrinol Invest 2004;27(1):31–6.

[88] Alexander EK, Hurwitz S, Heering JP, et al. Natural history of benign solid and cystic thyroid nodules. Ann Intern Med 2003;138(4):315–8.

[89] Schlinkert RT, van Heerden JA, Goellner JR, et al. Factors that predict malignant thyroid lesions when fine-needle aspiration is "suspicious for follicular neoplasm." Mayo Clin Proc 1997;72(10):913–6.

[90] MacDonald L, Yazdi HM. Nondiagnostic fine needle aspiration biopsy of the thyroid gland: a diagnostic dilemma. Acta Cytol 1996;40(3):423–8.

[91] Udelsman R, Westra WH, Donovan PI, et al. Randomized prospective evaluation of fro-zen-section analysis for follicular neoplasms of the thyroid. Ann Surg 2001;233(5):716–22.

[92] Meier DA, Brill DR, Becker DV, et al, Society of Nuclear Medicine. Procedure guideline for therapy of thyroid disease with (131)iodine. J Nucl Med 2002;43(6):856–61.

[93] Dietlein M, Dressler J, Grunwald F, et al. Guideline for radioiodine therapy for benign thyroid diseases (version 3) [German]. Nuklearmedizin 2004;43(6):217–20.

[94] Moser E. Radioiodine treatment of Plummer's disease. Exp Clin Endocrinol Diabetes 1998; 106(Suppl 4):S63–5.

[95] Nygaard B, Hegedus L, Nielsen KG, et al. Long-term effect of radioactive iodine on thyroid function and size in patients with solitary autonomously functioning toxic thyroid nodules. Clin Endocrinol (Oxf) 1999;50(2):197–202.

[96] Mariotti S, Martino E, Francesconi M, et al: Serum thyroid autoantibodies as a risk factor for development of hypothyroidism after radioactive iodine therapy for single thyroid 'hot' nodule. Acta Endocrinol (Copenh) 1986;113(4):500–7.

[97] Wallaschofski H, Muller D, Georgi P, et al. Induction of TSH-receptor antibodies in pa-tients with toxic multinodular goitre by radioiodine treatment. Horm Metab Res 2002; 34(1):36–9.

[98] Lazarus JH, Radioiodine Audit Subcommittee of the Royal College of Physicians Commit-tee on Diabetes and Endocrinology, and the Research Unit of the Royal College of Physi-cians. Guidelines for the use of radioiodine in the management of hyperthyroidism: a summary. J R Coll Physicians Lond 1995;29(6):464–9.

[99] Hegedus L, Hansen BM, Knudsen N, et al. Reduction of size of thyroid with radioactive iodine in multinodular non-toxic goitre. BMJ 1988;297(6649):661–2.

[100] Nygaard B, Hegedus L, Gervil M, et al. Radioiodine treatment of multinodular non-toxic goitre. BMJ 1993;307(6908):828–32.

[101] Huysmans DA, Hermus AR, Corstens FH, et al. Large, compressive goiters treated with radioiodine. Ann Intern Med 1994;121(10):757–62.

[102] de Klerk J, van Isselt JW, van Dijk A, et al. Iodine-131 therapy in sporadic nontoxic goiter. J Nucl Med 1997;38(3):372–6.

[103] Silva MN, Rubio IG, Knobel M, et al. Treatment of multinodular goiters in elderly patients with therapeutic doses of radioiodine preceded by stimulation with human recombinant TSH. Endocr J 2000;47(Suppl):144.

[104] Duick DS, Baskin HJ. Utility of recombinant human thyrotropin for augmentation of radioiodine uptake and treatment of nontoxic and toxic multinodular goiters. Endocr Pract 2003;9(3):204–9.

[105] Duick DS, Baskin HJ. Significance of radioiodine uptake at 72 hours versus 24 hours after pretreatment with recombinant human thyrotropin for enhancement of radioiodine ther-apy in patients with symptomatic nontoxic or toxic multinodular goiter. Endocr Pract 2004;10(3):253–60.

[106] Albino CC, Mesa CO Jr, Olandoski M, et al. Recombinant human thyrotropin as adjuvant in the treatment of multinodular goiters with radioiodine. J Clin Endocrinol Metab 2005; 90(5):2775–80. Epub 2005 Feb 15.

[107] Nielsen VE, Bonnema SJ, Hegedus L. Transient goiter enlargement after administration of 0.3 mg of recombinant human thyrotropin in patients with benign nontoxic nodular goiter: a randomized, double-blind, crossover trial. J Clin Endocrinol Metab 2006;91(4):1317–22. Epub 2006 Jan 24.

[108] Livraghi T, Paracchi A, Ferrari C, et al. Treatment of autonomous thyroid nodules with percutaneous ethanol injection: preliminary results: work in progress. Radiology 1990; 175(3):827–9.

[109] Verde G, Papini E, Pacella CM, et al. Ultrasound guided percutaneous ethanol injection in the treatment of cystic thyroid nodules. Clin Endocrinol (Oxf) 1994;41(6):719–24.

[110] Zingrillo M, Torlontano M, Chiarella R, et al. Percutaneous ethanol injection may be a definitive treatment for symptomatic thyroid cystic nodules not treatable by surgery: five-year follow-up study. Thyroid 1999;9(8):763–7.

[111] Kim JH, Lee HK, Lee JH, et al. Efficacy of sonographically guided percutaneous ethanol injection for treatment of thyroid cysts versus solid thyroid nodules. AJR Am J Roentgenol 2003;180(6):1723–6.

[112] Valcavi R, Frasoldati A. Ultrasound-guided percutaneous ethanol injection therapy in thyroid cystic nodules. Endocr Pract 2004;10(3):269–75.

[113] Guglielmi R, Pacella CM, Bianchini A, et al. Percutaneous ethanol injection treatment in benign thyroid lesions: role and efficacy. Thyroid 2004;14(2):125–31.

[114] Bennedbaek FN, Hegedus L. Treatment of recurrent thyroid cysts with ethanol: a randomized double-blind controlled trial. J Clin Endocrinol Metab 2003;88(12):5773–7.

[115] Papini E, Panunzi C, Pacella CM, et al. Percutaneous ultrasound-guided ethanol injection: a new treatment of toxic autonomously functioning thyroid nodules? J Clin Endocrinol Metab 1993;76(2):411–6.

[116] Bennedbaek FN, Nielsen LK, Hegedus L. Effect of percutaneous ethanol injection therapy versus suppressive doses of L-thyroxine on benign solitary solid cold thyroid nodules: a randomized trial. J Clin Endocrinol Metab 1998;83(3):830–5.

[117] Lippi F, Manetti L, Rago T. Percutaneous ultrasound-guided ethanol injection for treatment of autonomous thyroid nodules: results of a multicentric study [abstract]. J Endocrinol Invest 1994;17(Suppl 2):71.

[118] Zingrillo M, Collura D, Ghiggi MR, et al. Treatment of large cold benign thyroid nodules not eligible for surgery with percutaneous ethanol injection. J Clin Endocrinol Metab 1998; 83(11):3905–7.

[119] Zingrillo M, Modoni S, Conte M, et al. Percutaneous ethanol injection plus radioiodine versus radioiodine alone in the treatment of large toxic thyroid nodules. J Nucl Med 2003;44(2):207–10.

[120] Pacella CM, Bizzarri G, Guglielmi R, et al. Thyroid tissue: US-guided percutaneous interstitial laser ablation: a feasibility study. Radiology 2000;217(3):673–7.

[121] Dossing H, Bennedbaek FN, Karstrup S, et al. Benign solitary solid cold thyroid nodules: US-guided interstitial laser photocoagulation: initial experience. Radiology 2002;225(1): 53–7.

[122] Papini E, Guglielmi R, Bizzarri G, et al. Ultrasound-guided laser thermal ablation for treatment of benign thyroid nodules. Endocr Pract 2004;10(3):276–83.

[123] Pacella CM, Bizzarri G, Spiezia S, et al. Thyroid tissue: US-guided percutaneous laser thermal ablation. Radiology 2004;232(1):272–80. Epub 2004 May 20.

[124] Dossing H, Bennedbaek FN, Hegedus L. Effect of ultrasound-guided interstitial laser photocoagulation on benign solitary solid cold thyroid nodules: one versus three treatments. Thyroid 2006;16(8):763–8.

[125] Gazelle GS, Goldberg SN, Solbiati L, et al. Tumor ablation with radio-frequency energy. Radiology 2000;217(3):633–46.

[126] Kanauchi H, Mimura Y, Kaminishi M. Percutaneous radio-frequency ablation of the thyroid guided by ultrasonography. Eur J Surg 2001;167(4):305–7.

[127] Kim YS, Rhim H, Tae K, et al. Radiofrequency ablation of benign cold thyroid nodules: initial clinical experience. Thyroid 2006;16(4):361–7.

ELSEVIER
SAUNDERS

Endocrinol Metab Clin N Am
36 (2007) 737–751

ENDOCRINOLOGY
AND METABOLISM
CLINICS
OF NORTH AMERICA

Fine-Needle Aspiration of the Thyroid: Technique and Terminology

Yolanda C. Oertel, MD[a,b,c,*]

[a]Pathology Department (C-1219), Washington Hospital Center,
110 Irving Street, NW, Washington, DC 20010-2975, USA
[b]The George Washington University School of Medicine and Health Sciences,
2300 Eye Street NW, Washington, DC 20037, USA
[c]MCP Hahnemann University School of Medicine, 245 North 15th Street,
Philadelphia, PA 19102, USA

Fine-needle aspiration (FNA) is the accepted diagnostic test to determine whether a thyroid nodule is benign or malignant [1,2]. An accurate diagnosis depends on an adequate and representative sample interpreted correctly in the clinical context. There is no consensus among pathologists as to what represents an adequate sample. Although most cytopathologists are able to recognize an adequate specimen, we find it difficult to state the criteria that define what constitutes an adequate specimen. We are similar to Justice Potter Stewart when he referred to his ability to recognize pornography: "But I know it when I see it...."

Emphasis has been placed on having an experienced cytopathologist interpreting the smears. The pathologist's experience cannot substitute for a poor specimen. The pathologist is only as good as the sample he/she obtains or receives. Hence, we should address the fundamental issue of performing the procedure appropriately and handling the specimen well [3]. Based on over 30 years' experience as an "interventional pathologist," [4] and having trained many physicians (pathology residents and fellows, and endocrinologists, surgeons, radiologists, etc.) on how to perform FNA, I would like to share with you what I have learned. The technique is deceptively simple, but do not confuse simple with easy. The aspirator has to pay attention to multiple details to succeed. The two most important ones are (1) to put the patient at ease and (2) to apply very little suction when performing the procedure. I perform thyroidal aspirates on 100 to 120

* Pathology Department (C-1219), Washington Hospital Center, 110 Irving Street, NW, Washington, DC 20010-2975.
E-mail address: yolanda.c.oertel@medstar.net

0889-8529/07/$ - see front matter © 2007 Elsevier Inc. All rights reserved.
doi:10.1016/j.ecl.2007.05.001
endo.theclinics.com

patients per month. The patients tell me that the procedure is less painful than having blood drawn from their arms. We rarely have caused small hematomas and have not had major complications.

Equipment and technique

The equipment required is shown in (Fig. 1).

- A syringe handle or holder. I prefer the 10-mL Cameco Syringe Pistol (Belpro Medical Inc., Anjou, QC, Canada). If you prefer a lighter-weight holder, I recommend the Aspir Gun (Jorgensen Laboratories, Loveland, CO).
- Disposable syringes (10 mL)
- Disposable needles (with a clear hub), 22 gauge, 1 in and 1.5 in long
- Alcohol swabs, and gauze sponges

These are the items I use most frequently. We also have 20-mL syringes (and a syringe handle or holder); 23-gauge, 1-in and 1.5-in needles; 25 gauge, 5/8–in, 1-in, and 1.5-in needles.

We recommend having ice cubes available to numb the skin. We use 3"×5" plastic bags filled with tap water and kept in the freezer. We purchase these "liquid tight specimen bags" from Com-pac International (Carbondale, IL). Occasionally we use ethyl chloride spray for the same purpose.

We consider the syringe handle essential. It allows us to perform the aspiration with one hand while securing the lesion with the nondominant hand; hence, we know we are on target (ie, aspirating the intended lesion). The 22-gauge needle allows draining cystic lesions faster, and if there is thick colloid, it can be aspirated easily and with less pain. Using thinner needles takes longer to aspirate the fluid, the patient might need to swallow, and complications may arise. If the lesion has thick colloid, aspirating it through a 25-gauge needle is painful.

We advocate the use of ice cubes because they numb the skin and also cause vasoconstriction; there will be less hemodilution of the specimen.

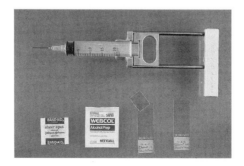

Fig. 1. Equipment needed to perform FNA.

Usually, we perform the first aspirate with the patient lying down (unless the patient is unable to climb onto the examining table or cannot lie down because of respiratory problems). The patient should be examined in a supine position and without hyperextending the neck muscles. I have learned from experience (trial and error) that small nodules are detected more easily when the patient is lying down rather than when the patient is sitting up and if the anterior neck muscles are relaxed. The latter is accomplished by asking the patient to tilt her chin down.

After cleaning the skin with alcohol and drying it with a gauze sponge, ask the patient to swallow. Then insert the needle into the lesion. While watching the needle hub, move the needle up and down with rapid movements and without applying suction. This "jiggling" of the needle dislodges the cells, and blood appears in the hub of the needle. Do not withdraw the needle until you see material in the hub. If this does not happen soon, start applying suction by gently pulling the plunger of the syringe. Withdraw the needle and prepare the smears as you would any blood smear. We use plain glass slides with one frosted end and smear the aspirated material on the glass slide using a hemacytometer cover glass (this is a thick piece of glass, narrower than the width of the regular glass microslide). If hemacytometers are not available, another glass slide can be used for this purpose. We prefer to use Diff-Quik stain for assessing adequacy of the specimen and for staining all available material. We rarely stain the smears with Papanicolaou stain. If the pathologist who will be reading the aspirates prefers to interpret Papanicolaou-stained material, the smears have to be fixed promptly in ethyl alcohol or sprayed with appropriate cytologic fixative. If the smears are going to be stained with Diff-Quik stain, they can be air-dried; there is no need for alcohol fixation. At some laboratories, the pathologists prefer the aspirated material to be submitted in RPMI or any other equivalent fluid. FNA requires team work and good communication among the members of the team [5].

The number of aspirates that should be performed depends on the size of the lesion. Most nodules (1–2 cm in diameter) can be sampled adequately with three aspirates.

The usefulness of a test depends on a low false-negative and a low false-positive rate. Most authorities agree that the false-negative rate of thyroidal FNA is less than or equal to 5% [6,7], and the false-positive rate ranges from 0% to 7.7%. Recently, disturbingly high figures have been reported: a false-negative rate of 25% and a false-positive rate of 9.9% [8]. The authors state that "The majority of errors occurred in poor quality specimens procured by radiologists or clinicians."

Another issue that has to be addressed by major professional organizations and credentialing boards is the percentage of unsatisfactory aspirates that should be allowed. It is my opinion that 5% of failures should be allowed. Ten percent should be the maximum. If your percentage of unsatisfactory aspirates exceeds 10%, you should get more training.

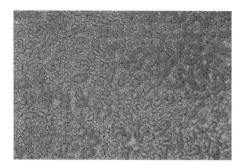

Fig. 2. Colloid admixed with blood. Low magnification; Diff-Quik stain.

Terminology

To accomplish proper management of patients, clinicians (endocrinologists) must have a diagnosis they understand. Clinicians and pathologists have to speak the same language. To compare findings from one study to another or from one medical institution to another requires that the terminology used be uniform.

The most common cytologic diagnoses comprise the following categories: (1) benign, (2) malignant, (3) follicular neoplasm, (4) inconclusive or indeterminate, and (5) suspicious for carcinoma. What follows are succinct definitions and illustrations of these entities. For more extensive descriptions, we refer the reader to two of our previous publications [9,10].

Benign

The majority of thyroid aspirates are diagnosed as benign, nonneoplastic—either adenomatoid nodules (with variable amounts of colloid or with an increased number of follicular epithelial cells) or as lymphocytic thyroiditis.

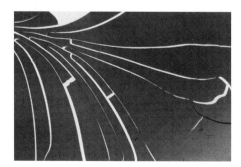

Fig. 3. Cracked colloid. Low magnification; Diff-Quik stain.

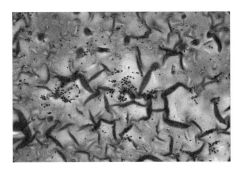

Fig. 4. Colloid and small groups of follicular epithelial cells. Low magnification; Diff-Quik stain.

Adenomatoid nodule: colloid rich or cellular/hyperplastic

The colloid-rich adenomatoid nodules contain abundant colloid (Figs. 2–5) and some follicular epithelial cells arranged in sheets, clusters, and spherules.

The hyperplastic or cellular adenomatoid nodules contain many follicular epithelial cells (arranged in sheets, clusters, spherules, rosettes, and tubules) and scant colloid (Figs. 6 and 7).

Either type of adenomatoid nodule may undergo cystic change. In such instances, there are mononucleated histiocytes (with foamy cytoplasm or with hemosiderin granules in their cytoplasm), some multinucleated histiocytes, and cholesterol crystals.

Lymphocytic thyroiditis (autoimmune thyroiditis, Hashimoto's thyroiditis)

Depending on the stage of the process, the number of cells and the type of cells varies. The initial stages show a predominance of lymphoid cells and

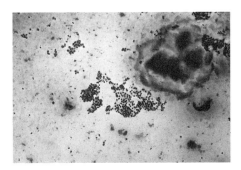

Fig. 5. Thin colloid in the background, particles of dense colloid (*upper right*), and clusters of follicular epithelial cells (*center*). Low magnification; Diff-Quik stain.

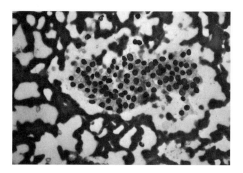

Fig. 6. Sheet of follicular epithelial cells. High magnification; Diff-Quik stain.

then follicular epithelial cells with oxyphilic cytoplasm (Hürthle cells) (Figs. 8–10), and later stages show extensive fibrosis. Frequently, skeletal muscle fibers are seen in the aspirates (Fig. 11).

Malignant

The most frequent malignant neoplasm is papillary carcinoma. There are several variants, most of which can be diagnosed on aspirates. The classic pattern of papillary carcinoma shows many neoplastic follicular epithelial cells ("tumor cellularity"). Papillary tissue fragments, with or without fibrovascular cores, are seen at low magnification (Fig. 12). The neoplastic follicular cells have moderate to abundant dense cytoplasm, well demarcated cellular borders, and enlarged nuclei that vary in size and shape. Intranuclear cytoplasmic pseudoinclusions (Fig. 13), psammoma bodies (Fig. 14), multinucleated histiocytes, and bubble-gum colloid are seen.

Cystic papillary carcinoma may be a source of false-negative diagnosis due to the lack of tumor cellularity. Smears contain numerous histiocytes (they have foamy cytoplasm or are laden with hemosiderin granules). There are cellular clusters with enlarged nuclei and pale to clear cytoplasm with

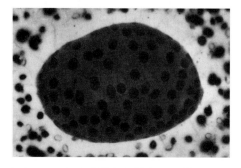

Fig. 7. Spherule (nonneoplastic follicles). High magnification; Diff-Quik stain.

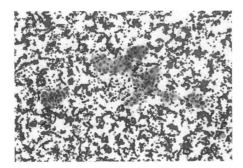

Fig. 8. Hashimoto's thyroiditis. Irregular clusters of oxyphilic follicular cells. Many lymphoid cells and red blood cells in the background. Low magnification; Diff-Quik stain.

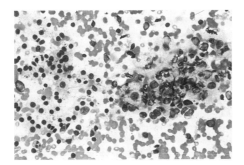

Fig. 9. Hashimoto's thyroiditis. Group of lymphoid cells (*right*) and sheet of follicular epithelial cells (*left*). Medium magnification; Diff-Quik stain.

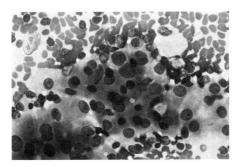

Fig. 10. Hashimoto's thyroiditis. Cluster of oxyphilic (Hürthle) cells surrounded by lymphoid cells and one histiocyte with foamy cytoplasm. High magnification; Diff-Quik stain.

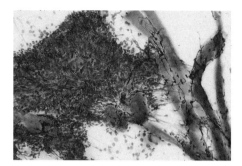

Fig. 11. Hashimoto's thyroiditis. Lymphoid tangles (*left*) and skeletal muscle fibers (*right*). Low magnification; Diff-Quik stain.

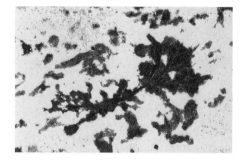

Fig. 12. Papillary carcinoma. Markedly cellular smear (tumor cellularity) with papillary tissue fragments. Low magnification; Diff-Quik stain.

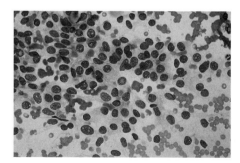

Fig. 13. Papillary carcinoma. Cluster of neoplastic cells. Note the intranuclear cytoplasmic pseudoinclusions. High magnification; Diff-Quik stain.

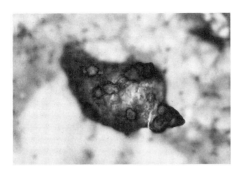

Fig. 14. Papillary carcinoma. Psammoma bodies. Low magnification; Diff-Quik stain.

smooth and well demarcated "scalloped" borders (Fig. 15). Dense colloid globules, which stain bright pink with Diff-Quik stain, are seen frequently (Fig. 16).

After draining a cystic lesion, if there is a palpable residual nodule, this should be aspirated. Frequently, the subsequent aspirate reveals more numerous neoplastic cells. Cystic lesions that recur (or refill after FNA) should make us suspect a cystic papillary carcinoma, even though the smears may not contain malignant cells.

Follicular variant of papillary carcinoma is another source of false-negative diagnosis. The smears are cell rich, but intranuclear cytoplasmic pseudoinclusions and psammoma bodies are seen infrequently.

Papillary carcinoma usually has an excellent prognosis. Some variants may behave more aggressively. The challenge for the pathologist is to find a better way to predict which of these neoplasms are more likely to recur or metastasize.

Medullary carcinoma originates from C cells and produces calcitonin. The smears are markedly cellular ("tumor cellularity") (Fig. 17).

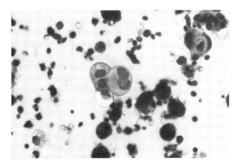

Fig. 15. Cystic papillary carcinoma. Two small groups of neoplastic cells (*center* and *upper right*) and many hemosiderin-laden macrophages. Medium magnification; Diff-Quik stain.

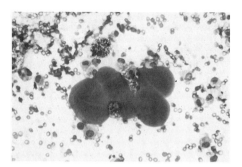

Fig. 16. Cystic papillary carcinoma. Globules of dense pink colloid. Medium magnification; Diff-Quik stain.

Frequently, the neoplastic cells have a plasmacytoid appearance and may appear singly or in small loose clusters. The nuclei vary in size and are situated eccentrically. Binucleation is common. Nucleoli are not conspicuous in most cases. Intranuclear cytoplasmic pseudoinclusions may be seen (Fig. 18). Bizarre mononucleated or multinucleated neoplastic cells are frequent. When the aspirates are stained with hematologic stains, calcitonin cytoplasmic granules may be seen. These granules may be stained using the immunoperoxidase technique (this works better on cellblock sections rather than on smears).

Smears from anaplastic carcinoma show abundant blood, necrotic debris, fragments of fibrocollagenous tissue, and markedly atypical cells. Two populations of neoplastic cells may be seen: spindled cells and large multinucleated cells. The latter may be of two types: pleomorphic tumor cells (with eosinophilic cytoplasm and several bizarre nuclei) and osteoclastoid cells (with multiple regular nuclei) (Figs. 19 and 20). Mitotic figures are present.

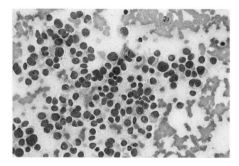

Fig. 17. Medullary carcinoma. Many loosely cohesive neoplastic cells with nuclei of varied sizes. Medium magnification; Diff-Quik stain.

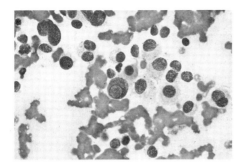

Fig. 18. Medullary carcinoma. Loosely cohesive neoplastic cells with plasmacytoid appearance. Note the intranuclear cytoplasmic pseudoinclusion.

Follicular neoplasm (follicular adenoma/follicular carcinoma)

Most cytopathologists agree that it is not possible to differentiate between a follicular adenoma and a follicular carcinoma in aspirated material. Hence, we make a diagnosis of follicular neoplasm and request that the lesion be excised surgically to determine whether it is benign (adenoma) or malignant (carcinoma). These lesions are a source of false-negative diagnosis because they bleed easily on aspiration and because the aspirates are hemodiluted and do not show tumor cellularity. The follicular epithelial cells are arranged in microfollicles with empty lumina or with dense inspissated colloid in their lumina (Figs. 21 and 22). The background of the smears is hemorrhagic and devoid of colloid.

Follicular neoplasms of Hürthle cell type cannot be diagnosed as Hürthle cell adenoma or Hürthle cell carcinoma on smears from thyroidal aspirates. These neoplasms usually show "tumor cellularity" (Fig. 23). Microfollicles with inspissated colloid in their lumina are seen more frequently (Fig. 24) than those with empty lumina (Fig. 25). These oxyphilic neoplasms tend to infarct spontaneously and after FNA.

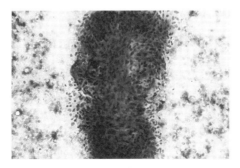

Fig. 19. Anaplastic carcinoma. Tissue fragment with spindled cells. Note the necrotic background. Low magnification; Diff-Quik stain.

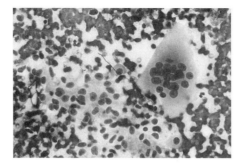

Fig. 20. Anaplastic carcinoma. Cluster of neoplastic cells and one osteoclastoid cell. Medium magnification; Diff-Quik stain.

Historically, the classification of thyroidal neoplasms has been based on their morphologic (histologic) appearance. More recently, emphasis has been placed on biochemical and molecular markers to help distinguish benign from malignant lesions. Studies performed on cytologic samples for Galectin-3 (expressed in thyroid malignancies) were initially optimistic. However, some cases of Hashimoto's thyroiditis were also positive [11]. Telomerase seemed to be a possible marker for malignancy, but assays have varied widely in sensitivity and specificity [12,13].

Inconclusive, indeterminate

An inconclusive or indeterminate diagnosis is the gray area when the cytopathologist cannot determine whether the lesion is neoplastic or not. This includes a cellular adenomatoid nodule versus a follicular neoplasm, a cellular adenomatoid nodule versus a follicular variant of papillary carcinoma, a cellular follicular lesion that is most likely neoplastic, or a hyperplastic

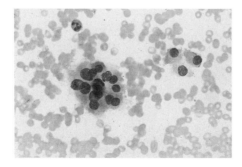

Fig. 21. Follicular neoplasm. Microfollicle with inspissated colloid (*center*) and three neoplastic cells (*right*). Background is hemorrhagic and devoid of colloid. High magnification; Diff-Quik stain.

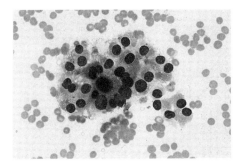

Fig. 22. Follicular neoplasm. Microfollicle (with inspissated colloid in the lumen) surrounded by loosely cohesive neoplastic follicular cells. Background is hemorrhagic and devoid of colloid. High magnification; Diff-Quik stain.

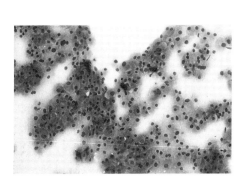

Fig. 23. Follicular neoplasm (Hürthle cell type). Irregular tissue fragments with numerous oxy-philic cells, (tumor cellularity). Low magnification; Diff-Quik stain.

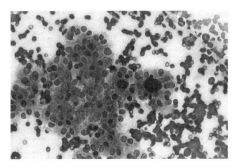

Fig. 24. Follicular neoplasm (Hürthle cell type). Two microfollicles with inspissated colloid in their lumina (*center*). Medium magnification; Diff-Quik stain.

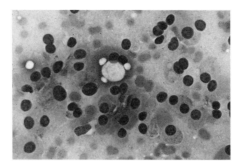

Fig. 25. Follicular neoplasm (Hürthle cell type). Note the microfollicle with empty lumen. High magnification; Diff-Quik stain.

oxyphilic cell nodule versus a Hürthle cell neoplasm. This area of diagnosis will benefit the most from ancillary immune techniques and molecular studies. Some success has been reported in distinguishing benign (follicular adenoma and hyperplastic nodules) from malignant (follicular variant of papillary carcinoma) ones [14–16] based on molecular profiling.

Suspicious for carcinoma

Another diagnostic category is that in which a malignancy is suspected but for which a definite diagnosis cannot be made due to a scant sample. In such instances, a repeat FNA might yield diagnostic material. Otherwise, these patients should undergo surgery. Intraoperative consultation, if it provides a diagnosis of malignancy, may allow a thyroidectomy (rather than a lobectomy with subsequent completion thyroidectomy).

Summary

FNA is a valuable diagnostic tool. When a thyroid nodule is detected, FNA is the right thing to do. But, are we doing it right? It is not only a matter of sticking a needle. You have to use clinical judgment and common sense. I hope this brief article is the beginning of a dialog, and I encourage you to e-mail (or mail) me specific questions regarding FNAs.

If you want to arrive at an accurate diagnosis and do right for your patient, you have to improve upon your palpatory skills and FNA technique. It is important to examine the patient when supine and without hyperextending the neck. The best pathologist in the world cannot provide a correct diagnosis if the smears show mostly blood because too much suction was applied. Excessive suction is the most common cause of unsatisfactory aspirates. This is easy to correct: Be gentle when aspirating thyroid lesions.

For over 15 years pathologists have been searching for the "magic marker" to identify malignant cells. Although progress has been made, our search continues. While we struggle in our daily practice to make the correct diagnosis, let us not neglect the basics.

References

[1] Gharib H, Papini E, Valcavi R. American Association of Clinical Endocrinologists and Associazione Medici Endocrinologi Medical Guidelines for clinical practice for the diagnosis and management of thyroid nodules. Endocr Pract 2006;12:63–102.

[2] Cooper DS, Doherty GM, Haugen BR, et al. Management guidelines for patients with thyroid nodules and differentiated thyroid cancer. The American Thyroid Association Guidelines Taskforce. Thyroid 2006;16:1–33.

[3] Oertel YC. Some thoughts about fine needle aspirations of thyroid nodules. Thyroid 2004;14:85–6.

[4] Oertel YC. Emerging role of the interventional pathologist. Diagn Cytopathol 2004;30: 295–6.

[5] Oertel YC, Burman KD, Boyle L, et al. Integrating fine-needle aspiration into a daily practice involving thyroid disorders: The Washington Hospital Center approach. Diagn Cytopathol 2001;27:120–2.

[6] Grant CS, Hay ID, Gough IR, et al. Long term followup of patients with benign thyroid fine needle aspiration cytologic diagnoses. Surgery 1989;106:980–6.

[7] Gharib H, Goellner JR. Fine-needle aspiration biopsy of the thyroid: an appraisal. Ann Intern Med 1993;118:282–9.

[8] Raab SS, Vrbin CM, Grzybicki DM, et al. Errors in thyroid gland fine-needle aspiration. Am J Clin Pathol 2006;125:873–82.

[9] Oertel YC, Oertel JE. Diagnosis of benign thyroid lesions: fine-needle aspiration and histopathologic correlation. Ann Diagn Pathol 1998;2:250–63.

[10] Oertel YC, Oertel JE. Diagnosis of malignant epithelial thyroid lesions: fine needle aspiration and histopathologic correlation. Ann Diagn Pathol 1998;2:377–400.

[11] Bartolazzi A, Gasbarri A, Papotti M, et al. Application of an immunodiagnostic method for improving preoperative diagnosis of nodular thyroid lesions. Lancet 2001;357:1644–50.

[12] Ito Y, Yoshida H, Tomoda C. Telomerase activity in thyroid neoplasms evaluated by the expression of human telomerase reverse transcriptase (hTERT). Anticancer Res 2005;25:509–14.

[13] Kammori M, Nakamura K, Hashimoto M. Clinical application of human telomerase reverse transcriptase gene expression in thyroid follicular tumors by fine-needle aspirations using in situ hybridization. Int J Oncol 2003;22:985–91.

[14] Mazzanti C, Zeiger MA, Costourous N, et al. Using gene expression profiling to differentiate benign versus malignant thyroid tumors. Cancer Res 2004;64:2898–903.

[15] Finley DJ, Arora N, Zhu B, et al. Molecular profiling distinguishes papillary carcinoma from benign thyroid nodules. J Clin Endocrinol Metab 2004;89:3214–23.

[16] Finley DJ, Lubitz CC, Wei C, et al. Advancing the molecular diagnosis of thyroid nodules: defining benign lesions by molecular profiling. Thyroid 2005;15:562–8.

ELSEVIER
SAUNDERS

Endocrinol Metab Clin N Am
36 (2007) 753–778

ENDOCRINOLOGY
AND METABOLISM
CLINICS
OF NORTH AMERICA

Papillary Thyroid Cancer: Monitoring and Therapy

R. Michael Tuttle, MD[a,b,*], Rébecca Leboeuf, MD[c], Andrew J. Martorella, MD[a,b]

[a]Joan and Sanford I. Weill Medical College of Cornell University,
525 E. 68th Street, New York, NY 10021, USA
[b]Memorial Sloan Kettering Cancer Center, Zuckerman Building, Room 834,
1275 York Avenue, New York, NY 10021, USA
[c]Sherbrooke University, Centre Hospitalier Universitaire de Sherbrooke,
3001 12th Avenue North, Sherbrooke, Quebec J1H 5N4, Canada

Thyroid cancer accounts for more than 90% of all endocrine malignancies but represents only about 1% of all human cancers. Although thyroid cancer is generally considered to be a rare tumor with exceptionally high long-term survival rates, the American Cancer Society [1] estimates that 30,180 new cases will be diagnosed in 2006. This is similar to the number of new cases of leukemia, pancreatic, and oropharynx cancer and exceeds the number of cases of ovarian, esophageal, cervical, and testicular cancer estimated to be diagnosed in the same time period (Table 1). The excellent long-term survival rates seen in patients who have thyroid cancer is reflected in the relatively small number of disease-specific deaths attributable to thyroid cancer anticipated in 2006 compared with other malignancies. As of January 1, 2003, there were approximately 347,424 thyroid cancer survivors living in the United States (268,149 women and 79,275 men) [2].

Differentiated thyroid cancer that arises from the thyroid follicular cells accounts for more than 90% of thyroid cancer cases diagnosed. Medullary thyroid cancer, arising from the neuroendocrine c-cells of the thyroid, accounts for about 3% of cases; the remaining cases are classified as anaplastic thyroid cancer (thought to arise from the differentiated thyroid cancers) or primary thyroid lymphoma. Within the differentiated thyroid cancer family, papillary thyroid cancer accounts for more than 90% of new cases, whereas

* Corresponding author. Memorial Sloan Kettering Cancer Center, Zuckerman Building, Room 834, 1275 York Avenue, New York, NY 10021.
E-mail address: tuttlem@mskcc.org (R.M. Tuttle).

0889-8529/07/$ - see front matter © 2007 Elsevier Inc. All rights reserved.
doi:10.1016/j.ecl.2007.04.004
endo.theclinics.com

Table 1
American cancer society estimated incidence and disease specific deaths in 2006

Site	Estimated incidence 2006	Estimated deaths 2006
Lung and bronchus	174,470	162,460
Breast	214,640	41,430
Prostate	234,460	27,350
Colon	106,680	55,170
Lymphoma	66,670	20,330
Uterine	41,200	7350
Kidney	38,890	12,840
Leukemia	35,070	22,280
Pancreas	33,730	32,300
Oral cavity and pharynx	30,990	7430
Thyroid	30,180	1500
Ovary	20,180	15,310
Multiple myeloma	16,570	11,310
Esophageal	14,550	13,770
Cervix	9710	3700
Testis	8250	370

Data from American Cancer Society. Cancer facts and figures 2006.

perhaps 10% of patients present with follicular thyroid cancer [3]. Analysis of 15,698 patients who had thyroid cancer followed in the SEER database (Surveillance Epidemiology and End Results; National Cancer Institute, http://www.seer.cancer.gov) demonstrate overall 10-year survival rates of 98% for papillary thyroid cancer, 92% for follicular thyroid cancer, 80% for medullary cancer, and 13% for anaplastic thyroid cancer [4]. Other retrospective studies have reported 40-year survival rates of 94% for papillary thyroid cancer and 84% for follicular thyroid cancer [5].

Although the mortality has remained rather stable over the last 25 years, the SEER data indicate a 52% rise in incidence of thyroid cancer between 1975 and 2001 [6]. Careful analysis shows that although there was no significant change in the incidence of the less common thyroid cancers such as follicular, medullary, and anaplastic, the increased incidence was almost completely explained by the dramatic increase in papillary thyroid cancer, which showed a 2.9-fold increase between 1988 and 2002 [7]. The incidence of thyroid cancer in women has risen from approximately 6 per 100,000 in the early 1970s to more than 12 per 100,000 by 2000 to 2003. A smaller, although statistically significant, rise has been seen in men over the same period (2.1 per 100,000 to 4.2 per 100,000). Based on these incidence rates, the life-time risk of developing thyroid cancer for men and women born in 2003 is 0.69% or 1 in 146 persons. The age adjusted-death rate remains low at 0.5 per 100,000 men and women per year [2].

Although radiation is the best known risk factor for development of thyroid cancer [8], it seems unlikely that that the low level fallout from the United States atomic weapons testing program is responsible for the dramatic rise in thyroid cancer because most of the patients diagnosed over the last several years were born many years after the above-ground testing ended in the United States in the late 1950s. Other risk factors for the development of thyroid cancer, such as occupational exposure, dietary habits, lifestyle, parity, and genetic predisposition, have been less well studied [9].

Since SEER began recording specific tumor characteristics in 1988, 49% of the increase in thyroid cancer cases was represented by tumors less than 1 cmat diagnosis, and 87% were 2 cm or smaller, suggesting that early detection of small tumors accounted for much of the rise in thyroid cancer incidence [7]. This early detection may be secondary the incidental finding of thyroid nodules on radiographic studies done for other indications but could also be due to diligent pathologists carefully searching the entire thyroid gland for microscopic evidence of small thyroid cancers even when the primary nodule is benign. Whether early detection secondary to wide-spread use of cross-sectional imaging of the neck, thyroid ultrasonography, and more wide-spread use of ultrasound-guided fine-needle aspiration can fully explain the dramatic increased incidence with stable disease specific mortality remains to be determined.

Regardless of the precise cause of this dramatic rise in incidence of thyroid cancer, endocrinologists, surgeons, and nuclear medicine physicians will be faced with a large number of patients who have thyroid cancer who need appropriate evaluation and treatment in the upcoming years. Many of these patients will be diagnosed with small tumors early in the course of their disease and will be expected to have nearly normal life expectancies. Our goal should be to offer the proper therapy, tailored to their individual risk of recurrence and death from disease, to ensure that these patients live as normal a life as possible with minimal treatment-related side effects.

Because the vast majority of thyroid cancer patients will be long-term survivors at low risk of recurrence and death from disease, it is imperative that we develop a strategy for long-term follow-up that minimizes testing to the greatest extent possible while providing adequate sensitivity to detect significant disease recurrence at an early stage. In this article, we define a treatment paradigm and a follow-up strategy that attempts to match the risk of recurrence and disease-specific mortality with the aggressiveness of primary treatment and intensity of follow-up studies.

Initial presentation

Thyroid cancer is diagnosed in women two to three times more often than in men. Although it can present at any age, the median age at diagnosis is close to 45 years of age. Most patients present with an asymptomatic painless mass in the thyroid that is detected by the patient or their health care provider. Thyroid function tests are almost uniformly normal [10].

Although fine-needle aspiration has the highest sensitivity and specificity for identification of malignant thyroid nodules, several clinical features, such as rapid growth, local compressive symptoms, male gender, suspicious criteria by ultrasonographic examination, vocal cord paralysis, family history of thyroid cancer (differentiated thyroid cancer or medullary thyroid cancer), prior history of radiation exposure during childhood, hard fixed nodule, or palpable cervical lymphadenopathy should raise the pretest probability of malignancy [11]. In addition, differentiated thyroid cancer can be associated with one of several rare syndromes, such as Gardner's syndrome, familial adenomatous polyposis, Carney complex, and Cowden's syndrome [12].

Tumor registry data indicate that, at the time of diagnosis, thyroid cancer is localized to the thyroid in 59% of cases, is spread to regional lymph nodes in 34%, and is present outside the neck as distant metastases in 5% [2]. This is consistent with the most published retrospective clinical series that report spread to regional lymph nodes in 20% to 50% of patients on routine clinical pathology examination [5,13–18]. With meticulous neck dissection and careful pathologic examination, as many as 80% to 90% of patients have microscopic lymph node involvement at the time of diagnosis [19,20]. In these clinical series, distant metastatic spread at diagnosis is seen in only 2% to 5% of cases [16,21,22].

Although most patients respond well to initial therapy with prolonged disease-specific survival, tumor recurrence rates remain high, particularly at both extremes of age. In the Ohio State series, 23.5% of the patients had a clinically evident recurrence at a median of 16.6 years after diagnosis. This included 17.8% who had local recurrence (74% had lymph node metastasis, 20% had thyroid bed recurrence, and 6% had recurrence in muscle or trachea) and 7.5% who had recurrence in sites outside the neck [5,22]. These data are similar to the Mayo clinic series where tumor recurrence was detected in 14% of patients with a follow-up period that extended beyond 40 years [23]. Clinically evident recurrences are not a trivial event, with 8% of the patients having local recurrence and 50% of the patients having distant recurrence dying of the disease [22]. With the increased sensitivity of serum thyroglobulin (Tg) and neck ultrasonography, it is clear that some of the cases that would have been classified as "recurrence" in older series are be considered persistent disease and hopefully detected at an earlier, more treatable stage using current follow-up paradigms.

Clinical guidelines

Over the last few years, several thyroid cancer specialist organizations around the world have published guidelines specifically addressing the pertinent management issues in thyroid cancer [11,24–28]. In the following sections, we explore the similarities and differences in the recommendations provided in these various guidelines to determine where there is uniform agreement and where we continue to have areas of controversy. Because each of the guidelines includes an exhaustive reference list, we do not cite all of the primary sources in our review but refer readers to the guidelines for additional references. The guidelines are referred to as ATA (American Thyroid Association [25]), ETA (European Thyroid Association [26]), AACE (American Association of Clinical Endocrinologists [27]), BTA (British Thyroid Association and Royal College of Surgeons [24]), or NCCN (National Comprehensive Cancer Network [11]) in the following discussion and tables.

Risk stratification

Risk stratification is the cornerstone of treatment and follow-up recommendations. Over the years, a relatively small group of clinical and histopathologic factors have been shown to be significant predictors of disease-specific mortality and usually risk of recurrence [29,30]. These include patient factors such as age at diagnosis and gender and tumor-related factors such as size of the primary tumor, extent of extrathyroidal invasion, specific tumor histology, and distant metastases (Table 2) [22, 31–37]. The MACIS system emphasizes the importance of adequate surgical resection by including a variable that reflects the completeness of resection based on the surgeons, intraoperative findings. Some series report lymph node involvement as a predictor of disease recurrence without impact on disease-specific survival [14], whereas others demonstrate that lymph node involvement can be a predictor of disease-specific mortality [5].

Table 2
Commonly used risk factors for stratification of risk of death from disease

Parameters	EORTC [31]	AGES [32]	AMES [33]	MACIS [34]	OSU [22]	MSKCC [35]	NTCTCS [36]	TNM [37]
Age	√	√	√	√	−	√	√	√
Gender	√	−	√	−	−	−	−	−
Size of primary tumor	−	√	√	√	√	√	√	√
Multicentricity	−	−	−	−	√	−	√	−
Tumor grade	−	√	−	−	−	√	−	−
Extrathyroidal extension	√	√	√	√	√	√	√	√
Lymph node involvement	−	−	−	−	√	√	√	√
Distant metastasis	√	√	√	√	√	√	√	√
Completeness of resection	−	−	−	√	−	−	−	−

Abbreviations: AGES, patient age, histologic grade of the tumor, tumor extent (extrathyroidal invasion or distant metastases), and size of the primary tumor; AMES, patient age, presence of distant metastases, extent and size of the primary tumor; EORTC, European Organization for Research on Treatment of Cancer; MACIS, metastasis, patient age, completeness of resection, local invasion, and tumor size; MSKCC, Memorial Sloan-Kettering Cancer Center; NTCTCS, National Thyroid Cancer Treatment Cooperative Study; OSU, Ohio State University; TNM, American Joint Committee on Cancer staging system of tumor size, nodal metastases (N), and distant metastases (M); √: variable used in defining risk group; −, variable not used.

Adapted from Dean DS, Hay ID. Prognostic indicators in differentiated thyroid carcinoma. Cancer Control 2000;7:229–39.

Although each of these staging systems reliably predicts disease-specific survival, they are less helpful at predicting disease recurrence [29,30]. None of the available staging systems includes a response-to-therapy variable, implicitly indicating that response to therapy has no impact on outcome. Therefore, patients who have an excellent response to initial therapy may be considered to be at a continued higher than would be appropriate because of potentially worrisome initial presenting features.

Because of the wide-spread use of American Joint Committee on Cancer (AJCC)/Union Internationale Contre le Cancer (UICC) staging systems throughout oncology [37] and their utility in predicting disease-specific mortality, the ATA and the ETA guidelines recommend using tumor/nodes/mestasis (TNM) staging for all differentiated thyroid cancer patients (Table 3) [25]. The ETA, the NCCN, and the ATA guidelines include the specifics of staging with the TNM system [25,26].

The newest TNM staging system (Version 6) [37] contains some substantial differences in clinical staging when compared with the older versions (see Ref. [26] for detailed comparison). The most important changes include the fact that tumors up to 2 cm are now considered T1 lesions, and the classification for lymph node metastasis has been changed to better reflect the biology of the disease with N1a referring to lymph node metastases in the central neck (pretracheal and paratracheal) and N1b referring to lymph nodes in the lateral neck and mediastinum. In addition, older patients who have minimal extrathyroidal extension are considered stage III, unless the extrathyroidal extension involve the subcutaneous soft tissues, larynx, trachea, esophagus, or recurrent laryngeal nerve, in which case they are upstaged to stage IVA. Regardless of the size of the primary tumor, if the extrathyroidal extension invades the prevertebral fascia, carotid artery, or mediastinal vessels, they are classified as stage IVB. Younger patients who have distant metastases continue to be stage II, whereas older patients who have distant metastases are classified as stage IVC.

Although the TNM staging system is useful for research purposes and epidemiologic studies and accurately identifies patients at risk for death from disease, most clinicians continue to use additional postoperative clinicopathologic staging to further refine the likely clinical course with respect to risk for recurrence, need for additional adjuvant therapy with radioactive iodine (RAI), and specific follow-up recommendations.

Goals of initial therapy

As outlined in the ATA guidelines [25], the goals of initial therapy are to surgically remove all evidence of gross disease in the neck while minimizing treatment and disease-related morbidity. In situations where radioactive iodine remnant ablation is required, complete surgical removal of the normal thyroid tissue facilitates the efficacy of RAI in destroying the remaining microscopic normal remnant and any metastatic disease that may be present. Furthermore, our initial therapies, if successful, should result in a decreased

Table 3
Tumor/node/metastasis classification system for differentiated thyroid carcinoma

Classification	Definition
T1	Tumor diameter ≤2 cm
T2	Primary tumor diameter >2–4 cm
T3	Primary tumor diameter >4 cm limited to the thyroid or with minimal extrathyroidal extension
T4$_a$	Tumor of any size extending beyond the thyroid capsule to invade subcutaneous soft tissues, larynx, trachea, esophagus, or recurrent laryngeal nerve
T4$_b$	Tumor invades prevertebral fascia or encases carotid artery or mediastinal vessels
TX	Primary tumor size unknown, but without extrathyroidal invasion
N0	No metastatic nodes
N1$_a$	Metastases to level VI (pretracheal, paratracheal, and prelaryngeal/Delphian lymph nodes)
N1$_b$	Metastasis to unilateral, bilateral, contralateral cervical, or superior mediastinal mode metastases
NX	Nodes not assessed at surgery
M0	No distant metastases
M1	Distant metastases
MX	Distant metastases not assessed

Stages	Patient age <45 yr	Patient aged ≥45 yr
Stage I	Any T, any N, M0	T1, N0, M0
Stage II	Any T, any N, M1	T2, N0, M0
Stage III		T3, N0, M0
		T1, N1$_a$, M0
		T2, N1$_a$, M0
		T3, N1$_a$, M0
Stage IVA		T4$_a$, N0, M0
		T4$_a$, N1$_a$, M0
		T1, N1$_b$, M0
		T2, N1$_b$, M0
		T3, N1$_b$, M0
		T4$_a$, N1$_b$, M0
Stage IVB		T4$_b$, Any N, M0
Stage IVC		Any T, Any N, M1

From AJCC cancer staging manual. 6th edition. New York: Springer-Verlag; 2002: with permission.

risk of recurrence and metastatic spread. Information obtained during the initial therapy (such as the intraoperative findings, histopathologic description, RAI scan results, and postoperative serum thyroglobulin) permit accurate staging of the disease and therefore facilitate proper risk stratification for further therapy and follow-up.

Primary surgical considerations regarding extent of thyroid resection

Because of the high prevalence of metastatic cervical lymph node involvement in differentiated thyroid cancer, several of the guidelines recommend routine preoperative ultrasonographic evaluation of neck lymph nodes to properly plan surgical intervention [11,25,26]. Preoperative ultrasound (US) identifies suspicious cervical adenopathy in 20% to 30% of cases and in some cases alters the planned surgical approach [38,39]. Because US is used in nearly all patients as routine follow-up in the postoperative period, it seems wise to use the US to identify clinically significant lymph nodes preoperatively so they can be addressed with the primary surgical procedure. We need to be careful that preoperative US does not lead to an overly aggressive surgical approach to small lateral neck lymph nodes that may be of little clinical consequence and are likely to be easily treated with subsequent radioactive iodine remnant ablation (RRA).

Routine preoperative use of other cross-sectional imaging studies or 2-(18F)fluoro-2-deoxy-D-glucose–positron emission tomography (18 FDG PET) scanning is not routinely warranted unless clinical features suggest locally invasive disease that may benefit from more careful preoperative planning [11,25,26]. Preoperative assessment of vocal cord function should be a mandatory part of the work-up of any patient who has thyroid cancer [11]. Finally, preoperative evaluation of serum thyroglobulin is not routinely recommended [25].

For more than 50 years, the debate regarding the optimal extent of surgical resection has raged. Potential arguments in support of total thyroidectomy usually include:

- Papillary thyroid cancer is often a bilateral, multifocal disease. Therefore, the remaining contralateral lobe is a potential site of recurrences after unilateral thyroid resection.
- Improved sensitivity for disease detection and ease of follow-up using serum Tg after RRA
- Lower local recurrence rates after bilateral resection even in low-risk patients in some [40] but not all series [41]

Potential arguments in favor of a unilateral thyroid procedure usually include:

- Lack of substantial survival benefit for total thyroidectomy, particularly in low-risk patients
- In low-risk patients, highly sensitive disease detection tools are not required because the overall prognosis is so excellent.
- Recurrences that develop in low-risk patients will probably be detected early with neck ultrasonography and treated effectively with no substantial impact on overall survival
- Lower risk of complications, such as hypoparathyroidism or recurrent laryngeal nerve damage with a unilateral procedure

The various published guidelines provide rather uniform recommendations in this regard. Each guideline gives several specific factors that should lead toward consideration for total thyroidectomy (compared in Table 4).

Table 4
Indications for total (near total) thyroidectomy for papillary thyroid cancer

Guideline	Age (yr)	History of radiation exposure	Family history DTC	Bilateral thyroid nodules	Bilateral thyroid cancer	Tumor size (cm)	Unfavorable histology	Multifocality	Extrathyroidal extension	Cervical metastasis	Distant metastasis
NCCN 2006	<15, >45	✓	✓	—	✓	>4	✓	—	✓	✓	✓
ATA 2006[a]	>45	✓	✓	✓	—	1–1.5	—	—	✓	✓	✓
ETA 2006[a]	—	✓	✓	—	—	>1	✓	✓	✓	✓	✓
BTA 2002	—	✓	✓	✓	✓	>1	—	✓	✓	✓	✓
AACE[a] 2001	—	—	—	—	—	—	—	—	✓	✓	✓

The presence of any one of worrisome features (✓) favors a total thyroidectomy over a unilateral procedure.

Abbreviations: AACE, American Association of Clinical Endocrinologists; ATA, American Thyroid Association; BTA, British Thyroid Association and Royal College of Surgeons; ETA, European Thyroid Association; NCCN, National Comprehensive Cancer Network; –, variable not used.

[a] Indications for total thyroidectomy include "high risk" in any of the usual staging systems, which could incorporate tumor size, age at diagnosis, and multifocality.

There is fairly uniform agreement that for papillary thyroid cancer, total (near total) thyroidectomy is generally the preferred operation unless the tumor is well differentiated, small, confined to the thyroid gland without unfavorable histology (eg, poorly differentiated, insular, tall cell variant), vascular invasion, or metastatic spread to regional lymph nodes or distant sites.

For follicular thyroid cancer (FTC), unilateral thyroid surgery is deemed acceptable for small tumors with minimal capsular invasion (Table 5). Total thyroidectomy and RRA are recommended for follicular thyroid cancer with significant capsular or vascular invasion.

Completion thyroidectomy should be recommended for patients in whom a total thyroidectomy would have been the proper surgery had the correct preoperative diagnosis been available [25]. This situation may arise if a unilateral surgery was done because the preoperative fine-needle aspiration was suspicious for malignancy, inadequate, or demonstrated follicular neoplasia. This situation can also arise if a small tumor, presumed to be a well differentiated papillary thyroid cancer in a low-risk patient who would have otherwise been effectively treated with a unilateral procedure, proves to have unfavorable histology, vascular invasion, microscopic extrathyroidal extension, or lymph node metastases in the final pathology report.

Primary surgical considerations regarding extent of lymph node resection

Compartment-oriented lymph node dissections are recommended in all the guidelines for patients who have known lymph node metastases detected on preoperative staging or intraoperatively. The guidelines uniformly agree that functional neck dissection is preferred over "berry picking" and that

Table 5
Patients who have follicular thyroid cancer

Guideline	Indications for total thyroidectomy	Less than total thyroidectomy considered acceptable
NCCN 2006	All FTC other than the minimally invasive tumor described to the right	Minimally invasive tumor with capsular invasion or a few foci of vascular invasion
ATA 2006[a]	No recommendations specific for FTC[a]	No recommendations specific for FTC[a]
ETA 2006[a]	No recommendations specific for FTC[a]	No recommendations specific for FTC[a]
BTA 2002	Primary tumor > 1 cm; widely invasive characteristics	Minimally invasive; primary tumor size < 1 cm
AACE 2001	All FTC with extensive capsular or any vascular invasion	Minimally invasive with only limited capsular invasion

Abbreviations: AACE, American Association of Clinical Endocrinologists; ATA, American Thyroid Association; BTA, British Thyroid Association and Royal College of Surgeons; ETA, European Thyroid Association; NCCN, National Comprehensive Cancer Network.
[a] Recommendations for differentiated thyroid cancer (papillary and follicular cancers considered as one group).

radical neck dissection is rarely indicated. All the guidelines note that this approach decreases the risk of recurrence in low-risk patients and may prolong survival in high-risk patients.

The BTA and the ATA argue that the potential increased risk of hypoparathyroidism and recurrent laryngeal nerve injury is small in experienced hands; therefore, a strong argument can be made that central-neck lymph nodes should be routinely dissected in all patients [24,25]. The ETA notes that routine central-neck dissection may also provide useful staging information that may guide subsequent treatment and follow-up [26]. The other guidelines recommend central compartment clearance only in patients who have documented metastatic disease because of the lack of proof that central-neck dissection prolongs survival and concerns regarding excessive morbidity, particularly in low-risk patients [11,26,27]. None of the guidelines recommends prophylactic lateral neck dissection for patients who have differentiated thyroid cancer.

Radioactive iodine remnant ablation

The use of radioactive iodine in the postthyroidectomy setting to destroy residual thyroid bed tissue has become known as radioactive iodine remnant ablation (RRA). Because RRA has been shown in selected patients to decrease recurrence rates [22,42–46] and decrease disease-specific mortality [22,42,44–46], it must also have a tumoricidal effect beyond destroying the microscopic residual thyroid cells remaining after a total thyroidectomy. Often, this microscopic disease is detected only on the posttherapy scan, thus improving the accuracy of initial staging of the patient [47]. Furthermore, destruction of all residual thyroid tissue increases the sensitivity and specificity of follow-up testing, such as serum thyroglobulin and RAI scanning.

Although there is agreement that RRA has a beneficial effect in high-risk patients, there continues to be controversy regarding the benefit of RAI in lower-risk patients (Table 6). Several studies have failed to demonstrate an improvement in recurrence or survival when RRA is restricted to low-risk patients [3,23,45,48–50]. When analyzed carefully the patients who seem to benefit the most from RRA in terms of decreased recurrence rate and possible disease-specific survival improvement have tumors greater than 1.5 cm or a high likelihood of residual microscopic disease remaining after appropriate surgery [5,23,42,51].

With regard to specific recommendations in low-risk patients, the guidelines generally agree that the lowest risk, small, intrathyroidal, well differentiated, papillary thyroid cancers do not require RRA (see Table 6). These are essentially the same tumors that are adequately treated with unilateral thyroid surgery without the requirement for total thyroidectomy.

Using a simple size criteria of greater than 1 to 1.5 cm of the primary tumor as recommended by the NCCN and the BTA [11,24] would subject

Table 6
Recommendations regarding selection of patients for radioactive iodine remnant ablation

Guideline	Very low risk[a]	Low risk	High risk
NCCN 2006	Not recommended	Recommended if postop diagnostic WBS shows thyroid bed uptake or metastatic disease or stimulated Tg >1 ng/mL	Recommended if postop diagnostic WBS shows thyroid bed uptake or metastatic disease or stimulated Tg >1 ng/mL
ATA 2006	Not recommended	Recommended for most TNM stage II, selected stage I[b]	Recommended for all TNM Stage III and IV[b]
ETA 2006	Not recommended	Probably if <18 yr old or if primary tumor is 1–4 cm confined to the thyroid, or unfavorable histology	Recommended if extrathyroidal invasion, lymph node or distant metastases, incomplete resection
BTA 2002	Not recommended	Majority of patients who have tumor >1 cm should receive RRA	Majority of patients who have tumor >1 cm should receive RRA
AACE 2001	–	Remains unsettled	All high risk

Abbreviations: AACE, American Association of Clinical Endocrinologists; ATA, American Thyroid Association; BTA, British Thyroid Association and Royal College of Surgeons; ETA, European Thyroid Association; NCCN, National Comprehensive Cancer Network; WBS, whole body scan.

[a] *Data from* Pacini F, Schlumberger M, Dralle H, et al. European consensus for the management of patients with differentiated thyroid carcinoma of the follicular epithelium. Eur J Endocrinol 2006;154:787–803.

[b] See Table 3 for TNM staging definitions.

many low-risk patients who have well differentiated intrathyroidal disease to the risks of RAI without a proven, tangible benefit beyond ease of follow-up for their clinician. Conversely, a few patients who have primary tumors less than 1.5 cm with aggressive features that should receive RRA would be undertreated. The ATA guidelines address this issue by noting that selected stage I (<2 cm primary) may also benefit if they demonstrate worrisome features such as multifocal disease, nodal metastases, extrathyroidal extension, vascular invasion, or more aggressive histologies [25]. Likewise, the ETA would consider RRA for small tumors with extrathyroidal extension or unfavorable histology [26].

The NCCN guidelines take a slightly different approach. They recommend consideration of RRA in most papillary thyroid cancers greater than 1 cm but would withhold the ablative dose of RAI if the postsurgical diagnostic scan obtained before RRA showed no uptake in the thyroid bed (or evidence of disease outside the thyroid bed) and the serum Tg was less than 1 ng/mL with thyroid-stimulating hormone (TSH) stimulation [11]. The logic is that if the primary utility of RRA in low-risk patients is to facilitate follow-up and early detection of disease and if surgery has rendered the RAI scan negative and the serum Tg undetectable, there is little reason to proceed with RAI. This approach seems sound, but in our experience, minor uptake in the thyroid bed (< 1%) is seen in the majority of patients evaluated for RRA at our institution. Therefore, this approach would avoid RRA in few of our patients.

Even though RRA is unlikely to improve the already excellent disease-specific survival rate in low-risk patients and the data indicating a significant decrease in recurrence is less than definitive, many continue to recommend RRA in these patients to improve the sensitivity and specificity of follow-up testing. This decision must be made on a case-by-case basis while weighing the risks of radioactive iodine administration with the likelihood of recurrence based on all available clinical data.

In summary, RRA is not recommended for small (< 1–2 cm), intrathyroidal, well differentiated papillary thyroid cancer without evidence for worrisome histologic features or evidence of metastases outside the thyroid. Similarly, RRA is routinely recommended for patients at high risk of death from disease as classified by any of the usual clinicopathologic staging systems. The utility of RRA in low-risk patients continues to be an area of intense debate. Given the lack of data demonstrating a survival benefit or a clear-cut decrease in recurrence, the primary benefit of RRA in low-risk patients seems to be improved sensitivity and specificity for disease detection during follow-up. The actual magnitude and the clinical importance of this potential benefit must be determined on a case-by-case basis with low-risk patients so that they clearly understand the controversies involved and the difficulty in assessing the risk-to-benefit ratio for their specific case.

Details of radioactive iodine remnant ablation

Most of the guidelines recommended a low iodine before RRA, but the duration varied from 1 to 4 weeks (Table 7). The ATA and ETA noted that thyroid hormone withdrawal or recombinant human TSH (rhTSH) stimulation was acceptable for routine RRA [25,26], whereas the NCCN, BTA, and AACE did not discuss the possible use of rhTSH as preparation for remnant ablation [11,24,27].

With regard to diagnostic whole-body scanning before ablation, there was general concern for stunning with higher doses of 131I and each of the guidelines recommended using low-dose 131I (1–3 mCi) or 123I as tracer dose to try to minimize any potential stunning. Although the NCCN noted that diagnostic whole-body scans were generally done by member institutions, the ATA, ETA, and AACE recommended only performing diagnostic

Table 7
Details surrounding radioactive iodine remnant ablation

Guideline	Low iodine diet	Method of thyroid-stimulating hormone stimulation	Diagnostic WBS	Administered activity	Posttherapy scan
NCCN 2006	–	THW recommended, rhTSH not addressed	Generally done by most institutions	Dose not specified	Recommended timing not specified
ATA 2006	1–2 wk	THW or rhTSH is acceptable	Should be used if needed to assess amount of thyroid remnant or if the results of scan would alter the decision to treat or the administered activity recommendation	30–100 mCi with higher doses (100–200 mCi) for more aggressive tumor histology	5–8 d after therapy
ETA 2006	3 wk	THW or rhTSH is acceptable	Only if needed to assess amount of thyroid remnant	30–100 mCi	3–5 d after therapy
BTA 2002	Recommended, duration not specified	THW recommended, rhTSH not addressed	Can be done, not required	100 mCi	3–5 d after therapy
AACE 2001	2–4 wk	TWH recommended, rhTSH not addressed	Done to determine administered activity	30–150 mCi	4–10 d after therapy

Abbreviations: AACE, American Association of Clinical Endocrinologists; ATA, American Thyroid Association; BTA, British Thyroid Association and Royal College of Surgeons; ETA, European Thyroid Association; NCCN, National Comprehensive Cancer Network; rhTSH, recombinant human TSH; THW, thyroid hormone withdrawal.

whole-body scans before RRA if the results of the scan were likely to change the administered activity of RAI administered or the need to perform RRA.

A posttherapy scan, done 3 to 8 days after RRA, was recommended by each guideline to detect metastatic lesions not seen on routine low dose diagnostic whole-body scans [47].

The recommended administered activities for routine RRA varied from 30 to 200 mCi, with a median value that approximates 100 mCi for the average patient. The ATA noted that higher doses may be considered for more aggressive tumor histologies [25].

Role for external beam irradiation in initial therapy

In the setting of initial therapy, external beam radiation is seldom necessary in patients who have papillary thyroid cancer [52]. The guidelines are in agreement that external beam radiation therapy (EBRT) is most often used for unresectable tumors that do not concentrate RAI or for older patients (>45 years) who have evidence of gross extrathyroidal extension of the tumor into surrounding structures that are likely to have microscopic or small-volume macroscopic disease that is not amenable to RAI therapy. The ETA provides guidance as to specific dosing, recommending a total dose of 50 to 60 Gy to the neck and upper mediastinum with a boost of 5 to 10 Gy to areas of gross residual disease [26].

Role of thyroid-stimulating hormone suppressive therapy

Suppression of TSH with supraphysiologic doses of levothyroxine to decrease the rate of progression and recurrence of thyroid cancer has been a cornerstone of treatment for more than 40 years [53,54]. Retrospective studies suggest that TSH suppression to less than 0.1 mU/L may be beneficial in high-risk patients [55,56], but the benefit of aggressive TSH suppression is much less clear in low-risk patients. Although all would agree that it is wise to avoid prolonged elevations in TSH, the precise level of TSH suppression required for low-risk patients has not been adequately defined.

Largely because the risk for atrial fibrillation and osteoporosis in older patients seems to rise when the TSH falls below 0.1 mU/L, the ATA and ACCE recommend a goal TSH of 0.1 to 0.4 mU/L for all patients except high-risk patients who have a goal TSH of less than 0.1 mU/L [25,27]. Although the NCCN does not give specific target goals, they note that low-risk patients should be titrated to achieve a TSH just below the lower bound of the reference range [11].

The ETA and the BTA recommend suppression of TSH to less than 0.1 mU/L in all patients, but the ETA notes that after 3 to 5 years of disease-free survival, the TSH suppression may be lessened even in high-risk patients. Similarly, low-risk patients who have had several years of disease-free survival can be titrated to a TSH between 0.5 and 1 mU/L [24,26].

Commonly used tests to detect recurrent/persistent disease

Serum thyroglobulin

As newer assays with improving sensitivities have become commercially available over the last 10 to 20 years, serum Tg determination has become the primary marker of differentiated thyroid cancer [57]. Although Tg is an excellent marker for well differentiated thyroid cancer, poorly differentiated tumors can produce Tg poorly and can evidence clinically significant recurrent disease with minimal Tg elevations [58]. Not all thyroid cancer recurrences that are detected with high-resolution US, without an associated rise in serum Tg, represent poorly differentiated thyroid cancer. For example, a careful neck US can identify metastatic well differentiated thyroid cancer in small cervical lymph nodes that are producing little, if any, measurable thyroglobulin [59].

The sensitivity for disease detection is improved with TSH stimulation with thyroid hormone withdrawal or rhTSH [60]. As more highly sensitivity Tg assays become available, additional studies will be required to determine if TSH stimulation improves the sensitivity for disease detection.

From a practical standpoint, it is critical that the Tg be measured serially in the same laboratory. Marked variations in serum Tg values are reported when the same blood samples are analyzed using different Tg assays [61].

The presence of anti-Tg antibodies continues to be a problem in at least 20% of patients who have thyroid cancer [62]. Because Tg antibodies can interfere with the measurement of Tg, most often causing false low Tg values in the commercially available assays, it is imperative the Tg antibodies be measured with every Tg determination. If the Tg antibodies are positive, the reliability of the Tg value is suspect and should be considered likely to be a falsely low value. Quantitative measurement of Tg antibodies as a surrogate tumor marker seems to have clinical validity because Tg antibodies usually decline over several years in patients who are free of disease and have been reported to rise before clinical detection of recurrent disease [62].

Routine diagnostic whole-body scan

The last 10 years has seen a marked paradigm shift away from routine diagnostic whole-body scanning and toward stimulated serum Tg and neck ultrasonography for the detection of thyroid cancer, especially in low-risk patients. Neither the ETA, the ATA, nor the NCCN recommend a routine diagnostic whole-body scan 1 year after RRA in low-risk patients who have a negative neck US and negative stimulated serum Tg [11,25,26]. They note that diagnostic whole-body scan may be of some utility in the follow-up of patients who have intermediate to high risk of having persistent disease [25,26]. From the European perspective, a diagnostic whole-body scan is unlikely to provide meaningful information in the absence of other evidence of recurrent disease and is therefore not routinely recommended as a screen for recurrent disease [26].

Cervical ultrasonography

Cervical ultrasonography is becoming the primary structural imaging modality in patients who have thyroid cancer [63]. Several of the guidelines note that a combination of serum Tg measurement and routine neck ultrasonography have excellent sensitivity and negative predictive value (NPV) in the follow-up of low-risk patients [11,25–27]. The ETA and the ATA recommend neck ultrasonography as part of routine follow-up care 6 and 12 months after RRA, and the ATA suggests to use US yearly for 3 to 5 years depending on the risk for recurrence and the Tg status of the individual patient [25].

Postoperative neck ultrasonography is user dependent, and dedicated ultrasonographers with a specific interest in thyroid disease and thyroid pathology are required to achieve the sensitivity reported in most of the large series. Postthyroidectomy US needs to evaluate not only the thyroid bed, but also the central and lateral cervical node compartments. Because of the marked dependence on the skill of the operator, many surgeons, endocrinologists, and nuclear medicine specialists are increasingly using intra-office US to achieve the high levels of sensitivity and specificity for the detection of recurrent disease.

(18F)fluoro-2-deoxy-D-glucose–positron emission tomography scanning

18 FDG PET scanning is seldom indicated in the initial therapy of patients who have well differentiated thyroid cancer [64,65]. A wealth of studies have demonstrated that 18 FDG PET scanning is best used to localize poorly differentiated thyroid cancer that is usually non-RAI avid. Even though 18 FDG PET scanning in thyroid cancer is generally reimbursed by insurance companies only for patients who have follicular-derived thyroid cancers with a serum Tg greater than 10 ng/mL (stimulated or suppressed is generally not specified) and a negative diagnostic whole-body scan, we also use 18 FDG PET scanning as an initial staging tool in poorly differentiated thyroid cancer and Hurthle cell thyroid cancers as an adjunct to RAI scanning, serum Tg, and other cross-sectional imaging studies. Additionally, 18 FDG PET scanning may help identify patients who would benefit from EBRT due to persistent FDG avid disease in the neck in the postoperative setting, even if all evidence of gross disease has been removed [52]. Finally, patients who have metastatic disease that is markedly FDG avid are unresponsive to high-dose RAI therapy [66] and have poor outcomes, with disease-free survival rates often less than 2 to 3 years [67].

Follow-up strategy for detecting persistent/recurrent disease

Follow-up paradigms for detecting recurrent disease are usually based on whether the patient is considered high risk or low risk for death from disease. Although these approaches are useful, it may be more instructive to base the follow-up strategy on an understanding of the biology of the tumor and likely sites of recurrence. For example, a 25-year-old woman with a 3-cm papillary thyroid cancer involving several lymph nodes at diagnosis is likely to have a well differentiated tumor that should concentrate RAI well, make considerable amounts of thyroglobulin, and have a high propensity for recurrence in cervical lymph nodes. Although the patient is AJCC stage I and at low risk of death from disease, her age at diagnosis, the size of the primary tumor, and the presence of lymph node metastasis places her at significant risk for recurrence. Therefore, after total thyroidectomy and RRA, a follow-up strategy that relies primarily on serum Tg (suppressed or stimulated) and neck ultrasonography is likely to have high sensitivity for the detection of disease and high negative predictive value (NPV) to identify patients likely to be cured and in need of less aggressive follow-up.

Conversely, a 65-year-old man who has a 5-cm papillary thyroid cancer with gross extrathyroidal extension involving the tracheal wall (AJCC stage IVA) at initial diagnosis is much more likely to have a more poorly differentiated thyroid cancer that may or may not produce significant amounts of thyroglobulin; is less likely to concentrate RAI; and could recur in the neck, lungs, bone, brain or other sites. Therefore, the follow-up strategy for this high-risk patient would include not only serum Tg and neck ultrasonography but also cross-sectional imaging of the brain, neck, and chest and probably 18 FDG PET scanning to detect metastatic lesions that are likely to be metabolic active and therefore seen on the 18 FDG PET scan but missed by RAI scanning.

Risk for recurrence should be reevaluated over time based on the length of disease-free interval since initial therapy and the cumulative NPV of the various follow-up tests. One of the problems of the staging systems is that they do not do include variables to modify the risk for death or risk for recurrence based on important additional clinical data accumulated over the years. Although all patients who have thyroid cancer require life-long follow-up because of the well known risk of late recurrences after as long as 30 to 40 years, the intensity of the follow-up can decrease as disease-free time passes.

The optimal follow-up strategy would emphasize studies that have a high sensitivity for early detection of recurrent disease and high NPVs for disease recurrence so that patients at low risk of recurrence can be identified as early as possible and followed with less aggressive testing.

There is general agreement among the various guidelines with respect to the general follow-up strategy, particularly in low-risk patients. Table 8 presents the essence of the follow-up recommendations across the various guidelines based on a typical risk stratification strategy. After total thyroidectomy and RRA, the primary follow-up in 6 to 12 months consists of neck ultrasonography and suppressed serum Tg. If either of these tests indicates

Table 8
Follow-up strategy based on risk stratification

	Very low risk	Low risk	Intermediate	High risk
General definition	<1 cm, probably treated with lobectomy [26]	No local or distant metastasis, all tumor resected, no extrathyroidal extension, no aggressive histology, and if RRA done, no uptake outside the thyroid bed [25]	Microscopic extrathyroidal extension at initial surgery, or aggressive histologies [25]	Gross extrathyroidal extension, incomplete tumor resection, uptake outside the thyroid bed on post-RRA scan, local or distant metastasis [25]
Suppressed Tg	6–12 mo, then periodically	Every 6–12 mo the first year, frequency after that not defined for those free of disease, probably yearly	Every 6–12 mo for first 1–2 yr, then yearly	Every 6–12 mo for first 3–5 yr, then yearly
Stimulated Tg	Not useful	At 12 mo if suppressed Tg is undetectable. No need for stimulated Tg alone if Tg is detectable	At 12 mo if suppressed Tg is undetectable. No need for stimulated Tg alone if Tg is detectable	At 12 mo if suppressed Tg is undetectable. No need for stimulated Tg alone if Tg is detectable
Neck ultrasonography	Yes, probably yearly or less frequently	6 mo, 12 mo, then yearly for 3–5 yr	6 mo, 12 mo, then yearly for 3–5 yr	6 mo, 12 mo, then yearly for 3–5 yr
Diagnostic whole-body scan	Not useful	Not required if stimulated Tg is negative and neck ultrasound is normal	May be helpful	May be helpful

Abbreviation: RRA, radioactive iodine remnant ablation.

persistent disease, then additional studies to localize and potentially treat the persistent disease with appropriate surgery, RAI, or EBRT is in order.

If the neck US is negative and the suppressed serum Tg is undetectable, low-risk patients can be followed with stimulated Tg alone (without diagnostic whole-body scanning), whereas intermediate- to high-risk patients may benefit from the addition of diagnostic whole-body scanning to the stimulated Tg testing. An undetectable stimulated serum Tg is reassuring and likely reflects the absence of detectable thyroid cancer.

The disease-free patient could then be followed with suppressed Tg every 6 to 12 months and neck US yearly for a period of time based on the risk of recurrence. Even in low-risk patients, the minimum follow-up would include physical examination and suppressed serum Tg on a yearly basis for the rest of their life. In high-risk patients who are likely to recur with poorly differentiated tumors that make little if any Tg and may or may not concentrate RAI, additional cross-sectional imaging or FDG PET scanning may be warranted.

Treatment options for persistent/recurrent disease

In the setting of clinically recurrent thyroid cancer, each of the guidelines endorses consideration of additional surgery if lesions are resectable and consideration of additional RAI if the lesions are likely to be RAI avid. Likewise, each guideline agrees that EBRT is usually only considered if the recurrent disease is not surgically resectable and is likely to be unresponsive to RAI. Therefore, initial investigations searching for persistent/recurrent disease should focus on neck US and cross-sectional imaging without iodinated contrast to identify structurally apparent disease that may require specific therapy (eg, surgery or EBRT) before additional RAI is contemplated. Once the structural imaging is complete, RAI scanning may be useful to localize small-volume disease and identify RAI avid lesions that may respond to additional RAI therapy.

In low- to moderate-risk patients, recurrence of thyroid cancer is usually heralded by a rising serum Tg (or failure of Tg to become undetectable after initial treatment) and is detected as small abnormal cervical lymph nodes on ultrasonography. In many of these patients, the diagnostic whole-body scan is negative; these are the so-called "Tg-positive, scan-negative" patients. For enlarging metastatic lymph nodes larger than 1 cm, we routinely recommend surgical resection because a single additional dose of RAI is unlikely to completely destroy lymph nodes of this size. For smaller lymph nodes, or for recurrent disease manifest only as rising serum Tg without corresponding structurally evident disease, we consider a second empiric dose of RAI (100–150 mCi) to localize the disease on posttherapy scan but also with hopes of having some therapeutic effect. If the abnormal lymph nodes resolve, then continued follow-up is in order. If the lymph nodes enlarge 6 months after RAI, surgical removal is considered.

These recommendations are consistent with ATA guidelines that recommend consideration of empiric RAI (100–200 mCi) for stimulated Tg values greater than 10 ng/mL after thyroid hormone withdrawal or greater than 5 ng/mL after rhTSH in an effort to localize disease on the posttherapy scan [25]. Similarly, the ETA recommends empiric RAI if the stimulated Tg is rising and above the "institutional cut off" after RRA [26], whereas the BTA reserves empiric RAI therapy for a "rising" Tg with a negative whole-body scan [24]. The NCCN guidelines recognize that this is a common clinical practice, but no study has demonstrated a decrease in morbidity or mortality from empiric RAI therapy of scan-negative patients [11]. The AACE guidelines note that there remains considerable controversy regarding the role of high-dose RAI in scan–negative, Tg-positive patients [27].

Over recent years, 18 FDG PET scanning has been demonstrated to have an important role in detecting non-RAI avid disease that is manifest primarily by persistent serum Tg levels [64,65]. In most studies, FDT PET scan identifies a metastatic lesion in 75% to 80% of Tg-positive, scan-negative patients. The sensitivity improves with suppressed Tg values greater than 10 ng/mL and in the setting of non–well differentiated tumors. Most insurance companies in the United States approve 18 FDG PET scanning for thyroid cancer provided the patient has a follicular-derived thyroid cancer, a Tg value great than 10 ng/mL (stimulated or suppressed not usually specified), and a negative diagnostic whole-body scan. The ATA endorses surgical resection of locally recurrent disease for palliation and prevention of gross invasion into the aero-digestive tract even in the presence of untreatable distant metastases [25].

As our tools for detection of persistent disease improve, we can find low-level Tg values in many patients who would have previously been thought to be disease free [25]. Often these low-risk patients have barely detectable level Tg values that are difficult to eradicate, even with aggressive surgery and repeated doses of RAI. Many patients who have low-level suppressed Tg values (less than about 5 ng/mL) with a negative diagnostic whole-body scan and negative neck ultrasonography see a gradual decline in Tg over a period of 5 to 10 years if they are followed with observation alone [68].

As discussed in the ATA guidelines, the clinical significance of these sub-centimeter neck lymph nodes and persistent low level Tg values without evidence of structural disease remains unknown [25]. Because our potential treatments may have significant side effects and because the benefit or aggressive treatment has yet to be proven, our practice is to use the highly sensitive detection tests, such as stimulated Tg and neck ultrasonography, to identify persistent/recurrent disease but to reserve active intervention for documented growth of small asymptomatic lymph nodes to at least 1 cm on serial US evaluations or evidence of rising serum Tg over time. In this way, we can identify patients who have clinically evident progressive disease and subject them to the risks and benefits of additional treatment while avoiding the risks of unnecessary treatment in many low-risk patients who have low-level disease that may or may not ever become clinically significant.

Treatment options for distant metastases

Although distant metastases are present in only 3% to 5% of patients who have papillary thyroid cancer at diagnosis, they can become evident in as many as 9% to 10% of patients who have papillary thyroid cancer and in as many as 20% of patients who have follicular thyroid cancer during the course of follow-up. In young patients, the pulmonary metastases often present as small, military, diffuse lesions throughout both lungs that usually respond well to repeated doses of RAI [69]. RAI is much less effective at destroying macroscopic pulmonary metastases, particularly when they arise in older patients who have less well differentiated disease. Often, even with continued TSH suppression, non-RAI avid macroscopic pulmonary metastases grow slowly over many years. 18 FDG PET scanning has been shown to accurately identify the non-RAI–responsive metastatic lesions that are metabolically active, destined to more rapid growth, and predictive of death from disease within a few years [66,67]. Patients who have structurally progressive macroscopic metastatic disease that is not responsive to RAI should be referred for consideration of a clinical trial or other systemic therapy (see article on novel therapies found elsewhere in this issue).

In the follow-up of patients who have distant metastases, it is important to pay particular attention to lesions that are in areas where continued growth into surrounding structures would result in serious morbidity. These include lesions in the brain, spinal column, weight-bearing bones, upper mediastinum near the great vessels, and in the tracheoesophageal groove. Progressive growth in individual metastatic lesions can result in acute neurovascular compromise, such as spinal cord compression, nerve root compression, superior vena cava syndrome, or an acute central nervous system event from brain metastases. Often the acute symptoms respond to high-dose glucocorticoid therapy followed by surgical resection or external beam irradiation. Usually, these medical emergencies are most rapidly palliated with surgical resection of the offending metastatic lesion. Depending on the clinical situation, the overall rate of disease progression, and other underlying medical conditions, urgent EBRT is also a reasonable palliative measure. Although resection or EBRT to these lesions in the setting of widespread distant metastases is not curative, appropriate treatment can avert serious neurovascular symptoms or prevent seriously morbid complications.

Summary

The last 10 years have seen a number of major paradigm shifts in the management of thyroid cancer. This is largely secondary to the more widespread use of highly sensitive detection tools, such as neck ultrasonography, highly sensitive Tg assays, and 18 FDG PET scanning in routine clinical practice. In addition, the ability to offer RAI studies, radioactive iodine remnant ablation, and stimulated Tg measurements with rhTSH rather than traditional thyroid hormone withdrawal has allowed many patients to obtain necessary studies and treatments without experiencing thyroid hormone withdrawal symptoms. More importantly, the last 5 years have seen a renewed focus on potential novel therapies for progressive non-RAI avid metastatic disease with a dramatic increase in preclinical studies and in the availability of clinical trials specifically for patients who have thyroid cancer.

Improvements in disease detection techniques result in a greater appreciation for low-level persistent disease in a great many patients. This creates anxiety for the patient and the treating physician to do something to make the Tg undetectable and remove all potentially abnormal neck lymph nodes. This pressure has led to many repeat neck surgeries and many additional doses of RAI over the last 10 years. Despite additional therapy, many patients are left with low-level persistent disease that cannot be easily eradicated using our current treatment approaches.

Our challenge over the next 10 years is to identify which of these patients who have low-level persistent disease is likely to have clinically significant disease progression during their lifetime. Proper identification of these patients is critical so that additional therapy can be offered to patients who are likely to have poor long-term outcomes while offering careful, thoughtful observation to patients who are likely to have excellent outcomes without the added risks of additional RAI or additional surgery.

Although an improved understanding of the molecular characteristics of the tumors at time of diagnosis is likely to provide additional prognostic information, proper ongoing risk stratification that is clinically meaningful requires novel risk stratification schemes. Staging systems that incorporate not only the usual tumor and patient risk factors available during initial therapy, but more importantly include variables that assess response to therapy, progression-free survival, trend in serum Tg over time, and the NPV of the various tests used in the follow-up of differentiated patients who have thyroid cancer, will greatly enhance our ability to tailor specific treatment and follow-up recommendations for individual patients.

References

[1] American Cancer Society. Cancer facts and figures 2006. 2006; Available at: www.cancer.org. Accessed November 1, 2006.
[2] Ries LA, Harkins D, Krapcho M, et al. SEER cancer statistics review, 1975–2003, based on November 2005 SEER data submission. 2006; Available at: http://seer.cancer.gov/csr/1975_2003/. Accessed November 1, 2006.
[3] Hundahl SA, Cady B, Cunningham MP, et al. Initial results from a prospective cohort study of 5583 cases of thyroid carcinoma treated in the United States during 1996. U.S. and German Thyroid Cancer Study Group. An American College of Surgeons Commission on Cancer Patient Care Evaluation study. Cancer 2000;89(1):202–17.
[4] Gilliland FD, Hunt WC, Morris DM, et al. Prognostic factors for thyroid carcinoma: a population-based study of 15,698 cases from the Surveillance, Epidemiology and End Results (SEER) program 1973–1991. Cancer 1997;79(3):564–73.

[5] Mazzaferri EL, Kloos RT. Clinical review 128: current approaches to primary therapy for papillary and follicular thyroid cancer. J Clin Endocrinol Metab 2001;86(4): 1447–63.

[6] Davies L, Welch HG. Epidemiology of head and neck cancer in the United States. Otolaryngol Head Neck Surg 2006;135(3):451–7.

[7] Davies L, Welch HG. Increasing incidence of thyroid cancer in the United States, 1973–2002. JAMA 2006;295(18):2164–7.

[8] Schneider AB, Sarne DH. Long-term risks for thyroid cancer and other neoplasms after exposure to radiation. Nat Clin Pract Endocrinol Metab 2005;1(2):82–91.

[9] Nagataki S, Nystrom E. Epidemiology and primary prevention of thyroid cancer. Thyroid 2002;12(10):889–96.

[10] Sherman SI. Thyroid carcinoma. Lancet 2003;361(9356):501–11.

[11] Sherman SI. National Comprehensive Cancer Network, Clinical Practice Guidelines in Oncology, Thyroid Cancer V.2.2006. 2006; Available at: http://www.nccn.org/professionals/physician_gls/PDF/thyroid.pdf. Accessed November 1, 2006.

[12] Malchoff CD, Malchoff DM. Familial nonmedullary thyroid carcinoma. Cancer Control 2006;13(2):106–10.

[13] Chow SM, Law SC, Chan JK, et al. Papillary microcarcinoma of the thyroid: prognostic significance of lymph node metastasis and multifocality. Cancer 2003;98(1):31–40.

[14] Grebe SK, Hay ID. Thyroid cancer nodal metastases: biologic significance and therapeutic considerations. Surg Oncol Clin N Am 1996;5(1):43–63.

[15] Ito Y, Uruno T, Nakano K, et al. An observation trial without surgical treatment in patients with papillary microcarcinoma of the thyroid. Thyroid 2003;13(4):381–7.

[16] McConahey WM, Hay ID, Woolner LB, et al. Papillary thyroid cancer treated at the Mayo Clinic, 1946 through 1970: initial manifestations, pathologic findings, therapy, and outcome. Mayo Clin Proc 1986;61(12):978–96.

[17] Nam-Goong IS, Kim HY, Gong G, et al. Ultrasonography-guided fine-needle aspiration of thyroid incidentaloma: correlation with pathological findings. Clin Endocrinol (Oxf) 2004; 60(1):21–8.

[18] Scheumann GF, Gimm O, Wegener G, et al. Prognostic significance and surgical management of locoregional lymph node metastases in papillary thyroid cancer. World J Surg 1994;18(4):559–67 [discussion: 567–8].

[19] Arturi F, Russo D, Giuffrida D, et al. Early diagnosis by genetic analysis of differentiated thyroid cancer metastases in small lymph nodes. J Clin Endocrinol Metab 1997;82(5): 1638–41.

[20] Qubain SW, Nakano S, Baba M, et al. Distribution of lymph node micrometastasis in pN0 well-differentiated thyroid carcinoma. Surgery 2002;131(3):249–56.

[21] Hay ID. Papillary thyroid carcinoma. Endocrinol Metab Clin North Am 1990;19(3): 545–76.

[22] Mazzaferri EL, Jhiang SM. Long-term impact of initial surgical and medical therapy on papillary and follicular thyroid cancer. Am J Med 1994;97(5):418–28.

[23] Hay ID, Thompson GB, Grant CS, et al. Papillary thyroid carcinoma managed at the Mayo Clinic during six decades (1940–1999): temporal trends in initial therapy and long-term outcome in 2444 consecutively treated patients. World J Surg 2002;26(8): 879–85.

[24] BTA. British Thyroid Association and Royal College of Physicians: guidelines for the management of thyroid cancer in adults 2002. Available at: www.british-thyroid-association.org. Accessed November 1, 2006.

[25] Cooper DS, Doherty GM, Haugen BR, et al. Management guidelines for patients with thyroid nodules and differentiated thyroid cancer. Thyroid 2006;16(2):109–42.

[26] Pacini F, Schlumberger M, Dralle H, et al. European consensus for the management of patients with differentiated thyroid carcinoma of the follicular epithelium. Eur J Endocrinol 2006;154(6):787–803.

[27] ThyroidCarcinomaTaskForce. AACE/AAES medical/surgical guidelines for clinical practice: management of thyroid carcinoma. American Association of Clinical Endocrinologists. American College of Endocrinology. Endocr Pract 2001;7(3):202–20.

[28] Watkinson JC. The British Thyroid Association guidelines for the management of thyroid cancer in adults. Nucl Med Commun 2004;25(9):897–900.

[29] Brierley JD, Panzarella T, Tsang RW, et al. A comparison of different staging systems predictability of patient outcome: thyroid carcinoma as an example. Cancer 1997;79(12): 2414–23.

[30] Dean DS, Hay ID. Prognostic indicators in differentiated thyroid carcinoma. Cancer Control 2000;7(3):229–39.

[31] Byar DP, Green SB, Dor P, et al. A prognostic index for thyroid carcinoma: a study of the E.O.R.T.C. Thyroid Cancer Cooperative Group. Eur J Cancer 1979;15(8):1033–41.

[32] Hay ID, Grant CS, Taylor WF, et al. Ipsilateral lobectomy versus bilateral lobar resection in papillary thyroid carcinoma: a retrospective analysis of surgical outcome using a novel prognostic scoring system. Surgery 1987;102(6):1088–95.

[33] Cady B, Rossi R. An expanded view of risk-group definition in differentiated thyroid carcinoma. Surgery 1988;104(6):947–53.

[34] Hay ID, Bergstralh EJ, Goellner JR, et al. Predicting outcome in papillary thyroid carcinoma: development of a reliable prognostic scoring system in a cohort of 1779 patients surgically treated at one institution during 1940 through 1989. Surgery 1993;114(6):1050–7 [discussion: 1057–8].

[35] Shaha AR, Loree TR, Shah JP. Prognostic factors and risk group analysis in follicular carcinoma of the thyroid. Surgery 1995;118(6):1131–6 [discussion: 1136–8].

[36] Sherman SI, Brierley JD, Sperling M, et al. Prospective multicenter study of thyroid carcinoma treatment: initial analysis of staging and outcome. National Thyroid Cancer Treatment Cooperative Study Registry Group. Cancer 1998;83(5):1012–21.

[37] AJCC Cancer Staging Manual. 6th edition. New York: Springer-Verlag; 2002.

[38] Shimamoto K, Satake H, Sawaki A, et al. Preoperative staging of thyroid papillary carcinoma with ultrasonography. Eur J Radiol 1998;29(1):4–10.

[39] Solorzano CC, Carneiro DM, Ramirez M, et al. Surgeon-performed ultrasound in the management of thyroid malignancy. Am Surg 2004;70(7):576–80 [discussion: 580–2].

[40] Hay ID, Grant CS, Bergstralh EJ, et al. Unilateral total lobectomy: is it sufficient surgical treatment for patients with AMES low-risk papillary thyroid carcinoma? Surgery 1998; 124(6):958–64 [discussion: 964–6].

[41] Shaha AR, Shah JP, Loree TR. Low-risk differentiated thyroid cancer: the need for selective treatment. Ann Surg Oncol 1997;4(4):328–33.

[42] DeGroot LJ, Kaplan EL, McCormick M, et al. Natural history, treatment, and course of papillary thyroid carcinoma. J Clin Endocrinol Metab 1990;71(2):414–24.

[43] Mazzaferri EL, Jhiang SM. Differentiated thyroid cancer long-term impact of initial therapy. Trans Am Clin Climatol Assoc 1994;106:151–68 [discussion: 168–70].

[44] Samaan NA, Schultz PN, Hickey RC, et al. The results of various modalities of treatment of well differentiated thyroid carcinomas: a retrospective review of 1599 patients. J Clin Endocrinol Metab 1992;75(3):714–20.

[45] Sawka AM, Thephamongkhol K, Brouwers M, et al. Clinical review 170: a systematic review and metaanalysis of the effectiveness of radioactive iodine remnant ablation for well-differentiated thyroid cancer. J Clin Endocrinol Metab 2004;89(8):3668–76.

[46] Taylor T, Specker B, Robbins J, et al. Outcome after treatment of high-risk papillary and non-Hurthle-cell follicular thyroid carcinoma. Ann Intern Med 1998;129(8):622–7.

[47] Sherman SI, Tielens ET, Sostre S, et al. Clinical utility of posttreatment radioiodine scans in the management of patients with thyroid carcinoma. J Clin Endocrinol Metab 1994;78(3): 629–34.

[48] Kim S, Wei JP, Braveman JM, et al. Predicting outcome and directing therapy for papillary thyroid carcinoma. Arch Surg 2004;139(4):390–4 [discussion: 393–4].

[49] Sanders LE, Cady B. Differentiated thyroid cancer: reexamination of risk groups and outcome of treatment. Arch Surg 1998;133(4):419–25.

[50] Sugitani I, Fujimoto Y. Symptomatic versus asymptomatic papillary thyroid microcarcinoma: a retrospective analysis of surgical outcome and prognostic factors. Endocr J 1999;46(1):209–16.

[51] Mazzaferri EL. Thyroid remnant 131I ablation for papillary and follicular thyroid carcinoma. Thyroid 1997;7(2):265–71.

[52] Lee N, Tuttle RM. External beam radiation for differentiated thyroid cancer. Endocr Relat Cancer 2006;13(4):971–7.

[53] Biondi B, Filetti S, Schlumberger M. Thyroid-hormone therapy and thyroid cancer: a reassessment. Nat Clin Pract Endocrinol Metab 2005;1(1):32–40.

[54] McGriff NJ, Csako G, Gourgiotis L, et al. Effects of thyroid hormone suppression therapy on adverse clinical outcomes in thyroid cancer. Ann Med 2002;34(7–8):554–64.

[55] Cooper DS, Specker B, Ho M, et al. Thyrotropin suppression and disease progression in patients with differentiated thyroid cancer: results from the National Thyroid Cancer Treatment Cooperative Registry. Thyroid 1998;8(9):737–44.

[56] Pujol P, Daures JP, Nsakala N, et al. Degree of thyrotropin suppression as a prognostic determinant in differentiated thyroid cancer. J Clin Endocrinol Metab 1996;81(12):4318–23.

[57] Spencer CA. Serum thyroglobulin measurements: clinical utility and technical limitations in the management of patients with differentiated thyroid carcinomas. Endocr Pract 2000;6(6):481–4.

[58] Robbins RJ, Srivastava S, Shaha A, et al. Factors influencing the basal and recombinant human thyrotropin-stimulated serum thyroglobulin in patients with metastatic thyroid carcinoma. J Clin Endocrinol Metab 2004;89(12):6010–6.

[59] Pacini F, Molinaro E, Castagna MG, et al. Recombinant human thyrotropin-stimulated serum thyroglobulin combined with neck ultrasonography has the highest sensitivity in monitoring differentiated thyroid carcinoma. J Clin Endocrinol Metab 2003;88(8):3668–73.

[60] Mazzaferri EL, Robbins RJ, Spencer CA, et al. A consensus report of the role of serum thyroglobulin as a monitoring method for low-risk patients with papillary thyroid carcinoma. J Clin Endocrinol Metab 2003;88(4):1433–41.

[61] Spencer CA, Bergoglio LM, Kazarosyan M, et al. Clinical impact of thyroglobulin (Tg) and Tg autoantibody method differences on the management of patients with differentiated thyroid carcinomas. J Clin Endocrinol Metab 2005;90(10):5566–75.

[62] Spencer CA. Challenges of serum thyroglobulin (Tg) measurement in the presence of Tg autoantibodies. J Clin Endocrinol Metab 2004;89(8):3702–4.

[63] Wong KT, Ahuja AT. Ultrasound of thyroid cancer. Cancer Imaging 2005;5:157–66.

[64] Larson SM, Robbins R. Positron emission tomography in thyroid cancer management. Semin Roentgenol 2002;37(2):169–74.

[65] Stokkel MP, Duchateau CS, Dragoiescu C. The value of FDG-PET in the follow-up of differentiated thyroid cancer: a review of the literature. Q J Nucl Med Mol Imaging 2006;50(1):78–87.

[66] Wang W, Larson SM, Tuttle RM, et al. Resistance of [18f]-fluorodeoxyglucose-avid metastatic thyroid cancer lesions to treatment with high-dose radioactive iodine. Thyroid 2001;11(12):1169–75.

[67] Robbins RJ, Wan Q, Grewal RK, et al. Real-time prognosis for metastatic thyroid carcinoma based on 2-[18F]fluoro-2-deoxy-D-glucose-positron emission tomography scanning. J Clin Endocrinol Metab 2006;91(2):498–505.

[68] Pacini F, Agate L, Elisei R, et al. Outcome of differentiated thyroid cancer with detectable serum Tg and negative diagnostic (131)I whole body scan: comparison of patients treated with high (131)I activities versus untreated patients. J Clin Endocrinol Metab 2001;86(9):4092–7.

[69] Durante C, Haddy N, Baudin E, et al. Long-term outcome of 444 patients with distant metastases from papillary and follicular thyroid carcinoma: benefits and limits of radioiodine therapy. J Clin Endocrinol Metab 2006;91(8):2892–9.

ELSEVIER
SAUNDERS

Endocrinol Metab Clin N Am
36 (2007) 779–806

ENDOCRINOLOGY
AND METABOLISM
CLINICS
OF NORTH AMERICA

Thyroid Cancer in Children

Catherine Dinauer, MD[a], Gary L. Francis, MD, PhD[b],*

[a]Department of Pediatrics, Yale School of Medicine, P.O. Box 208081, 464 Congress Avenue,
New Haven, CT 06520-8081, USA
[b]Division of Endocrinology and Metabolism, Department of Pediatrics, Medical College
of Virginia, Virginia Commonwealth University, P.O. Box 980140,
Richmond, VA 23298, USA

In 1996, we were asked to review the subject of thyroid cancer in children [1]. Over the subsequent decade, much has been learned about the treatment and outcome of these uncommon tumors. We now recognize quantitative and perhaps qualitative differences in genetic mutations and growth factor expression patterns in childhood thyroid cancers compared with those of adults [2–21]. We also know that thyroid cancers induce a robust immune response in children that might contribute to their longevity [22–25]. Very young patients (those under 10 years of age) probably represent a unique subset of children at particularly high risk for persistent or recurrent disease; the management of these patients is under evaluation [26]. We remain limited in our knowledge of how to stratify children into low- and high-risk categories for appropriate long-term follow-up and in our knowledge of how to treat children with detectable serum thyroglobulin (Tg) but negative imaging studies. In this article, we update our understanding of thyroid cancers in children with special emphasis on how these data relate to the current guidelines for management of thyroid cancer developed by the American Thyroid Association (ATA) Taskforce [27]. We also review the limited data regarding management of children who have detectable serum Tg but negative whole-body scans (WBS).

Thyroid cancers are the third most common solid tumor in children and adolescents, with an annual incidence of 1.75/100,000 [28,29]. They are one of the few malignant disorders in adults for which the incidence and mortality are increasing [28]. The ATA Taskforce recently published guidelines for managing patients who have differentiated thyroid cancer, but these did not

* Corresponding author.
E-mail address: glfrancis@vcu.edu (G.L. Francis).

0889-8529/07/$ - see front matter © 2007 Elsevier Inc. All rights reserved.
doi:10.1016/j.ecl.2007.04.002
endo.theclinics.com

specifically address all aspects of the management of children who have this disease [27].

Assessment of thyroid nodules in children

Our discussion begins with an update on thyroid nodules in children. Thyroid nodules are reported to occur in about 1 to 1.5% of children [30], and palpable thyroid nodules have been reported in as many as 7 out of 1000 (0.7%) children in the Southwestern United States [31]. As in adults, the majority of thyroid nodules in children are benign, but very young age [30], iodine deficiency [32], radiation therapy to the head and neck [33–35], and possibly autoimmune thyroiditis [36–38] increase the risks that a lesion will prove to be malignant.

Previous studies reported a high prevalence of malignant disease among thyroid nodules in children (30%–50%) [39], but contemporary studies by Hung [40] found that only 19.9% of solitary thyroid nodules in children were malignant. Whether this represents a change in the incidence of malignant disease or improved ascertainment of benign lesions cannot be determined from these data. In adults, nonpalpable or small thyroid nodules seem to carry the same malignant potential as do palpable lesions of similar size [41]. We believe this is true for children, as shown by Corrias and colleagues [42], who found a similar prevalence of malignant lesions among thyroid nodules in children irrespective of nodule size, tumor growth, or the number of nodules present, but their study only reported on 42 cases, which limits the statistical power of this observation.

The ATA Taskforce recommends that patients who have a thyroid nodule larger than 1 to 1.5 cm in any dimension first have a serum thyrotropin (TSH) measurement [27]. If the TSH is suppressed, indicating a hyperfunctioning nodule, a radionuclide scan should be performed. If the TSH is not suppressed, a thyroid ultrasound (US) should be performed along with fine-needle aspiration (FNA) using US guidance [27]. Few centers have adequate experience to document the positive and negative predictive value of FNA for children. However, Gharib and colleagues [43,44] performed 57 FNAs on patients younger than 17 years of age. Thirteen percent were nondiagnostic. There were no false-positive results, but there was one false-negative result (1/7 malignant lesions, 14%). Corrias and colleagues used FNA to evaluate thyroid nodules in 41 children [42]. There were no false-negative results, but all patients were at low risk for malignant disease. Based on these and other published observations totaling over 100 children with thyroid nodules, FNA seems to have similar specificity and sensitivity in children as in adults [42,45].

The use of US is commonplace in the evaluation of thyroid nodules, providing an anatomic characterization, identifying suspicious lymph nodes, and guiding FNA. By US, a translucent halo, homogenous echo-texture, and lack of internal calcifications are more commonly identified in benign lesions [42,46]. In contrast, indistinct margins, internal calcifications, and variable echo-texture are more characteristic of malignant lesions [46]. Neither these criteria nor the presence of central blood flow on power Doppler is sufficiently unique to allow reliable distinction between benign and malignant lesions [42,47].

An area of controversy is the management of "inadequate" or "nondiagnostic" FNA. Most clinicians would repeat the FNA [48]. The ATA Taskforce recommends repeat FNA for nondiagnostic samples and close observation or surgical removal for lesions that continue to yield inadequate material [27]. Attempts to improve diagnosis from nondiagnostic specimens have focused on molecular markers that are upregulated in thyroid cancers. Although these procedures remain experimental, they are worth mentioning. The first is based on the expression of telomerase, a ribonucleoprotein polymerase that replaces TTAGGG nucleotide repeats onto the ends of chromosomes (telomeres), allowing the cells to replicate [49]. In normal somatic cells, telomerase is repressed, and these terminal nucleotide repeats are successively lost with each cell division. Cells eventually reach critically shortened telomeric length, at which point senescence and cell death occur. In immortal or malignant cells, telomerase is reactivated, allowing cells to perpetually divide. Telomerase activity can be detected using TRAP (Telomeric Repeat Amplification Protocol) analyses. TRAP analyses were positive in 86% of invasive papillary thyroid cancer (PTC) [50], leading Lerma and Mora [51] to examine telomerase activity in patients who had nonconclusive FNA cytology. Detection of telomerase activity helped to confirm neoplasia in 6 of 23 (26%) suspicious nodules. Telomerase analyses have also been used to distinguish FTC from benign adenomas. Kammori and colleagues [52] detected telomerase activity in six of six (100%) FTC and five of 15 (33%) follicular adenomas. Management of cystic lesions is also controversial because cysts may harbor occult PTC. Immunohistochemical staining for galectin-3 showed that almost all cystic PTC (29/30, 97%) were positive for galectin-3 [53]. Similar studies have not been performed in childhood thyroid cancers, and such analyses remain experimental. We are concerned with the higher probability of malignancy among thyroid nodules in children, and until these or other molecular markers are proven to have adequate sensitivity and specificity, it is our opinion that nondiagnostic findings on FNA in children warrant concern. In low-risk adolescents, we support the recommendations to repeat the FNA or to remove the lesions, but we recommend surgical removal for younger children (< 10 years of age) and for those who have high-risk lesions as defined by the US characteristics, family history, or exposure to ionizing radiation [26].

Another controversial area is the follow-up of patients who have benign lesions on FNA. Orlandi and colleagues [54] performed annual FNA on 306 patients (14–84 years of age) with benign initial FNA. Over the subsequent 2 to 12 years, 97.7% continued to have benign cytology, but three patients (0.98%) developed suspicious findings and four (1.3%) developed PTC. The authors suggested that at least three annual FNAs should be performed to reduce the risk of missing PTC. Despite these suggestions, most adult endocrinologists perform repeat FNA only for large nodules, nodules that increase in size, or nodules that develop suspicious US findings. Although some patients in their study were adolescents (14 years of age and older), we do not know how commonly children will have PTC detected by repeat FNA. We use several clinical features in deciding whether to follow or remove an apparently benign nodule. These include (1) patient age, (2) past history of ionizing radiation, (3) family history of thyroid nodules or thyroid cancer, (4) US characteristics, and (5) FNA cytology [55]. We believe the probability of malignant disease is greater in children under 10 years of age, and we are less inclined to follow benign-appearing lesions in this age group [26]. For low-risk patients, such as the adolescent who has no history of ionizing radiation exposure, benign US features, and benign FNA cytology, we have been willing to follow these lesions over time with serial US examination. Nodules that increase in size are re-evaluated with FNA or surgically removed [56–58].

Surgical management of childhood differentiated thyroid cancer

According to the ATA Taskforce, initial therapy for PTC is designed to remove the primary lesion and any local invasive disease or involved cervical lymph nodes because these are the most common sites of recurrence [27]. Therapy should minimize treatment- and disease-related morbidity, permit accurate staging for prognosis and follow-up, facilitate postoperative treatment with radioactive iodine when appropriate, permit accurate long-term surveillance for recurrence, and minimize the risk of recurrence.

Preoperative staging helps in this process. Using standard pathologic techniques, lymph node involvement has been reported in 20% to 50% of adults who have PTC [59]. For this reason, the ATA Taskforce recommends preoperative US of the contralateral lobe and the cervical nodes for all patients undergoing thyroidectomy when based on a malignant FNA [27]. The roles of CT, MRI, and positron emission tomography (PET) in this context were questioned by the ATA Taskforce. To our knowledge, no study has specifically addressed these issues in children. The higher prevalence of cervical node involvement in children (50%–80%) [60,61] and the high prevalence of distant metastases (mainly lung, in 20%–30%) [61] lead us to strongly support the use of preoperative US in the evaluation of children. A recent study by Vierhapper and colleagues [62] showed that routine determination of serum calcitonin (Ct) levels in patients who have thyroid nodules facilitates early diagnosis of medullary thyroid carcinoma (MTC). They suggested that routine serum Ct levels should be determined in all patients. Despite the fact that Ct measurements have not been shown to benefit children who have thyroid nodules, we recommend serum Ct in the evaluation of children who have thyroid nodules showing unusual cytology on

FNA [55]. Concerns regarding assay specificity, the possibility of false-positive Ct values, and the unavailability of pentagastrin stimulation to confirm a positive Ct result warrant additional study before we can recommend serum Ct measures for all children who have thyroid nodules [63–65].

The ATA Taskforce recommends a variety of primary surgical procedures for patients who have thyroid cancer, based on the results of the FNA, tumor size, and extent of disease [27]. They recommend total or near- total thyroidectomy for patients who have PTC detected by FNA if the tumor is 1.0 to 1.5 cm or larger in size, if there are contralateral nodules, regional or distant metastases, a history of radiation exposure, a positive family history of thyroid cancer, or age greater than 45 years. Total thyroidectomy is also recommended for patients who have cellular atypia or patients who have FNA findings suspicious for PTC. Lobectomy is the recommended procedure of choice for patients with indeterminate FNA, based on a 20% risk of cancer. Lobectomy is also listed as possibly the procedure of choice for small, low-risk, isolated PTC in the absence of cervical lymph node involvement. The ATA Taskforce acknowledges that central compartment lymph node dissection might reduce the risk of recurrence for PTC but might not be required for FTC [27]. Lateral compartment dissection is recommended for patients who have lymph node involvement. The ATA Taskforce does not specifically address these issues for children [27].

Hung and Sarlis [26] stratified children with thyroid cancer into two age groups, those younger than 10 years of age, in whom the risks of recurrence and mortality are high, and those older than 10 years of age, in whom mortality and recurrence risks are similar to those seen in young adults. They recommended total or near-total thyroidectomy as the initial surgical procedure for several reasons. First, 40% of children who have PTC have multifocal disease and a higher recurrence risk if less than total thyroidectomy is performed [60]. Second, many children who have PTC have disseminated disease and require radioactive iodine therapy [60]. Third, sensitive assays for serum thyroglobulin (Tg) are used as a marker for persistent or recurrent disease [66] and are most useful in patients who have undergone total thyroidectomy and radioactive iodine ablation [66].

Although retrospective studies have generally failed to show survival advantage after total thyroidectomy in children, many studies document a lower recurrence risk for children after total or near-total thyroidectomy. Welch Dinauer [67] showed that recurrence risks were significantly greater (odds ratio, 8.7; 95% confidence interval, 1.4–54) for children treated with lobectomy (even if PTC was believed to be a unilateral, solitary nodule) when compared with children treated with subtotal or total thyroidectomy. Similar findings were reported by Borson-Chazot and colleagues [68] in a cohort of 74 patients. Several of their patients were believed to be free from nodal disease but when treated with lobectomy developed recurrent disease (10%) in the contralateral lobe. In the largest series, Ian Hay evaluated 189 patients

(3–20 years of age) [69]. The risk of recurrence was reduced by more than 50% if a bilateral thyroid resection was performed compared with a unilateral resection (P = .0049). Based on these data, we recommend total thyroidectomy for children who have differentiated thyroid cancer.

The ATA Taskforce acknowledges that cervical lymph node involvement is present in 20% to 90% of adults who have PTC but perhaps fewer patients who have other histologies [27]. They recommend routine central compartment (level VI) neck dissection for all patients who have PTC or Hürthle cell carcinoma. The value of lymph node dissection for children who have PTC has not been well studied. However, Demidchek and Kontratovich [70] published follow-up data on 110 children who required reintervention for persistent or recurrent disease. Seventy-five (68%) required reintervention for lymph node metastasis, and 12 (11%) required reintervention for pulmonary metastasis. The risk for reintervention was significantly reduced if bilateral lymph node dissection was performed as part of the initial surgical treatment (7.2% versus 20.6%). Their data support performing lymph node dissection in children, but they did not report on any preoperative neck US in their evaluation. It is possible that preoperative US might have detected patients who had lymph node involvement, possibly limiting the value of neck dissection. Further study is required to address this question.

Postoperative staging using the tumor-node-metastasis classification system is strongly recommended by the ATA Taskforce for all patients based on fact that staging helps to identify those at low and high risk for mortality [27]. In addition, other tumor staging systems specific to thyroid cancer, such as the age-metastasis-extent of disease-size of tumor (AMES), metastasis-age-completeness of resection-invasion-size, and others are recommended to help determine the risk of recurrence, but none is deemed superior. Because of their young age, all children who do not have distant metastases will be in the favorable AMES category, limiting the ability of the AMES system to stratify children into risk of recurrence. The metastasis-age-completeness of resection-invasion-size system has been applied to children and is useful, although a lower cutoff score is used in children compared with adults [71,72].

Radioactive iodine treatment for childhood differentiated thyroid cancer

Radioactive iodine remnant ablation (RRA) is increasingly used for adults who have PTC. Large retrospective cohorts show improved recurrence risk and reduced disease specific mortality when RRA is provided [73–75]. This primarily benefits adults who have tumors greater than 1.5 cm and adults who have residual disease after surgery. Low-risk adults have no benefit in terms of morbidity or mortality, although some investigators argue that RRA in low-risk patients results in the absence of radioactive iodine uptake and undetectable Tg, thereby providing benefit through reassuring the patient that they are free from disease. The ATA Taskforce recommends RRA for patients who have stage III and IV disease; all patients younger than 45 years of age who have stage II disease; most patients who have stage II disease who are older than 45 years of age; and selected patients who have stage I disease (those with multifocal disease) and patients who have nodal metastases, extrathyroidal invasion, vascular invasion, or aggressive histologies [27].

The use of radioactive iodine ablation for the treatment of children who have thyroid cancer continues to be debated. Hung and Sarlis indicate that despite surgery, significant uptake ($>0.3\%$) is usually found in the thyroid bed [26]. For this reason, they suggest that children should receive a 30 mCi ablative dose after initial surgery. Data by Chow and colleagues [76] strongly support the use of radioactive iodine ablation in children who have thyroid cancer. They reported 60 naive and 14 recurrent children (8.6–20.9 years of age) diagnosed with differentiated thyroid cancer (DTC) over a 37-year span. Radioactive iodine ablation was prescribed if any of the following were present: tumor size greater than 1 cm, cervical lymph node disease, extrathyroidal extension, residual postoperative disease in situ, or distant metastasis. Although their study was not prospective, it was unique in that radioactive iodine ablation was standardized. They gave 80 mCi to patients who did not have distant metastasis and 150 mCi to those who had distant metastasis. Thirty-six of the 60 (60%) patients received radioactive iodine. Local recurrence rates for patients who did not receive radioactive iodine were significantly higher (42%) than for patients who received radioactive iodine (6.3%, $P = .001$). In patients who did not have distant metastases at presentation and who underwent total thyroidectomy (n = 56), 5 of the 24 (20.8%) patients who did not receive radioactive iodine developed pulmonary metastasis, and none of the 32 patients who received radioactive iodine developed pulmonary metastasis. The number of patients who had pulmonary metastases was too small to achieve statistical significance ($P = .1$).

The Chow study sheds light on the changing trends in the management of children with DTC. Children diagnosed between 1960 and 1986 were less likely than those treated between 1986 and 1997 to undergo total thyroidectomy (67% versus 93.5%) and less likely to receive radioactive iodine (RAI) treatment (44.8% versus 74.2%). The children diagnosed before 1986 were more likely to develop local recurrence (37.9% versus 3.2%) and distant metastasis (17.2% versus 0%). In addition, all the patients treated after 1986 were disease-free at last follow-up.

Another observation from their study relates to the management of children who have small (<1 cm) PTC [76]. Only two patients who had small thyroid cancers (<1 cm) were included in their study: One presented with cervical lymph node involvement and the other with pulmonary metastases. These and similar observations from other investigators suggest that even small PTC (<1 cm) have the potential to metastasize in children. Whether or not these data pertain to individual patients who have isolated small PTC discovered incidentally at surgery or CT imaging for other reasons is not clear, it has led us to be cautious in the management of these patients and to consider RRA for all children who have differentiated thyroid cancer, including those who have small tumors.

For successful remnant ablation, serum TSH levels must be elevated to allow for maximal radioactive iodine uptake. In adults, optimal TSH levels need to be greater than 35 mU/L [77]. Such levels can usually be achieved with thyroid hormone withdrawal for 3 to 4 weeks. The ATA Taskforce recommends that radioactive iodine scanning ([131]Iodine-WBS) be done before RRA if remnant size cannot be ascertained by US or surgical reports or if the results would alter therapy [27]. They also recommend that a low iodine diet should be followed for 1 to 2 weeks before RRA and that the lowest possible dose of radioactive iodine should be used unless microscopic disease or more aggressive histologies are present. All patients undergoing RRA should have posttherapy scintigraphic images because approximately 10% of patients have abnormal uptake seen in new areas, leading to unexpected alterations in clinical management.

There are few data specific to children that allow us to describe a standard protocol for pre-RRA scanning or [131]Iodine dosing for RRA. A recent study by Lau and colleagues [78] suggested that diagnostic whole-body radioactive iodine scans were useful in directing management of 37.5% of children at their institution, and they support the use of diagnostic radioactive iodine WBS for children who have PTC. The data from Chow and colleagues [76] strongly support the use of RRA in children, but the doses used were 80 mCi for those without distant metastasis and 150 mCi for those with distant metastasis. It is not clear from their data if lower doses would confer a similar recurrence-free advantage. Hung and Sarlis [26] suggested that children should receive a 30 mCi RRA dose 6 weeks after the initial surgery. For some small children (3–5 years of age), this may represent a rather large dose of [131]Iodine; therefore, others suggest that children should be treated with [131]Iodine based on body weight (1.0–1.5 mCi/kg body weight) [79,80]. To our knowledge, there are no comparative studies to evaluate the efficacy of either of these strategies. In our opinion, if one were to prescribe doses for radioactive iodine ablation based on body weight (1–1.5 mCi/kg), preablation scanning might be omitted in adolescents. However, we have encountered several young children (3–5 years of age) who had significant uptake in the neck after total thyroidectomy and might have developed radiation-induced thyroiditis had they been treated without additional surgery before RRA. For that reason, we recommend pre-RRA diagnostic scans for children younger than 10 years of age despite the possibility of stunning [81,82]. We also advocate the use of [123]Iodine for pre-RRA scanning to further reduce this risk [83].

For young patients, dosimetry might be helpful in selecting appropriate doses of radioactive iodine [84]. Benua and Leeper [84] showed that doses providing less than2 Gy to bone marrow and retention of less than 120 mCi at 48 hours did not induce permanent bone marrow suppression. However,

Dorn and colleagues [85] found the "dose-limiting organ" to be bone marrow in only 46% of cases and the lung in almost 10% of cases. We do not know the frequency with which the lung is the "dose-limited organ" in children, and therefore we reserve dosimetry for guiding therapy of "high-risk" patients (very young children, children who ave pulmonary metastases, and children requiring multiple RAI treatments).

Radioactive iodine therapy is associated with short- and long-term risks. In the short-term, nausea (frequently managed with antiemetics), sialadenitis (within 2–4 days, but also up to 6 months after therapy with ^{131}Iodine), xerostomia, thrombocytopenia (platelet nadir of 50–100,000) and leukopenia (white blood count nadir of 2000–4500 approximately 4–6 weeks after ^{131}Iodine) are common [55,85,86].

In the long-term (months to years), transient increases in follicle stimulating hormone occur in adolescent boys [87–89], whereas ovarian function tends to be preserved in women, and pregnancy outcomes seem to be normal [90–94]. A conservative recommendation is to avoid pregnancy for at least 6 to 12 months after treatment [95]. Pulmonary fibrosis is a concern in children treated with ^{131}Iodine particularly for those receiving multiple doses and those with intertreatment intervals of 6 months or less [61].

Of more serious concern are follow-up data from Ian Hay regarding the long-term safety of ^{131}Iodine treatment [69]. He followed 188 patients who were younger than 21 years of age at diagnosis for a median of 28 years and up to 60 years in some cases. Recurrent disease developed in 27% at 20 years and in 33% at 40 years. Although cause-specific mortality was low (approximately 1%), overall survival was reduced, and 88% of the excess mortality was causally related to second malignancy. Fourteen patients died of non-PTC related cancers; 79% of patients had received some form of radiation (external beam, radium implant, radioactive iodine, or combinations of these) for treatment of PTC. Although 94% of children who received ^{131}Iodine alone did not die from non-PTC related cancers, there were four non-PTC cancer-related deaths among the children who received ^{131}Iodine, three among children who received external beam radiation therapy (XRT) or radium implants, and four among children who received XRT/radium implants and ^{131}Iodine. The data suggest that the combination of ^{131}Iodine plus external beam radiation therapy or radium implants is associated with an increased risk of second malignancy and suggest the possibility that ^{131}Iodine alone might be a risk factor.

Thyroid hormone suppression

After initial surgery and RRA, Biondi and colleagues [96] recommend suppression of TSH into the low-normal range (0.5–2.5 mU/L) for patients who have low-risk disease and suppression of TSH to subnormal levels only in patients who have high-risk PTC or FTC. The ATA Taskforce recommends that serum TSH be suppressed to 0.1 to 0.5 in low-risk patients and to levels below 0.1 mU/L in high-risk patients [27].

Neither group defines children as low- or high-risk patients. Despite low risks for mortality, children are at high risk for recurrence [60]. Baudin and colleagues [79] recommended initial suppression of TSH to less than 0.1 µIU/mL followed by relaxation of TSH suppression to 0.5 mU/L once children enter remission. The long-term outcome of these approaches is not known especially with regard to effects of thyroid hormone suppression on bone mineral density (BMD) [97]. A recent study by Karga and colleagues [98] suggests that reductions in BMD might be reversible, particularly in young patients. They showed that BMD was reduced by hyperthyroidism for up to 3 years after treatment but then recovered, particularly in younger women (13–30 years of age). Life-long TSH suppression is not equivalent to shorter courses of hyperthyroidism from Graves' disease. In the absence of data to the contrary, the recommendation of Baudin and colleagues [79] (initial suppression of TSH to less than 0.1 mU/L followed by relaxation to 0.5 mU/L once patients enter remission) seems to be reasonable for children because 90% of recurrent PTC in some series develops in the first 10 years after initial therapy [60].

Follow-up of differentiated thyroid cancer in children

The ATA Taskforce recommends that surveillance for recurrent disease be stratified according to risk [27]. The most stringent definition of absence of persistent disease would include all of the following criteria: (1) no clinical evidence of disease, (2) no imaging evidence of disease (ie, no uptake outside the thyroid bed on initial post-RRA scan images or no sign of disease on US and recent diagnostic WBS), and (3) undetectable serum Tg (baseline and after stimulation) in the absence of Tg antibodies [27].

Initial follow-up of low-risk adults (85%) who are treated with total thyroidectomy and RRA should include suppressed serum Tg measures and cervical US followed by stimulated Tg determination. Approximately 20% of adults who have suppressed Tg levels below 1 ng/mL will have Tg levels above 2 ng/mL after rhTSH or thyroid hormone withdrawal stimulation, indicating disease [99]. According to the ATA Taskforce, the clinical importance of such low-level disease burden is not clear [79,99]. A serial increase in serum Tg levels is indicative of disease that might achieve clinical importance in adults [79,99].

It is not clear if similar cutoffs in serum Tg values apply to children, and our lack of knowledge in this area is of profound importance. Children generally have well differentiated disease, and essentially all the retrospective survival data for children with PTC are based on undetectable [131]Iodine uptake on diagnostic (2–5 mCi) WBS. Undectable uptake on WBS has been the gold standard for cure over several decades for children [55]. Using that criterion, long-term survival approaches 100% [69]. We do not know the serum Tg levels of these children, and therefore we do not know how aggressive we should be in treating persistent disease that is based solely on a detectable serum Tg level without clinical or imaging evidence for disease.

Such deficiencies have led to the concept of "treat-to-negative-[131]Iodine whole body scan" for young patients who have thyroid cancer [100]. In a large series, Durante and colleagues reported outcomes for 444 patients who had distant metastases. Patients were treated with [131]Iodine (100 mCi) every 3 to 9 months for 2 years and then annually until disappearance of metastatic uptake. Thyroxine treatment was given at suppressive doses between [131]Iodine treatments. Negative [131]Iodine WBS and radiographs were attained in 43% of the patients, especially those who were younger and had well differentiated tumors with limited disease. To achieve negative scans, 96% of the patients required multiple treatments with [131]Iodine (100–600 mCi), and almost half required more than 5 years of treatment. Only 7% of patients who achieved negative imaging experienced a subsequent tumor recurrence, and overall survival was 92% at 10 years. From these data, a negative WBS seems to be a strong indicator of lengthy recurrence-free and overall survival.

Included in their study were 37 patients under 19 years of age [100]. With this "treat-to-negative-whole-body-scan" approach, 79% of young patients achieved remission, 100% achieved 10-year survival, 87% achieved 20-year survival, and the relative mortality risk was 1.0. Based on these data, the authors recommended that young patients should be treated until disappearance of any [131]Iodine uptake or until a cumulative dose of 22 GBq (600 mCi) has been administered. For patients who have persistent disease after 600 mCi [131]Iodine, the decision to treat should be individualized because the risks for leukemia and other cancers increase with administration of more than 600 mCi [101]. Powers and colleagues [71,72,102] made similar observations for children who had primary or recurrent thyroid cancer.

Several pediatric series show that approximately 50% of children who have pulmonary metastases develop stable but persistent disease after [131]Iodine therapy [33]. Given the favorable long-term survival in children who have unknown Tg levels and the stable but persistent disease in almost half with pulmonary metastases, it would seem prudent to be cautious in our treatment of Tg-positive, WBS-negative children for whom the benefit of additional therapy is unknown.

The ATA Taskforce suggests that such patients can be managed with empiric radioactive iodine therapy (100–200 mCi) followed by whole-body imaging [27]. This approach might localize disease in 50% of patients and has led to a decline in serum Tg levels in some studies [103,104]. Serum Tg levels might decline over time in such patients without therapy [103,105].

There are several critical issues that must be included in any attempt to use serum Tg as the sole indicator of disease or disease progression in children. First, not all laboratories use the same standard for Tg determination leading to variations in the absolute Tg level and in the Tg cutoff for disease detection. Pacini and colleagues [66,106] showed that 71.4% of patients who had undetectable serum Tg levels after thyroid hormone withdrawal had negative WBS. Over time, 89.2% showed complete remission. Cailleux and colleagues [107] found that serum Tg levels above 10 ng/mL (off thyroid hormone suppression) were highly predictive of residual disease. Mazzaferri and Kloos [108] showed that recombinant human thyrotropin (rhTSH)-stimulated serum Tg levels above 2 ng/mL was indicative of disease. Haugen and colleagues [109] found that rhTSH-stimulated Tg levels below 4 ng/mL rarely required additional evaluation, whereas Robbins and colleagues [110] found that a rhTSH-stimulated Tg ≤ 2 ng/mL was highly predictive (91.7%) of freedom-from-disease.

Second, we do not know the absolute value of suppressed or stimulated serum Tg that correlates with freedom-from-disease in children. Hoe and colleagues [111] reported stimulated-Tg levels in two children who were free from disease (both had stimulated-Tg ≤ 2.1 ng/mL) and in one child who had disease (stimulated-Tg, 15 ng/mL). Lau and colleagues [78] reported their experience with stimulated-Tg values in five children. Three had undetectable stimulated-Tg levels, and all three had negative WBSs. One child who had minimal neck uptake had undetectable stimulated-Tg, but that child had positive Tg antibodies that might have interfered. Finally, one child had a stimulated-Tg level of 80 to 90 pmol/L but a negative WBS and negative CT. From these data, we cannot determine the absolute value of stimulated-Tg indicative of disease requiring therapy in children, but, as in adults, it seems that serum Tg values in the vicinity of 2 ng/mL strongly suggest freedom from disease. We believe that serial Tg measurements are a sensitive method by which to detect disease in children and use this for the negative predictive value [112]. In theory, children who have been treated with total thyroidectomy and radioactive iodine ablation should have undetectable serum Tg (≤0.5 ng/mL in the absence of circulating thyroglobulin antibodies) while on thyroid hormone suppression. Undectable stimulated-Tg seems to be a robust indicator of freedom from disease [55,66].

Third, we do not know the natural history of detectable serum Tg in children who have negative WBSs. Wang and colleagues [105] showed that the majority of adults who have rhTSH-stimulated serum Tg ranging from 2 to 10 ng/mL had stable or decreasing rhTSH-stimulated Tg values when followed without additional RAI or surgery. Empiric therapy with 150 to 200 mCi of RAI did not seem to lower serum Tg levels.

The decision of whether or not to treat an child based on serum Tg alone is made on the basis of risk for recurrence, magnitude of serum Tg, serial changes in Tg values, and history of prior response to therapy [33]. No study has defined the lower limit of serum Tg that would indicate disease of sufficient magnitude to warrant therapy in children, and the possibility of false-positive serum Tg values, particularly at the lower limits of detection, remains a concern [113,114]. Furthermore, the safety of continuing to treat such low-level disease burden is unknown. Data from Ian Hay have generated concern regarding the long-term safety of such treatments [69]. Among the 188 patients in his cohort, 14 died of non-PTC–related cancers, and 79% of patients had received some form of radiation (external beam, radium implant, radioactive iodine, or combinations of these) for treatment of PTC. Although 94% of children who received ^{131}Iodine alone did not die from non-PTC–related cancers, there were four non-PTC cancer related deaths among the children who received ^{131}Iodine, three among children who received XRT or radium implants and four among children who received XRT/radium implants and ^{131}Iodine. The data suggest that the combination of ^{131}Iodine plus XRT or radium implants is associated with an increased risk of second malignancy and the possibility that ^{131}Iodine alone might be a risk factor. We do not know the total cumulative doses received by these patients and cannot address a potential threshold effect.

One approach to this conundrum is to empirically treat Tg-positive, WBS-negative children with a single dose of radioactive iodine. Diffuse microscopic disease might be successfully treated with this dose, and disease that is localized on posttherapy WBS might be amenable to surgical removal. Serial measures of serum Tg and neck US could then be used to determine the response to therapy. Declining serum Tg levels would suggest a potential benefit from treatment, whereas stable Tg levels might support a course of observation without additional radioactive iodine. Over time, Tg levels might further decline, indicating disease resolution. If Tg levels increase, there would be need for repeat evaluation and consideration of additional radioactive iodine therapy.

In an informal survey, most pediatric endocrinologists fail to find benefit from [18F]-2-fluoro-2-deoxy-D-glucose PET scans in attempts to localize disease in such Tg-positive, WBS-negative children. This and the favorable long-term survival for children who have persistent disease support the contention that children who have positive but low-level Tg measures have low-level, well differentiated disease and not dedifferentiated thyroid cancer [115,116].

The optimal means and frequency with which to detect disease in children are not well defined. Hung and Sarlis [26] suggested that radioactive iodine WBS and serum Tg levels should be determined at 6-month intervals for the first 18 months and then at 3- to 5-year intervals. A recent study by Lau and colleagues [78] suggested that diagnostic whole-body radioactive iodine scans were useful in directing management of 37.5% of children at their institution, and they support the use of diagnostic radioactive iodine WBSs for children who have PTC. Similar approaches are commonly used but might not take full advantage of thyroid US. Antonelli and colleagues [117] compared the results of WBS, serum Tg, and thyroid US in children. Overall, 23% had disease detected by US but not by Tg or WBS, whereas 46% had disease that was not detected by US. This suggests that some combination of WBS, serum Tg, and US might be optimal for children, but the frequency of surveillance remains unknown. Chest CT does not seem to be as sensitive for detecting disease in children. Bal and colleagues compared findings from WBS (2–3 mCi), chest radiograph, and chest CT [118]. Only 25% to 30% of chest radiographs and chest CT identified disease, and the routine 2- to 3-mCi radioactive iodine-WBS found disease in only slightly more than half of the patients.

The ATA Taskforce recommends that rhTSH should be considered for Tg-stimulation [27], but rhTSH has not been approved for use in children, and the data pertaining to its utility in children are sparse. Iorcansky and colleagues [119] showed that rhTSH-stimulation, using the typical adult dose (0.9 mg × 2 doses given 24 hours apart) seems to be safe and to generate TSH levels in children that are similar to those induced by thyroid hormone withdrawal. Hoe and colleagues [111] reported their experience with seven children who were treated with total thyroidectomy and radioactive iodine ablation. The children received rhTSH (0.9 mg intramuscularly) on days 1 and 2. TSH levels were 224 ± 93 mIU/l on day 2 and 13 ± 5 mIU/l on day 5. Serum Tg levels and WBS were performed on day 5. Five children were free from disease. All had negative WBS but only two had serum Tg values that could be interpreted. Both had Tg ≤ 2.1 ng/mL. Two children had disease detected. One had a negative WBS and Tg of 15 ng/mL, and one had a positive WBS but no Tg measurement. There were no adverse effects. The data are limited but in general agree with findings in adults that stimulated Tg values above 2 ng/mL are indicative of disease [109,110].

rhTSH has been used in preparing patients for radioactive iodine ablation but is not approved for this indication in the United States [120–122]. Lau and colleagues [78] reported their experience with rhTSH stimulation for radioactive iodine ablation in eight children. Seven of the eight underwent diagnostic iodine scans with rhTSH stimulation and received radioiodine treatment with doses of [131]Iodine ranging from 39 to 100 mCi. Older children were prepared by rhTSH stimulation using two intramuscular doses of 0.9 mg, whereas the youngest children (5 and 7 years of age) received two intramuscular doses of 0.6 mg. Seven of eight patients had significant uptake in the neck on diagnostic scan, and two had pulmonary uptake. Six months after therapy, six patients were evaluated with WBS and serum Tg levels, and five of them showed a partial or complete response. Three (50%) had undetectable serum Tg and negative WBS, one had minimal neck uptake (<1%) and undetectable serum Tg but positive Tg-antibodies, and one (5 years of age) had improvement but required a second dose of [131]Iodine. The remaining patient (12 years of age) had a serum Tg level that was initially 80 to 90 pmol/L but a negative WBS and CT. Subsequent Tg levels increased to 2980 pmol/L but the [18F]-2-fluoro-2-deoxy-D-glucose PET scan was negative. Neck dissection revealed a small focus of PTC in the neck that was removed. Follow-up Tg declined to 131 pmol/L.

The optimal frequency with which to perform stimulated-Tg testing (in response to thyroid hormone withdrawal or rhTSH) is unknown for children, but it is our clinical practice to assess serum Tg responses on an annual basis and to treat patients who have persistent or recurrent disease based on the results of these annual tests. The requirement for annual surveillance will be relaxed over time, but the ideal time at which to lengthen the intervals between examinations is not clear. We found that 90% of recurrences develop within 7 years after diagnosis, but others have found equal probability of recurrence in the first and second decades after diagnosis [60,123].

Children who have unusual pathology might be at higher risk for recurrence and mortality, but there are few data pertaining to this question. In children, 40% of PTC are typical PTC, 30% are the follicular variant, 10% to 35% are the solid variant, and 20% to 30% are the mixed variant [124]. The solid variant is thought to occur more commonly in radiation-induced tumors. The columnar variant is uncommon but is more aggressive in adults and probably in children. Cribriform PTC; PTC with focal, insular, squamous, or anaplastic components; diffuse-sclerosing; and oxyphilic-cell, clear-cell, and encapsulated variants of PTC are rare in children, and their clinical significance is debated [124]. With few exceptions, such as the recombinant ret oncogene rearrangement of papillary thyroid cancer (ret/PTC-3) in radiation-induced disease [103,125,126], correlations between molecular alterations and histology are inconsistent [124]. Rearrangements generating ret/PTC and transversions in Braf transforming gene are the most frequent molecular alterations found in PTC (10%–80%) [4,21]. tyrosine receptor kinase oncogene rearrangements occur in 10% of PTC, and mutations in neuroblastoma RAS viral oncogene homolog are found in the follicular variant of PTC [118]. PTC with solid patterns of growth are more likely to develop metastases (75% of cases). Other features associated with low-risk disease in adults, such as microcarcinomas (PTC measuring <1 cm), are frequently associated with invasive or metastatic disease in children [76].

FTC are generally subdivided into those with gross invasion and those with macroscopic encapsulation [124]. Another grossly encapsulated angioinvasive form has been recently introduced [124]. The risks of local recurrence and distant metastasis are higher when vascular invasion is present. Genetic studies suggest involvement of genes located on chromosomes 2, 3p, 6, 7q, 8, 9, 10q, 11, 13q, 17p, and 22 in FTC [127,128]. Rearrangements of the peroxisome proliferator-activated receptor gamma ($PPAR\gamma$) are found in 25% to 50% of FTC [129], and recombination between this and the paired homeobox gene-8 ($PAX8$-$PPAR\gamma$) is common in low–stage, angio-invasive FTC [130].

Medullary thyroid cancer in children

MTCs account for 3% to 5% of thyroid cancers and 15% of thyroid cancer deaths [131–133]. These malignant tumors arise from the parafollicular

C-cells, which are of neuroendocrine origin. Immunohistochemical staining for chromogranin, calcitonin (Ct), and carcinoembryonic antigen may be useful for diagnosis in uncertain cases. MTCs may occur as a sporadic isolated disease but are generally inherited alone (familial MTC [FMTC]) or as part of the multiple endocrine neoplasia (MEN) syndromes [132,133]. These include MEN 2A (associated with pheochromocytoma) and hyperparathyroidism and MEN type 2B (associated with pheochromocytoma, intestinal ganglioneuromatosis, mucosal neuromas, and marfanoid habitus) [134,135].

Inherited forms of MTC contain activating mutations of the *RET* proto-oncogene that can be detected by conventional genetic analysis in 95% of cases [134,135]. Full gene sequencing has identified additional mutations in some of the remaining cases [136–140]. Constitutive activation of the *RET* receptor results in the development of sequential C-cell hyperplasia, Ct hypersecretion, malignant transformation, and metastasis. FMTC is commonly associated with mutations at codons 618 and 620 and with non-cysteine mutations at codons 768 and 804 [136,141]. Patients who have MEN 2A have germline mutations in exons 10 and 11 of the RET gene 98% of the time, with a cys 634 → arg substitution present in over 80% of cases [136,142]. Modern RET mutation analysis also includes exons 13 through 16, allowing identification of RET mutations in 99% of MEN 2 families [143]. In rare families who have FMTC, the commonly identified RET mutations might not be detected by conventional screening, and for them, extended screening of exon 8 is recommended [144]. Two uncommon variants of MEN 2A exist, one associated with Hirschsprung disease (exons 609, 618, 620) [145,146] and the other with cutaneous lichen amyloidosis (exon 634) [142,147,148]. In MEN 2B, a single mutation at codon 918 (met 918 → thr) is found in 92% to 95% of patients [149]. Family history may be less informative in MEN 2B because these mutations more frequently arise de novo [149]. Somatic (nongerm-line) mutations of the 918 codon have been reported and are associated with a more aggressive form of sporadic MTC [136,150].

In adults, sporadic MTC accounts for 50% to 75% of cases and is most commonly associated with somatic *RET* mutations [151]. Although sporadic MTC was previously considered a disease restricted to adults, 24% of patients with sporadic MTC harbor germline *RET* mutations that place their kindred at potential heritable risk [139,140,142,152].

MTC is the first endocrine neoplasm to appear in most patients who have the MEN 2 syndromes, and because MTC exhibits almost complete penetrance, essentially all gene carriers develop MTC unless prophylactic thyroidectomy is performed. All children who have a family history of MEN 2 and any child who has a diagnosis of MTC even without an informative family history should undergo *RET* mutation analysis [142,153]. The optimal age at which to perform thyroidectomy is determined according to the *RET* proto-oncogene mutation [141,154]. Current guidelines stratify *RET* mutations into three classes based on genotype-phenotype correlations

[154]. Class 1 mutations (mutations in codons 768, 790, 791, 804, and 891) have the least risk of aggressive MTC and warrant prophylactic thyroidectomy before the age of 10 years [154–158]. Class 2 mutations (codons 609, 611, 618, 620, and 634) generally warrant prophylactic thyroidectomy before the age of 5 years. Class 3 mutations (mutations at codons 883, 918, and 922) have the highest risk of aggressive MTC and warrant prophylactic thyroidectomy within the first few months of life. Some families may have difficulty with the ethical issues raised by contemplating surgery in asymptomatic children who have positive test results [159]. Most centers with genetic testing programs are well versed in addressing these issues.

Screening should be performed to detect other endocrine manifestations of the MEN syndromes. MEN 2A accounts for more than 75% of MEN 2 [160,161]. Approximately 50% of patients who have MEN 2A and a mutation at codon 634 develop pheochromocytoma, and 20% to 30% develop hyperparathyroidism [160,162]. For patients who have MEN 2A and for children over 5 years of age who have a family history of MEN 2A, screening for pheochromocytoma and hyperparathyroidism should begin preoperatively and continue on an annual basis. In patients who have MEN 2A associated with Hirschsprung disease, gastrointestinal disease may be diagnosed years before any other manifestations of MEN 2 [163–165]. Therefore, patients who have inherited forms of Hirschsprung disease (and their family members) should undergo *RET* mutation testing and biochemical screening for the associated MEN 2A endocrinopathies [155].

MEN 2B is less common but presents at a much earlier age and is the most aggressive form of MTC, giving rise to metastatic disease as early as 1 year of age [166–169]. Physical features may include elongated facies, mucosal ganglioneuromas, hyperextensibility, and marfanoid body habitus. Prophylactic thyroidectomy should be performed in the first few months of life [155]. In rare individuals who have noninformative *RET* mutational analysis, full *RET* sequencing should be obtained. Children who have typical features and a positive family history of MEN 2B should undergo thyroidectomy within the first few months of life, regardless of *RET* gene analysis.

In *RET* carriers, the goal of surgery is to remove the thyroid before the onset of MTC [154]. Thirty percent of patients who have inherited forms of MTC develop bilateral, multifocal disease and regional metastasis, particularly those who have tumors greater than 1 cm [151,154,170,171]. Even with microscopic MTC (<0.5 cm), regional metastasis to the central and lateral cervical lymph nodes has been reported [172]. Once lymph node metastasis occurs in MTC, survival is poor. For these reasons, total thyroidectomy with central compartment lymph node dissection are well accepted standards for any child harboring a *RET* mutation, with the timing of surgery based on the specific RET mutation [154,159,173]. Not all centers recommend surgery based on the RET mutation and the assigned risk class. Instead, they advocate for prophylactic thyroidectomy between the ages 5 and 8 years in all MEN 2A carriers [174]. In addition, there is debate about the need for central neck dissection in young children who have normal Ct levels [173–175]. Recent outcomes for prophylactic thyroidectomy in familial cohorts report overall disease-free 5- to 10-year survival rates of almost 90% and 100% disease-free status in some class 1 cohorts [158,174]. As more long-term data become available, recommendations regarding the timing of prophylactic thyroidectomy and the extent of lymph node surgery will be further refined.

In the uncommon situation where a child without a positive family history is discovered to have MTC in a thyroid nodule or cervical lymph node(s), there is a much greater risk for regional metastases, persistent, and recurrent disease [176]. Serum Ct should be determined, and complete radiologic evaluation of the neck, chest, and abdomen should be performed [177]. Aggressive surgery, including bilateral dissection of the central compartment lymph nodes, is indicated, and more extensive lymph node dissection (ipsilateral or bilateral modified radical neck dissection) may be warranted [36].

With the availability of *RET* mutation analysis, biochemical screening to diagnose MTC is less commonly used [89,154,178,179]. Ct measurements are useful in the initial evaluation of *RET* gene carriers because mild elevations in Ct are suspicious for C-cell hyperplasia or MTC and should result in immediate thyroidectomy irrespective of genotypic recommendations [154,180]. After surgery for MTC, serum Ct should be determined at 6 months and every 6 to 12 months thereafter. Undetectable serum Ct (biochemical cure) is associated with a 5-year recurrence rate of only 5% and a 10-year survival rate of 97.7% [181]. Thyroid hormone replacement, but not suppression, is required because C cells are not responsive to TSH. There is no role for radioactive iodine imaging or treatment.

Radiologic studies, including CT, MRI, US, and nuclear medicine scans (octreotide or dimercaptosuccinic acid), should be performed to evaluate new cervical adenopathy and persistent or increasing Ct levels [172]. Technetium 99m methoxyisobutyl isonitrile (sestamibi) and [18F]-2-fluoro-2-deoxy-D-glucose scans (PET) are also useful [182]. Adjunctive chemotherapy, external-beam radiation therapy, radioimmunotherapy, and tyrosine-kinase inhibitors have induced disease stabilization, reduced morbidity, and reduced the incidence of cervical recurrence, but no regimen routinely results in cure [36,183–192].

Summary

Thyroid cancers are uncommon pediatric tumors, but an updated understanding of the molecular biology and treatment of these conditions will assist the clinician in selecting specific treatment and follow-up programs for individual patients. In general, children who have thyroid cancers may have a modest decline in life expectancy, but they continue to be at risk for recurrent disease through many decades. Optimal surveillance techniques and intervals have yet to be determined, and we hope that this article will stimulate interest in collaborative studies designed to answer questions such as the optimal level of TSH suppression for children who have thyroid cancer, the optimal interval for serum Tg measurements and WBS, and the use of rhTSH stimulation. For children who have MTC, RET mutation detection allows for proactive evaluation and treatment, but this is a relatively new and still evolving science. Novel scanning techniques and newer therapies that focus on tyrosine kinase inhibitors are clearly indicated.

References

[1] McClellan DR, Francis GL. Thyroid cancer in children, pregnant women, and patients with Graves' disease. Endocrinol Metab Clin North Am 1996;25(1):27–48.

[2] Fenton CL, Patel A, Tuttle RM, et al. Autoantibodies to p53 in sera of patients with auto-immune thyroid disease. Ann Clin Lab Sci 2000;30(2):179–83.

[3] Fenton C, Patel A, Dinauer C, et al. The expression of vascular endothelial growth factor and the type 1 vascular endothelial growth factor receptor correlate with the size of papillary thyroid carcinoma in children and young adults. Thyroid 2000;10(4):349–57.

[4] Fenton CL, Lukes Y, Nicholson D, et al. The ret/PTC mutations are common in sporadic papillary thyroid carcinoma of children and young adults. J Clin Endocrinol Metab 2000; 85(3):1170–5.

[5] Fenton C, Anderson J, Lukes Y, et al. Ras mutations are uncommon in sporadic thyroid cancer in children and young adults. J Endocrinol Invest 1999;22(10):781–9.

[6] Patel A, Fenton C, Ramirez R, et al. Tyrosine kinase expression is increased in papillary thyroid carcinoma of children and young adults. Front Biosci 2000;5:A1–9.

[7] Tuttle RM, Patel A, Francis G, et al. Vascular endothelial growth factor (VEGF) and Type 1 VEGF receptor (Flt-1) are highly expressed in Russian papillary thyroid carcinomas. Paper presented at the 12th International Thyroid Congress. Kyoto (Japan), October 22–27, 2000.

[8] Tuttle RM, Fenton C, Lukes Y, et al. Activation of the ret/PTC oncogene in papillary thyroid cancer from Russian children exposed to radiation following the Chernobyl accident. Paper presented at: 12th International Thyroid Congress. Kyoto (Japan), October 22–27, 2000.

[9] Fenton CPA, Burch HB, Tuttle RM, et al. Nuclear localization of thyroid transcription factor-1 correlates with serum thyrotropin activity and may be increased in differentiated thyroid carcinomas with aggressive clinical course. Ann Clin Lab Sci 2001 2001;31:245–52.

[10] Ramirez R, Hsu D, Patel A, et al. Over-expression of hepatocyte growth factor/scatter factor (HGF/SF) and the HGF/SF receptor (cMET) are associated with a high risk of metastasis and recurrence for children and young adults with papillary thyroid carcinoma. Clin Endocrinol (Oxf) 2000;53(5):635–44.

[11] Straight A, Patel A, Fenton C, et al. Thyroid carcinomas that express telomerase follow a more aggressive clinical course for children and adolescents. J Endocrinol Invest 2002; 25:302–8.

[12] Tuttle RMFM, Francis GL, Robbins RJ. Serum vascular endothelial growth factor levels are elevated in metastatic differentiated thyroid cancer but not increased by short term TSH stimulation. J Clin Endocrinol Metab 2002;87:1737–42.

[13] Patel A, Jhiang S, Dogra S, et al. Differentiated thyroid carcinoma that express sodium-iodide symporter have a lower risk of recurrence for children and adolescents. Pediatr Res 2002;52(5):737–44.

[14] Eccles T, Patel AR, Michael Tuttle, et al. Erythropoietin and the erythropoietin receptor are expressed by papillary thyroid carcinoma from children and adolescents: expression of erythropoietin receptor might be a favorable prognostic indicator. Ann Clin Lab Sci 2003;33(4):411–22.

[15] Shah R, Banks K, Patel A, et al. Intense expression of the b7-2 antigen presentation coactivator is an unfavorable prognostic indicator for differentiated thyroid carcinoma of children and adolescents. J Clin Endocrinol Metab 2002;87(9):4391–7.

[16] Patel A, Fenton C, Terrell R, et al. Nitrotyrosine, inducible nitric oxide synthase (iNOS), and endothelial nitric oxide synthase (eNOS) are increased in thyroid tumors from children and adolescents. J Endocrinol Invest 2002;25(8):675–83.

[17] Patel A, Straight AM, Mann H, et al. Matrix metalloproteinase (MMP) expression by differentiated thyroid carcinoma of children and adolescents. J Endocrinol Invest 2002;25(5): 403–8.

[18] Gydee H, O'Neill JT, Patel A, et al. Differentiated thyroid carcinomas from children and adolescents express insulin-like growth factor-1 (IGF-1) and the IGF-1 receptor (IGF-1-R): cancers with the most intense IGF-1-R expression may be more aggressive. Pediatr Res 2004;55(3):1–7.

[19] Costello A, Rey-Hipolito C, Patel A, et al. Thyroid cancers express CD-40 and CD-40 ligand: cancers that express CD-40 ligand may have a greater risk of recurrence in young patients. Thyroid 2005;15(2):105–13.

[20] Yates CM, Patel A, Oakley K, et al. Erythropoietin in thyroid cancer. J Endocrinol Invest 2006;29(4):320–9.

[21] Penko K, Livezey J, Fenton C, et al. BRAF mutations are uncommon in papillary thyroid cancer of young patients. Thyroid 2005;15(4):320–5.

[22] Gupta S, Patel A, Folstad A, et al. Infiltration of differentiated thyroid carcinoma by proliferating lymphocytes is associated with improved disease-free survival for children and young adults. J Clin Endocrinol Metab 2001;86(3):1346–54.

[23] Loh KC, Greenspan FS, Dong F, et al. Influence of lymphocytic thyroiditis on the prognostic outcome of patients with papillary thyroid carcinoma. J Clin Endocrinol Metab 1999; 84(2):458–63.

[24] Patel A, Fenton C, Dogra S, et al. Infiltration of childhood thyroid carcinoma by proliferating lymphocytes is associated with increased expression of the FAS receptor and the Bax Pro-apoptotic peptide. Paper presented at the Endocrine Society. San Francisco (CA), June 19–22, 2002.

[25] Modi J, Patel A, Terrell R, et al. Papillary thyroid carcinoma from children and adolescents contain a mixture of lymphocytes. J Clin Endocrinol Metab 2003;88:4418–25.

[26] Hung W, Sarlis NJ. Current controversies in the management of pediatric patients with well- differentiated nonmedullary thyroid cancer: a review. Thyroid 2002;12(8):683–702.

[27] Cooper DS, Doherty GM, Haugen BR, et al. Management guidelines for patients with thyroid nodules and differentiated thyroid cancer. Thyroid 2006;16(2):109–42.

[28] SEER. Surveillance, epidemiology and end results. nih.gov. 2002.

[29] Feinmesser R, Lubin E, Segal K, et al. Carcinoma of the thyroid in children: a review. J Pediatr Endocrinol Metab 1997;10(6):561–8.

[30] Wartofsky L. The thyroid nodule. In: Wartofsky L, editor. Thyroid cancer: a comprehensive guide to clinical management. Totowa (NJ): Humana Press; 2000. p. 3–7.

[31] Rallison ML, Dobyns BM, Keating FR Jr, et al. Thyroid nodularity in children. JAMA 1975;233(10):1069–72.

[32] Moretti F, Nanni S, Pontecorvi A. Molecular pathogenesis of thyroid nodules and cancer. Baillieres Best Pract Res Clin Endocrinol Metab 2000;14(4):517–39.

[33] LaQuaglia M, Black T, Holcomb G 3rd, et al. Differentiated thyroid cancer: clinical characteristics, treatment, and outcome in patients under 21 years of age who present with distant metastases: a report from the Surgical Discipline Committee of the Children's Cancer Group. J Pediatr Surg 2000;35(6):955–9.

[34] Boulad F, Bromley M, Black P, et al. Thyroid dysfunction following bone marrow transplantation using hyperfractionated radiation. Bone Marrow Transplant 1995;15(1):71–6.

[35] Sklar CA, Mertens AC, Mitby P, et al. Risk of disease recurrence and second neoplasms in survivors of childhood cancer treated with growth hormone: a report from the Childhood Cancer Survivor Study. J Clin Endocrinol Metab 2002;87(7):3136–41.

[36] Kebebew E, Clark OH. Differentiated thyroid cancer: "complete" rational approach. World J Surg 2000;24(8):942–51.

[37] Tamimi DM. The association between chronic lymphocytic thyroiditis and thyroid tumors. Int J Surg Pathol 2002;10(2):141–6.

[38] Holm LE, Blomgren H, Lowhagen T. Cancer risks in patients with chronic lymphocytic thyroiditis. N Engl J Med 1985;312(10):601–4.

[39] Hung W. Nodular thyroid disease and thyroid carcinoma. Pediatr Ann 1992;21(1):50–7.

[40] Hung W. Solitary thyroid nodules in 93 children and adolescents: a 35-years experience. Horm Res 1999;52(1):15–8.

[41] Hagag P, Strauss S, Weiss M. Role of ultrasound-guided fine-needle aspiration biopsy in evaluation of nonpalpable thyroid nodules. Thyroid 1998;8(11):989–95.

[42] Corrias A, Einaudi S, Chiorboli E, et al. Accuracy of fine needle aspiration biopsy of thyroid nodules in detecting malignancy in childhood: comparison with conventional clinical, laboratory, and imaging approaches. J Clin Endocrinol Metab 2001;86(10): 4644–8.

[43] Gharib H. Fine-needle aspiration biopsy of thyroid nodules: advantages, limitations, and effect. Mayo Clin Proc 1994;69(1):44–9.

[44] Gharib H, Goellner JR. Fine-needle aspiration biopsy of the thyroid: an appraisal. Ann Intern Med 1993;118(4):282–9.

[45] Gharib H, Zimmerman D, Goellner JR, et al. Fine-needle aspiration biopsy: use in diagnosis and management of pediatric thyroid diseases. Endocr Pract 1995;1(1):9–13.

[46] James EM, Charboneau JW, Hay ID. The thyroid. In: Rumack CM, Wilson SR, Charboneau JW, editors. Diagnostic ultrasound, vol 1St. Louis (MO): Mosby Year Book; 1991. p. 507–23.

[47] De Nicola H, Szejnfeld J, Logullo AF, et al. Flow pattern and vascular resistive index as predictors of malignancy risk in thyroid follicular neoplasms. J Ultrasound Med 2005; 24(7):897–904.

[48] Orija IB, Hamrahian AH, Reddy SS. Management of nondiagnostic thyroid fine-needle aspiration biopsy: survey of endocrinologists. Endocr Pract 2004;10(4):317–23.

[49] Ahn MJ, Noh YH, Lee YS, et al. Telomerase activity and its clinicopathological significance in gastric cancer. Eur J Cancer 1997;33(8):1309–13.

[50] Haugen BR, Nawaz S, Markham N, et al. Telomerase activity in benign and malignant thyroid tumors. Thyroid 1997;7(3):337–42.

[51] Lerma E, Mora J. Telomerase activity in "suspicious" thyroid cytology. Cancer 2005; 105(6):492–7.

[52] Kammori M, Takubo K, Nakamura K, et al. Telomerase activity and telomere length in benign and malignant human thyroid tissues. Cancer Lett 2000;159(2):175–81.

[53] Papotti M, Volante M, Saggiorato E, et al. Role of galectin-3 immunodetection in the cytological diagnosis of thyroid cystic papillary carcinoma. Eur J Endocrinol 2002;147(4): 515–21.

[54] Orlandi A, Puscar A, Capriata E, et al. Repeated fine-needle aspiration of the thyroid in benign nodular thyroid disease: critical evaluation of long-term follow-up. Thyroid 2005; 15(3):274–8.

[55] Bauer AJ, Tuttle RM, Francis G. Thyroid nodules and thyroid carcinoma in children. In: Pescovitz O, Eugster E, editors. Pediatric endocrinology: mechanisms, manifestations, and management. Philadelphia: Lippincott, Inc; 2004.

[56] Gharib H, Mazzaferri EL. Thyroxine suppressive therapy in patients with nodular thyroid disease. Ann Intern Med 1998;128(5):386–94.

[57] Gharib H. Changing concepts in the diagnosis and management of thyroid nodules. Endocrinol Metab Clin North Am 1997;26(4):777–800.

[58] Giuffrida D, Gharib H. Controversies in the management of cold, hot, and occult thyroid nodules. Am J Med 1995;99(6):642–50.

[59] Scheumann GF, Gimm O, Wegener G, et al. Prognostic significance and surgical management of locoregional lymph node metastases in papillary thyroid cancer. World J Surg 1994;18(4):559–67.

[60] Welch Dinauer CA, Tuttle RM, Robie DK, et al. Clinical features associated with metastasis and recurrence of differentiated thyroid cancer in children, adolescents and young adults. Clin Endocrinol (Oxf) 1998;49(5):619–28.

[61] Reiners C, Demidchik YE. Differentiated thyroid cancer in childhood: pathology, diagnosis, therapy. Pediatr Endocrinol Rev 2003;1(Suppl 2):230–5 [discussion: 235–6].

[62] Vierhapper H, Niederle B, Bieglmayer C, et al. Early diagnosis and curative therapy of medullary thyroid carcinoma by routine measurement of serum calcitonin in patients with thyroid disorders. Thyroid 2005;15(11):1267–72.

[63] Hodak SP, Burman KD. The calcitonin conundrum: is it time for routine measurement of serum calcitonin in patients with thyroid nodules? J Clin Endocrinol Metab 2004;89(2): 511–4.

[64] Martinetti A, Seregni E, Ferrari L, et al. Evaluation of circulating calcitonin: analytical aspects. Tumori 2003;89(5):566–8.

[65] Papi G, Corsello SM, Cioni K, et al. Value of routine measurement of serum calcitonin concentrations in patients with nodular thyroid disease: a multicenter study. J Endocrinol Invest 2006;29(5):427–37.

[66] Pacini F, Capezzone M, Elisei R, et al. Diagnostic 131-iodine whole-body scan may be avoided in thyroid cancer patients who have undetectable stimulated serum Tg levels after initial treatment. J Clin Endocrinol Metab 2002;87(4):1499–501.

[67] Welch Dinauer CA, Tuttle RM, Robie DK, et al. Extensive surgery improves recurrence-free survival for children and young patients with class I papillary thyroid carcinoma. J Pediatr Surg 1999;34(12):1799–804.

[68] Borson-Chazot F, Causeret S, Lifante JC, et al. Predictive factors for recurrence from a series of 74 children and adolescents with differentiated thyroid cancer. World J Surg 2004; 28(11):1088–92.

[69] Hayashi N, Nakamori S, Hiraoka N, et al. Antitumor effects of peroxisome proliferator activate receptor gamma ligands on anaplastic thyroid carcinoma. Int J Oncol 2004;24(1): 89–95.

[70] Demidchik Iu E, Kontratovich VA. [Repeat surgery for recurrent thyroid cancer in children]. Vopr Onkol 2003;49(3):366–9 [in Russian].

[71] Powers PA, Dinauer CA, Tuttle RM, et al. The MACIS score predicts the clinical course of papillary thyroid carcinoma in children and adolescents. J Pediatr Endocrinol Metab 2004; 17(3):339–43.

[72] Powers PA, Dinauer CA, Tuttle RM, et al. Tumor size and extent of disease at diagnosis predict the response to initial therapy for papillary thyroid carcinoma in children and adolescents. J Pediatr Endocrinol Metab 2003;16(5):693–703.

[73] DeGroot LJ, Kaplan EL, McCormick M, et al. Natural history, treatment, and course of papillary thyroid carcinoma. J Clin Endocrinol Metab 1990;71(2):414–24.

[74] Mazzaferri EL. Long-term outcome of patients with differentiated thyroid carcinoma: effect of therapy. Endocr Pract 2000;6(6):469–76.

[75] Samaan NA, Schultz PN, Hickey RC, et al. The results of various modalities of treatment of well differentiated thyroid carcinomas: a retrospective review of 1599 patients. J Clin Endocrinol Metab 1992;75(3):714–20.

[76] Chow S, Law S, Mendenhall W, et al. Differentiated thyroid carcinoma in childhood and adolescence–clinical course and role of radioiodine. Pediatr Blood Cancer 2004;42:176–83.

[77] Torres MS, Ramirez L, Simkin PH, et al. Effect of various doses of recombinant human thyrotropin on the thyroid radioactive iodine uptake and serum levels of thyroid hormones and thyroglobulin in normal subjects. J Clin Endocrinol Metab 2001;86(4):1660–4.

[78] Lau WF, Zacharin MR, Waters K, et al. Management of paediatric thyroid carcinoma: recent experience with recombinant human thyroid stimulating hormone in preparation for radioiodine therapy. Intern Med J 2006;36(9):564–70.

[79] Baudin E, Do Cao C, Cailleux AF, et al. Positive predictive value of serum thyroglobulin levels, measured during the first year of follow-up after thyroid hormone withdrawal, in thyroid cancer patients. J Clin Endocrinol Metab 2003;88(3):1107–11.

[80] Reynolds JC. Comparison of I-131 Absorbed radiation doses in children and adults: a tool for estimating therapeutic I-131 doses in children. In: Robbins J, editor. Treatment of thyroid cancer in childhood. Washington DC: US Departments of Energy and Commerce; 1993. p. 127–35.

[81] Kao CH, Yen TC. Stunning effects after a diagnostic dose of iodine-131. Nuklearmedizin 1998;37(1):30–2.

[82] Leger FA, Izembart M, Dagousset F, et al. Decreased uptake of therapeutic doses of iodine-131 after 185-MBq iodine-131 diagnostic imaging for thyroid remnants in differentiated thyroid carcinoma. Eur J Nucl Med 1998;25(3):242–6.

[83] Mandel SJ, Shankar LK, Benard F, et al. Superiority of iodine-123 compared with iodine-131 scanning for thyroid remnants in patients with differentiated thyroid cancer. Clin Nucl Med 2001;26(1):6–9.

[84] Benua R, Leeper R. A method and rationale for treating thyroid carcinoma with the largest safe dose of I-131. In: Meideros-Neto G, Gaitan E, editors. Frontiers in thyroidology, vol. II. New York: Plenum; 1986. p. 1317–21.

[85] Dorn R, Kopp J, Vogt H, et al. Dosimetry-guided radioactive iodine treatment in patients with metastatic differentiated thyroid cancer: largest safe dose using a risk-adapted approach. J Nucl Med 2003;44(3):451–6.

[86] Sweeney D, Johnston G. Radioiodine treatment of thyroid cancer. In: Wartofsky L, editor. Thyroid cancer: a comprehensive guide to clinical management. Totowa (NJ): Humana Press; 2000. p. 155–62.

[87] Handelsman DJ, Turtle JR. Testicular damage after radioactive iodine (I-131) therapy for thyroid cancer. Clin Endocrinol (Oxf) 1983;18(5):465–72.

[88] Ahmed SR, Shalet SM. Radioactive iodine and testicular damage. N Engl J Med 1984; 311(24):1576.

[89] Pacini F, Gasperi M, Fugazzola L, et al. Testicular function in patients with differentiated thyroid carcinoma treated with radioiodine. J Nucl Med 1994;35(9):1418–22.

[90] Casara D, Rubello D, Saladini G, et al. Pregnancy after high therapeutic doses of iodine-131 in differentiated thyroid cancer: potential risks and recommendations. Eur J Nucl Med 1993;20(3):192–4.

[91] Balan KK, Critchley M. Outcome of pregnancy following treatment of well-differentiated thyroid cancer with 131iodine. Br J Obstet Gynaecol 1992;99(12):1021–2.

[92] Kulakov VI, Sokur TN, Volobuev AI, et al. Female reproductive function in areas affected by radiation after the Chernobyl power station accident. Environ Health Perspect 1993; 101(Suppl 2):117–23.

[93] Lin JD, Wang HS, Weng HF, et al. Outcome of pregnancy after radioactive iodine treatment for well differentiated thyroid carcinomas. J Endocrinol Invest 1998; 21(10):662–7.

[94] Schlumberger M, De Vathaire F, Ceccarelli C, et al. Outcome of pregnancy in women with thyroid carcinoma. J Endocrinol Invest 1995;18(2):150–1.

[95] Smith MB, Xue H, Takahashi H, et al. Iodine 131 thyroid ablation in female children and adolescents: long-term risk of infertility and birth defects. Ann Surg Oncol 1994;1(2): 128–31.

[96] Biondi B, Filetti S, Schlumberger M. Thyroid-hormone therapy and thyroid cancer: a reassessment. Nat Clin Pract Endocrinol Metab 2005;1(1):32–40.

[97] Toft AD. Clinical practice: subclinical hyperthyroidism. N Engl J Med 2001;345(7):512–6.

[98] Karga H, Papapetrou PD, Korakovouni A, et al. Bone mineral density in hyperthyroidism. Clin Endocrinol (Oxf) 2004;61(4):466–72.

[99] Mazzaferri EL, Robbins RJ, Spencer CA, et al. A consensus report of the role of serum thyroglobulin as a monitoring method for low-risk patients with papillary thyroid carcinoma. J Clin Endocrinol Metab 2003;88(4):1433–41.

[100] Durante C, Haddy N, Baudin E, et al. Long-term outcome of 444 patients with distant metastases from papillary and follicular thyroid carcinoma: benefits and limits of radioiodine therapy. J Clin Endocrinol Metab 2006;91(8):2892–9.

[101] Rubino C, de Vathaire F, Dottorini ME, et al. Second primary malignancies in thyroid cancer patients. Br J Cancer 2003;89(9):1638–44.

[102] Powers PA, Dinauer CA, Tuttle RM, et al. Treatment of recurrent papillary thyroid carcinoma in children and adolescents. J Pediatr Endocrinol Metab 2003;16:1033–40.

[103] Pacini F, Agate L, Elisei R, et al. Outcome of differentiated thyroid cancer with detectable serum Tg and negative diagnostic (131)I whole body scan: comparison of patients treated with high (131)I activities versus untreated patients. J Clin Endocrinol Metab 2001;86(9):4092–7.

[104] Pineda JD, Lee T, Ain K, et al. Iodine-131 therapy for thyroid cancer patients with elevated thyroglobulin and negative diagnostic scan. J Clin Endocrinol Metab 1995;80(5):1488–92.

[105] Wang L, Robbins R, Feldman E, et al. Management of low measurable thyroglobulin (Tg) levels in thyroid cancer survivors who have negative whole body scans. Paper presented at the 76th Annual Meeting American Thyroid Association, Vancouver (BC), September 30–October 1, 2004.

[106] Pacini F, Molinaro E, Castagna MG, et al. Recombinant human thyrotropin-stimulated serum thyroglobulin combined with neck ultrasonography has the highest sensitivity in monitoring differentiated thyroid carcinoma. J Clin Endocrinol Metab 2003;88(8):3668–73.

[107] Cailleux AF, Baudin E, Travagli JP, et al. Is diagnostic iodine-131 scanning useful after total thyroid ablation for differentiated thyroid cancer? J Clin Endocrinol Metab 2000;85(1):175–8.

[108] Mazzaferri EL, Kloos RT. Is diagnostic iodine-131 scanning with recombinant human TSH useful in the follow-up of differentiated thyroid cancer after thyroid ablation? J Clin Endocrinol Metab 2002;87(4):1490–8.

[109] Haugen BR, Ridgway EC, McLaughlin BA, et al. Clinical comparison of whole-body radioiodine scan and serum thyroglobulin after stimulation with recombinant human thyrotropin. Thyroid 2002;12(1):37–43.

[110] Robbins RJ, Chon JT, Fleisher M, et al. Is the serum thyroglobulin response to recombinant human thyrotropin sufficient, by itself, to monitor for residual thyroid carcinoma? J Clin Endocrinol Metab 2002;87(7):3242–7.

[111] Hoe FM, Charron M, Moshang T Jr. Use of the recombinant human TSH stimulated thyroglobulin level and diagnostic whole body scan in children with differentiated thyroid carcinoma. J Pediatr Endocrinol Metab 2006;19(1):25–30.

[112] Ceccarelli C, Pacini F, Lippi F, et al. Thyroid cancer in children and adolescents. Surgery 1988;104(6):1143–8.

[113] Fenton C, Anderson JS, Patel AD, et al. Thyroglobulin messenger ribonucleic acid levels in the peripheral blood of children with benign and malignant thyroid disease. Pediatr Res 2001;49(3):429–34.

[114] Ringel MD, Balducci-Silano PL, Anderson JS, et al. Quantitative reverse transcription-polymerase chain reaction of circulating thyroglobulin messenger ribonucleic acid for monitoring patients with thyroid carcinoma. J Clin Endocrinol Metab 1999;84(11):4037–42.

[115] Helal BO, Merlet P, Toubert ME, et al. Clinical impact of (18)F-FDG PET in thyroid carcinoma patients with elevated thyroglobulin levels and negative (131)I scanning results after therapy. J Nucl Med 2001;42(10):1464–9.

[116] Wang W, Macapinlac H, Larson SM, et al. [18F]-2-fluoro-2-deoxy-D-glucose positron emission tomography localizes residual thyroid cancer in patients with negative diagnostic (131)I whole body scans and elevated serum thyroglobulin levels. J Clin Endocrinol Metab 1999;84(7):2291–302.

[117] Antonelli A, Miccoli P, Fallahi P, et al. Role of neck ultrasonography in the follow-up of children operated on for thyroid papillary cancer. Thyroid 2003;13(5):479–84.

[118] Frattini M, Ferrario C, Bressan P, et al. Alternative mutations of BRAF, RET and NTRK1 are associated with similar but distinct gene expression patterns in papillary thyroid cancer. Oncogene 2004;23(44):7436–40.

[119] Iorcansky S, Herzovich V, Qualey RR, et al. Serum thyrotropin (TSH) levels after recombinant human TSH injections in children and teenagers with papillary thyroid cancer. J Clin Endocrinol Metab 2005;90(12):6553–5.

[120] Robbins RJ, Larson SM, Sinha N, et al. A retrospective review of the effectiveness of recombinant human TSH as a preparation for radioiodine thyroid remnant ablation. J Nucl Med 2002;43(11):1482–8.

[121] Pacini F, Molinaro E, Castagna MG, et al. Ablation of thyroid residues with 30 mCi (131)I: a comparison in thyroid cancer patients prepared with recombinant human TSH or thyroid hormone withdrawal. J Clin Endocrinol Metab 2002;87(9):4063–8.

[122] Barbaro D, Boni G, Meucci G, et al. Radioiodine treatment with 30 mCi after recombinant human thyrotropin stimulation in thyroid cancer: effectiveness for postsurgical remnants ablation and possible role of iodine content in L-thyroxine in the outcome of ablation. J Clin Endocrinol Metab 2003;88(9):4110–5.

[123] Schlumberger M, De Vathaire F, Travagli JP, et al. Differentiated thyroid carcinoma in childhood: long term follow-up of 72 patients. J Clin Endocrinol Metab 1987;65(6): 1088–94.

[124] Vasyl Vasko, Andrew J, Bauer R, et al. Thyroid neoplasia in children. Basel (Switzerland): S. Karger AG; in press.

[125] Nikiforov Y, Gnepp DR, Fagin JA. Thyroid lesions in children and adolescents after the Chernobyl disaster: implications for the study of radiation tumorigenesis [see comments]. J Clin Endocrinol Metab 1996;81(1):9–14.

[126] Thomas GA, Bunnell H, Cook HA, et al. High prevalence of RET/PTC rearrangements in Ukrainian and Belarussian post-Chernobyl thyroid papillary carcinomas: a strong correlation between RET/PTC3 and the solid-follicular variant. J Clin Endocrinol Metab 1999; 84(11):4232–8.

[127] Snijders AM, Nowee ME, Fridlyand J, et al. Genome-wide-array-based comparative genomic hybridization reveals genetic homogeneity and frequent copy number increases encompassing CCNE1 in fallopian tube carcinoma. Oncogene 2003;22(27): 4281–6.

[128] Wreesmann VB, Ghossein RA, Hezel M, et al. Follicular variant of papillary thyroid carcinoma: genome-wide appraisal of a controversial entity. Genes Chromosomes Cancer 2004;40(4):355–64.

[129] McIver B, Grebe SK, Eberhardt NL. The PAX8/PPAR gamma fusion oncogene as a potential therapeutic target in follicular thyroid carcinoma. Curr Drug Targets Immune Endocr Metabol Disord 2004;4(3):221–34.

[130] Foukakis T, Au AY, Wallin G, et al. The ras effector NORE1A is suppressed in follicular thyroid carcinomas with a PAX8-PPAR{gamma} fusion. J Clin Endocrinol Metab 2005; 91(3):1143–9.

[131] Oertel J, Oertel Y. Medullary thyroid cancer. In: Wartofsky L, editor. Thyroid cancer: a comprehensive guide to clinical management. Totowa (NJ): Humana Press; 2000. p. 383–8.

[132] Chi DD, Moley JF. Medullary thyroid carcinoma: genetic advances, treatment recommendations, and the approach to the patient with persistent hypercalcitoninemia. Surg Oncol Clin N Am 1998;7(4):681–706.

[133] Jensen MH, Davis RK, Derrick L. Thyroid cancer: a computer-assisted review of 5287 cases. Otolaryngol Head Neck Surg 1990;102(1):51–65.

[134] Manie S, Santoro M, Fusco A, et al. The RET receptor: function in development and dysfunction in congenital malformation. Trends Genet 2001;17(10):580–9.

[135] Takahashi M, Cooper GM. ret transforming gene encodes a fusion protein homologous to tyrosine kinases. Mol Cell Biol 1987;7(4):1378–85.

[136] Learoyd DL, Marsh DJ, Richardson AL, et al. Genetic testing for familial cancer: consequences of RET proto-oncogene mutation analysis in multiple endocrine neoplasia, type 2 [see comments]. Arch Surg 1997;132(9):1022–5.

[137] Shimotake T, Iwai N, Inoue K, et al. Germline mutations of the RET proto-oncogene in pedigree with MEN type 2A: DNA analysis and its implications for pediatric surgery. J Pediatr Surg 1996;31(6):779–81.

[138] Mulligan LM, Kwok JB, Healey CS, et al. Germ-line mutations of the RET proto-oncogene in multiple endocrine neoplasia type 2A. Nature 1993;363(6428):458–60.

[139] Zedenius J, Wallin G, Hamberger B, et al. Somatic and MEN 2A de novo mutations identified in the RET proto-oncogene by screening of sporadic MTC:s. Hum Mol Genet 1994; 3(8):1259–62.

[140] Wohllk N, Cote GJ, Evans DB, et al. Application of genetic screening information to the management of medullary thyroid carcinoma and multiple endocrine neoplasia type 2. Endocrinol Metab Clin North Am 1996;25(1):1–25.

[141] Eng C, Clayton D, Schuffenecker I, et al. The relationship between specific RET proto-oncogene mutations and disease phenotype in multiple endocrine neoplasia type 2. International RET mutation consortium analysis. JAMA 1996;276(19):1575–9.

[142] Selgas R, Jimenez-Heffernan J, Lopez-Cabrera M. On the epithelial-mesenchymal transition of mesothelial cells. Kidney Int 2004;66(2):866–7.

[143] Cote GJ, Gagel RF. Lessons learned from the management of a rare genetic cancer. N Engl J Med 2003;349(16):1566–8.

[144] Kaldrymides P, Mytakidis N, Anagnostopoulos T, et al. A rare RET gene exon 8 mutation is found in two Greek kindreds with familial medullary thyroid carcinoma: implications for screening. Clin Endocrinol (Oxf) 2006;64(5):561–6.

[145] Edery P, Lyonnet S, Mulligan LM, et al. Mutations of the RET proto-oncogene in Hirschsprung's disease. Nature 1994;367(6461):378–80.

[146] Romeo G, Ronchetto P, Luo Y, et al. Point mutations affecting the tyrosine kinase domain of the RET proto-oncogene in Hirschsprung's disease. Nature 1994;367(6461):377–8.

[147] Gagel RF, Levy ML, Donovan DT, et al. Multiple endocrine neoplasia type 2a associated with cutaneous lichen amyloidosis. Ann Intern Med 1989;111(10):802–6.

[148] Kousseff BG, Espinoza C, Zamore GA. Sipple syndrome with lichen amyloidosis as a paracrinopathy: pleiotropy, heterogeneity, or a contiguous gene? J Am Acad Dermatol 1991; 25(4):651–7.

[149] Hofstra RM, Landsvater RM, Ceccherini I, et al. A mutation in the RET proto-oncogene associated with multiple endocrine neoplasia type 2B and sporadic medullary thyroid carcinoma. Nature 1994;367(6461):375–6.

[150] Zedenius J, Larsson C, Bergholm U, et al. Mutations of codon 918 in the RET proto-oncogene correlate to poor prognosis in sporadic medullary thyroid carcinomas. J Clin Endocrinol Metab 1995;80(10):3088–90.

[151] Raue F, Frank-Raue K, Grauer A. Multiple endocrine neoplasia type 2: clinical features and screening. Endocrinol Metab Clin North Am 1994;23(1):137–56.

[152] Eng C, Mulligan LM, Smith DP, et al. Low frequency of germline mutations in the RET proto-oncogene in patients with apparently sporadic medullary thyroid carcinoma. Clin Endocrinol (Oxf) 1995;43(1):123–7.

[153] Gagel RF, Cote GJ, Martins Bugalho MJ, et al. Clinical use of molecular information in the management of multiple endocrine neoplasia type 2A. J Intern Med 1995;238(4):333–41.

[154] Machens A, Ukkat J, Brauckhoff M, et al. Advances in the management of hereditary medullary thyroid cancer. J Intern Med 2005;257(1):50–9.

[155] Brandi ML, Gagel RF, Angeli A, et al. Guidelines for diagnosis and therapy of MEN type 1 and type 2. J Clin Endocrinol Metab 2001;86(12):5658–71.

[156] Sansom BF. An assessment of the risks to the health of grazing animals from the radioactive contamination of pastures. Br Vet J 1989;145(3):206–11.

[157] Simon S, Pavel M, Hensen J, et al. Multiple endocrine neoplasia 2A syndrome: surgical management. J Pediatr Surg 2002;37(6):897–900.

[158] Frank-Raue K, Buhr H, Dralle H, et al. Long-term outcome in 46 gene carriers of hereditary medullary thyroid carcinoma after prophylactic thyroidectomy: impact of individual RET genotype. Eur J Endocrinol 2006;155(2):229–36.

[159] Learoyd DL, Gosnell J, Elston MS, et al. Experience of prophylactic thyroidectomy in multiple endocrine neoplasia type 2A kindreds with RET codon 804 mutations. Clin Endocrinol (Oxf) 2005;63(6):636–41.

[160] Gagel RF, Tashjian AH Jr, Cummings T, et al. The clinical outcome of prospective screening for multiple endocrine neoplasia type 2a: an 18-year experience. N Engl J Med 1988; 318(8):478–84.

[161] Ponder BA, Ponder MA, Coffey R, et al. Risk estimation and screening in families of patients with medullary thyroid carcinoma. Lancet 20 1988;1(8582):397–401.

[162] Schuffenecker I, Virally-Monod M, Brohet R, et al. Risk and penetrance of primary hyperparathyroidism in multiple endocrine neoplasia type 2A families with mutations at codon 634 of the RET proto-oncogene. Groupe D'etude des Tumeurs a Calcitonine. J Clin Endocrinol Metab 1998;83(2):487–91.

[163] Cohen MS, Phay JE, Albinson C, et al. Gastrointestinal manifestations of multiple endocrine neoplasia type 2. Ann Surg 2002;235(5):648–54.

[164] Decker RA, Peacock ML. Occurrence of MEN 2a in familial Hirschsprung's disease: a new indication for genetic testing of the RET proto-oncogene. J Pediatr Surg 1998; 33(2):207–14.

[165] Decker RA, Peacock ML, Watson P. Hirschsprung disease in MEN 2A: increased spectrum of RET exon 10 genotypes and strong genotype-phenotype correlation. Hum Mol Genet 1998;7(1):129–34.

[166] Duh QY, Sancho JJ, Greenspan FS, et al. Medullary thyroid carcinoma: the need for early diagnosis and total thyroidectomy. Arch Surg 1989;124(10):1206–10.

[167] Telander RL, Zimmerman D, Kaufman BH, et al. Pediatric endocrine surgery. Surg Clin North Am 1985;65(6):1551–87.

[168] O'Riordain DS, O'Brien T, Crotty TB, et al. Multiple endocrine neoplasia type 2B: more than an endocrine disorder. Surgery 1995;118(6):936–42.

[169] Wells GB, Lasner TM, Yousem DM, et al. Lhermitte-Duclos disease and Cowden's syndrome in an adolescent patient. Case report. J Neurosurg 1994;81(1):133–6.

[170] Gagel RF, Robinson MF, Donovan DT, et al. Clinical review 44: medullary thyroid carcinoma: recent progress. J Clin Endocrinol Metab 1993;76(4):809–14.

[171] Saad MF, Ordonez NG, Rashid RK, et al. Medullary carcinoma of the thyroid: a study of the clinical features and prognostic factors in 161 patients. Medicine (Baltimore) 1984; 63(6):319–42.

[172] Ball DW. Medullary Thyroid Carcinoma. In: Wartofsky L, editor. Thyroid cancer, a comprehensive guide to clinical management. Totowa (NJ): Humana Press, Inc.; 2000. p. 365–81.

[173] Gosnell JE, Sywak MS, Sidhu SB, et al. New era: prophylactic surgery for patients with multiple endocrine neoplasia-2a. ANZ J Surg 2006;76(7):586–90.

[174] Skinner MA, Moley JA, Dilley WG, et al. Prophylactic thyroidectomy in multiple endocrine neoplasia type 2A. N Engl J Med 2005;353(11):1105–13.

[175] Heizmann O, Haecker FM, Zumsteg U, et al. Presymptomatic thyroidectomy in multiple endocrine neoplasia 2a. Eur J Surg Oncol 2006;32(1):98–102.

[176] Telander RL, Moir CR. Medullary thyroid carcinoma in children. Semin Pediatr Surg 1994;3(3):188–93.

[177] Wang PW, Wang ST, Liu RT, et al. Levothyroxine suppression of thyroglobulin in patients with differentiated thyroid carcinoma. J Clin Endocrinol Metab 1999;84(12):4549–53.

[178] Lamb EJ, Heddle RM, Ellis A. Spuriously elevated plasma calcitonin in a patient with a thyroid nodule not associated with medullary thyroid carcinoma. Postgrad Med J 1999; 75(883):289–90.

[179] Niccoli P, Wion-Barbot N, Caron P, et al. Interest of routine measurement of serum calcitonin: study in a large series of thyroidectomized patients. The French Medullary Study Group. J Clin Endocrinol Metab 1997;82(2):338–41.

[180] Ozgen AG, Hamulu F, Bayraktar F, et al. Evaluation of routine basal serum calcitonin measurement for early diagnosis of medullary thyroid carcinoma in seven hundred seventy-three patients with nodular goiter. Thyroid 1999;9(6):579–82.

[181] Vannelli GB, Barni T, Modigliani U, et al. Insulin-like growth factor-I receptors in nonfunctioning thyroid nodules. J Clin Endocrinol Metab 1990;71(5):1175–82.

[182] Roelants V, Michel L, Lonneux M, et al. Usefulness of [99mTC]MIBI and [18F]fluorodeoxyglucose for imaging recurrent medullary thyroid cancer and hyperparathyroidism in MEN 2a syndrome. Acta Clin Belg 2001;56(6):373–7.

[183] Carlomagno F, Vitagliano D, Guida T, et al. ZD6474, an orally available inhibitor of KDR tyrosine kinase activity, efficiently blocks oncogenic RET kinases. Cancer Res 2002;62(24): 7284–90.

[184] Cohen MS, Hussain HB, Moley JF. Inhibition of medullary thyroid carcinoma cell proliferation and RET phosphorylation by tyrosine kinase inhibitors. Surgery 2002;132(6):960–6 [discussion: 966–7].

[185] Croyle ML, Knauf JA, Traxler P, et al. Specific inhibition of kinase activity of ret-oncoproteins and of ret-induced cell growth by PKI166. Paper presented at the 84th Annual Meeting of the Endocrine Society.San Francisco (CA), June 19–22, 2002.

[186] Kikumori T, Hayashi H, Cote G. STI 571 (gleevec) inhibits growth of a human medullary thyroid carcinma cell line with an activating RET proto-oncogene mutation. Paper presented at the 8th International Workshop on MEN. Grand Rapids (MI), June 15–18, 2002.

[187] O'Doherty MJ, Coakley AJ. Drug therapy alternatives in the treatment of thyroid cancer. Drugs 1998;55(6):801–12.

[188] Skinner MA, Safford SD, Freemerman AJ. RET tyrosine kinase and medullary thyroid cells are unaffected by clinical doses of STI571. Anticancer Res 2003;23(5A):3601–6.

[189] Guba M, von Breitenbuch P, Steinbauer M, et al. Rapamycin inhibits primary and metastatic tumor growth by antiangiogenesis: involvement of vascular endothelial growth factor. Nat Med 2002;8(2):128–35.

[190] Strock C, Ball D, Denmeade S. RET tyrosine kinase inhibitors in medullary thyroid carcinoma. Paper presented at.the 8th International Workshop on MEN. Grand Rapids (MI), June 15–18, 2002.

[191] Traugott A, Moley JF. Medullary thyroid cancer: medical management and follow-up. Curr Treat Options Oncol 2005;6(4):339–46.

[192] Yamazaki M, Zhang R, Straus FH, et al. Effective gene therapy for medullary thyroid carcinoma using recombinant adenovirus inducing tumor-specific expression of interleukin-12. Gene Ther 2002;9(1):64–74.

ELSEVIER
SAUNDERS

Endocrinol Metab Clin N Am
36 (2007) 807–822

ENDOCRINOLOGY
AND METABOLISM
CLINICS
OF NORTH AMERICA

Radioiodine in the Treatment of Thyroid Cancer

Douglas Van Nostrand, MD, FACP, FACNP[a,c,*],
Leonard Wartofsky, MD, MACP[b,c]

[a]Division of Nuclear Medicine, Washington Hospital Center, 110 Irving Street,
NW, Washington, DC 20010, USA
[b]Department of Medicine, Washington Hospital Center, 110 Irving Street,
NW, Washington, DC 20010, USA
[c]Georgetown University Medical Center, Washington, DC, USA

The first report of treating patients who had thyroid cancer with radioactive iodine (131-I) was in 1946 [1]. Since then, 131-I has been an important and well accepted component in the armamentarium for the treatment of patients who have well differentiated thyroid cancer (WDTC). This article presents an overview of the use of 131-I in the treatment of patients who have WDTC. We review (1) definitions; (2) staging; (3) the two-principal methods for selection of a dosage of 131-I for ablation and treatment; (4) the objectives of ablation and treatment; (5) the indications for ablation and treatment; (6) the recommendations for the use of 131-I for ablation and treatment contained in the Guidelines of the American Thyroid Association (ATA), the European Consensus, the Society of Nuclear Medicine, and the European Association of Nuclear Medicine; (7) the dosage recommendations and selection of dosage for 131-I by the these organizations; and (8) the Washington Hospital Center approach.

Definitions

"Ablation" is the first-time administration of 131-I to a patient who has WDTC. This is typically within 4 to 8 weeks after the patient's initial diagnosis and thyroidectomy. Even after total thyroidectomy, some thyroid tissue usually remains, and the primary objective of ablation is to destroy

* Corresponding author. Division of Nuclear Medicine, Washington Hospital Center, 110 Irving Street, NW, Washington, DC 20010.
 E-mail address: douglas.van.nostrand@medstar.net (D. Van Nostrand).

doi:10.1016/j.ecl.2007.04.006

this normal residual thyroid tissue. Ablation may have other objectives, which are discussed in the section entitled "The Objectives of Radioiodine Ablation and Treatment."

"Treatment" is the term applied to the administration of 131-I for recurrent or metastatic WDTC. Although many physicians may argue that this distinction in the definitions is not a requirement, we argue that differential use of the two terms helps communicate "time" and the "primary objective" of the therapeutic intervention and helps with the development and application of guidelines.

"Dosage" refers to the amount of 131-I administered in millicuries or Becquerels, and the term may be used interchangeably with the term "activity." The term "dose" expresses the amount of the radiation absorbed dose in rads or grays to the patient.

Staging

A large number of staging systems exist, including the AMES (*A*ge, *M*etastases, *E*xtent of tumor, and *S*ize of tumor), the TNM (*T*umor, *N*ode, *M*etastases), the Ohio State Scoring system, AGES system (*A*ge, *G*rade of histology, *E*xtent, *S*ize of tumor), the MACIS system (*M*etastases, *A*ge, *C*ompleteness of resection, *I*nvasion, *S*ize of tumor), and the NTCTCS system (*N*ational *T*hyroid *C*ancer *T*reatment *C*ooperative *S*tudy). The TNM system was developed by the American Joint Commission on Cancer and is used by the ATA for the management guidelines for WDTC (Table 1). The European Consensus did not use "stages" but used levels of risk (ie, "very low," "low," and "high"), which are defined elsewhere in this article.

Approaches for the selection of radioiodine dosage (activity) for ablation or treatment

A dosage of 131-I may be selected by one of two methods: empiric or dosimetric (Fig. 1).

The empiric approach is the administration of a fixed dosage of 131-I that has been recommended over the years by various physicians [2–7] based typically on the physician's experience and modified by that physician's weighting of various factors, such as (1) whether or not the dosage is being given for ablation versus treatment, (2) the extent of tumor, (3) the grade of histology, (4) the patient's age, (5) the presence of distant metastases, and (6) whether or not the patient is a child or adult (Box 1). Several empiric approaches for the selection of dosages of 131-I for the treatment of metastatic WDTC [2–7] are illustrated in Fig. 2.

Selection of a fixed dosage by the empiric approach has the advantages of ease of dosage selection, a long history of use, and an acceptable frequency and severity of complications. An additional potential advantage is that

Table 1
American Joint Commission on Cancer TNM staging system

Tumor size	
TX	Primary tumor cannot be assessed
TO	No evidence of primary tumor
T1	Tumor ≤2 cm in greatest dimension limited to thyroid
T2	Tumor >2 cm but <4 cm in greatest dimension and limited to the thyroid
T3	Tumor >4 cm in greatest dimension limited to the thyroid or tumor of any size with minimal extrathyroid extension (eg, to sternothyroid muscle or perithyroid soft tissues)
T4a	Tumor of any size extending beyond the thyroid capsule and invading local soft tissues, larynx, trachea, esophagus, or recurrent laryngeal nerve
T4b	Tumor invading prevertebral fascia, mediastinal vessels, or encasing carotid artery in the neck
Nodes	
NX	Regional nodes cannot be assessed
N0	No metastases to regional nodes
N1	Metastases to regional nodes are present
N1A	To level 6 (pretracheal, paratracheal, prelaryngeal, and Delphian lymph nodes)
Metastases	
MX	Presence of distant metastases cannot be assessed
M0	No distant metastases
M1	Distant metastases

a "one-size-fits-all" approach permits the elimination of the diagnostic or dosimetric scan(s), thereby avoiding the potential of "stunning" secondary to the diagnostic use of 131-I (see below). The concept of stunning is controversial, as is the value of a preablation or pretreatment scan, in altering management before the administration of an empiric fixed dosages [8–11]. These controversies are beyond the scope of this article. In our view, the major disadvantage of the empiric approach is its failure to allow determination of whether or not the dosage administered may have a therapeutic effect or exceed a predetermined maximal radiation absorbed dose to a critical organ, such as the bone marrow. In other words, empiric fixed dosages make no attempt to determine the minimal amount of 131-I that delivers a lethal dose to the tumor or the maximum allowable reasonably safe dose. When a given empiric dosage is not sufficiently effective and one or more subsequent dosages are required, an additional potential limitation is that such multiple empiric fixed dosages fractionated over time may not be equivalent to the same total dosimetrically determined dosage of 131-I given at one time. This may be the case for two reasons. First, dose rates (rads/h) may be important because fractionated dosages give lower dose rates. Second, previous nonlethal dosages may reduce the effectiveness of subsequent dosages. For example, two 100-mCi (3.7 GBq) dosages administered 3 or 6 months apart may not deliver the same radiation absorbed dose as 200 mCi (11.1 GBq) administered as one single dosage because the dose rate is lower by the former approach and by partially destroying

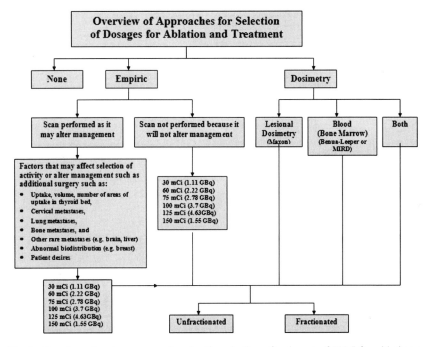

Fig. 1. Overview of various approaches for the selection of a dosage of 131-I for ablation or treatment of patients who have WDTC. (*Modified from* Van Nostrand D. Radioiodine ablation. In: Wartofsky L, Van Nostrand D, editors. Thyroid cancer: a comprehensive guide to clinical management. 2nd edition. Totowa (NJ): Humana Press; 2006. p. 277; with permission.)

the target lesion, the first 100-mCi dosage may significantly reduce the uptake of the second 100-mCi dosage. The dosimetric approach has been reviewed previously in detail [12] and may be lesional or whole-body dosimetry.

Lesional dosimetry has been well described by Maxon and colleagues [13,14] and attempts to determine the dosage of radioiodine to be administered, which is based on the radiation absorbed dose (rads or grays) that is needed to be delivered to destroy a metastasis. The advantages of lesional dosimetry are potentially improving outcomes by selecting and administering higher radioiodine dosages that have a greater chance of having a tumoricidal effect, potentially selecting and administering lower and safer radioiodine dosages that will still have a tumoricidal effect while reducing side effects, or potentially avoiding unnecessary costs and untoward effects in patients in whom tumoricidal doses cannot be achieved. The disadvantages of the dosimetric approach include increased cost and inconvenience to perform the dosimetry and the difficulty in performing lesional dosimetry for locoregional and distant metastases.

Whole-body dosimetry, as described by Benua and colleagues [15], attempts to determine the maximum allowable activity (MTA) that would deliver a maximum tolerable dose (MTD) to a critical organ to prevent or

Box 1. Various factors affecting selection of radioiodine dosages for ablation and treatment

- Stage (or risk)
- Convenience
- Cost
- Facilities
- Governmental regulations
- Age
- Histology
- Extent of surgery
- Percent uptake of 131-I in residual thyroid tissue
- Volume of residual thyroid tissue
- Effective half-life of 131-1 in the residual thyroid tissue
- Geometrical shape of residual thyroid tissue,
- Patient's compliance with low-iodine diet
- Level of TSH
- Location of metastases (eg, lung, bone, or brain)
- Number of metastases
- Size of metastasis(es)
- Number of organs involved
- Patient signs and symptoms secondary to metastases
- Uptake of 131-I in metastases
- Radiologic evidence of disease (eg, macronodular versus micronodular pulmonary disease on chest radiograph or CT)
- Potential for surgical excision
- Response of metastases to previous 131-I treatment (such as indicated by physical examination, 131-I scan, chest radiograph, CT, MRI, ultrasound, or serum thyroglobulin levels)
- Total accumulative dosage of 131-I
- Baseline CBC and differential pretreatment with special attention to neutrophils, lymphocytes, and platelets
- Response of absolute neutrophil and platelet count during the 3 to 6 weeks after the previous treatment
- Change in baseline absolute neutrophil and platelet count after previous treatment
- Pulmonary function tests pretreatment
- Change in pulmonary function tests since previous treatment
- Bone marrow biopsy for assessment of percent cellularity and adipose tissue in the bone marrow
- Concomitant disease(s)
- Patient desire(s)

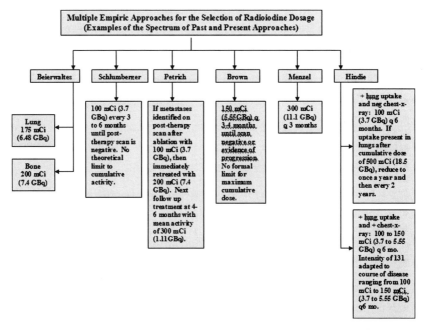

Fig. 2. Various physicians' empiric approaches to the selection of 131-I activity for the treatment of patients who have WDTC. (*From* Van Nostrand D. Radioiodine treatment for distant metastases. In: Thyroid cancer: a comprehensive guide to clinical management. Wartofsky L, Van Nostrand D, editors. Totowa (NJ): Humana Press; 2006. p. 419; with permission.)

minimize unacceptable results. The MTD is typically 200 rads (cGy) to the blood, the latter serving as a surrogate for the bone marrow. Using the medical internal radiation dose approach, 300 rads (cGy) to the blood has been proposed as the MTD [16,17]. The advantages of whole-body dosimetry include (1) the ability to determine in each patient the MTA of radioiodine based on a MTD, (2) the identification of the up to 20% of patients whose MTA is less than the empiric fixed dosage that may have been given [18–20], (3) the ability to administer a one-time higher radiation absorbed dose to metastases instead of multiple lower-radiation absorbed doses from multiple lower fractionated empiric dosages, (4) a long history of use, and (5) reasonable frequency and severity of complications relative to the sites and the severity of the extent of distant metastatic disease. The limitations of the whole body dosimetric approach include (1) increased cost and inconvenience; (2) the failure to estimate the radiation dose to the metastasis, thereby administering the MTA but not having any therapeutic effect; (3) the potential for stunning from the diagnostic dosage of 131-1, which may result in reduced therapeutic radiation dose delivered to the metastasis; and (4) the failure to measure MTD to organs other than the blood, such as the salivary glands.

Many physicians who support the empiric approach argue that there is no evidence-based literature to support improved outcomes with dosages of

radioiodine determined by the dosimetric approach relative to empiric dosages. As a result, they submit that empiric dosages should be used. Because
we know that empiric doses satisfactorily destroy remnant thyroid tissue,
this is an acceptable argument for the use of empiric dosages for ablation.
However, there are no definitive studies evaluating outcomes of empiric dosages in the treatment of distant metastases. In addition, there is no agreement
among physicians who advocate empiric dosage regarding what the empiric
dosage should be, and there is no evidence-based literature to support improved outcomes with dosages based upon one empiric approach versus another empiric approach. Physicians who support the dosimetric approach
have argued that until evidence-based literature is obtained that demonstrates
the superiority of one of the many empiric approaches or one of the several
dosimetric approaches, the use of any one of the dosimetric approaches helps
select dosages that are based upon logical objectives of maximizing the radiation absorbed dose delivered to the metastases or helping to assure that
one does not exceed the maximum safe dose to the blood. One can argue
further that the empiric approaches achieve neither goal of therapy.

In patients who have WDTC, good prospective outcome trials comparing
the various empiric and dosimetric approaches are difficult if not impossible
to perform. Until further data are available, the practicing physician must
select one of the empiric approaches, dosimetric approaches, or a combination of both. Our facility uses a combination of empiric and dosimetric
methods, and this approach is discussed below.

The objectives of radioiodine ablation and treatment

Multiple objectives for 131-1 ablation have been proposed and include (1)
ablating residual thyroid tissue, thereby increasing the sensitivity of detecting metastatic disease on subsequent follow-up radioiodine whole-body
scans; (2) ablating residual thyroid tissue, thereby facilitating the interpretation of follow-up serum thyroglobulin levels; (3) potentially treating residual
postoperative microscopic tumor foci; (4) decreasing the rate of recurrence;
(5) increasing survival; and (6) obtaining postablation whole-body scans,
which have higher sensitivity than diagnostic scans. The ATA guidelines
state that the objectives of ablation are "… to eliminate the post surgical
remnant in an effort to decrease the risk for recurrent locoregional disease
and to facilitate long-term surveillance with whole body iodine scan and/
or stimulated thyroglobulin measurements' [8]. The objectives as noted by
the European Consensus are "… (1) 131-I treatment of residual postoperative microscopic tumor foci, [which] may decrease the recurrence rate and
possibly the mortality rate, (2) 131-I treatment of residual normal thyroid
tissue [facilitating] the early detection of recurrence based on serum TG
measurement and eventually on 131-I WBS, and (3) a high activity of
131-I permits a highly sensitive post-therapy WBS 2-5 days after the administration, and this may reveal previously undiagnosed tumors" [9]. The

evidence-based literature regarding the success of radioiodine ablation for many of these objectives has been reviewed elsewhere [21,22]. The objectives for 131-1 treatment include (1) improved survival, (2) reduced rate of recurrence, (3) palliation, or (4) reduced morbidity.

The indications of radioiodine ablation

The ATA and the European Consensus have published their guidelines regarding the indications for ablation [8,9]. The ATA recommendations are based upon the American Joint Commission on Cancer TNM staging system (see Table 1). The ATA rates its recommendations on the basis of the strength of the evidence; these ratings are shown in Box 2. The European Consensus recommendations are based upon risk: very low, low, and high. A comparison of the ATA and European Consensus recommendations are noted in Table 2.

In summary, the ATA and the EC would ablate all patients with the exceptions of selected stage I patients and patients in the very low risk group. Stage I patients in whom it is deemed appropriate to forego ablation include patients lacking characteristics such as multifocal disease, nodal metastases, and extrathyroidal or vascular invasive or more aggressive histology. The very low risk group includes patients who have had complete surgery (total thyroidectomy), favorable histology, unifocal T < 1 cm (microcarcinoma), N0, M0, and no extrathyroid extension.

The indications of radioiodine treatment

Comparisons of the ATA and European Consensus guidelines for the indications of 131-I treatment for locoregional disease, pulmonary metastases, bone metastases, and brain metastases are shown in Table 3.

Box 2. American Thyroid Association definitions of recommendations

Recommendation A: Strongly recommends and based on good evidence
Recommendation B: Recommends based on fair evidence
Recommendation C: Recommends based on expert opinion
Recommendation D: Recommends against and based on expert opinion
Recommendations E: Recommends against and based on fair evidence
Recommendations F: Strongly recommends against and based on good evidence
Recommendations I: Recommends neither for nor against
Definitions have been abbreviated.

Table 2

Comparison of American Thyroid Association and European Consensus recommendations for ablation

Stage	Risk	Recommendations
ATA		
Stage I	For patients <45 yr old, any T, any N, MO For patients ≥45 yr old, T1, any NO, MO	Radioiodine (131-I) ablation is recommended in selected patients who have Stage I disease, especially those who have multifocal disease, nodal metastases, extrathyroidal or vascular invasive, or more aggressive histology; Recommendation B
Stage II	For patients <45 yr old, any T, any N, M1; For patients ≥45 years old, T2, any NO, MO	131-I ablation is recommended for all patients who have Stage II disease <45 years old and most patients ≥45 years old; Recommendation B
Stage III	For patients ≥45 yr old, T3: any NO, MO; T1: N1a, MO; T2: N1a, MO; T3: N1a, MO	131-I ablation is recommended for all patients who have stage III disease; Recommendation B
Stage IV	For patients ≥45 years old, T4a: any NO, MO; T4a: N1a, MO; T1: N1b, MO; T2, N1b, MO; T3, N1b, MO; T4a: N1b, MO; T4b: any N, MO; Any T: any N, M1	131-I ablation is recommended for patients who have tage IV disease; Recommendation B
EC		
Very low risk	Complete surgery; favorable histology; unifocal T ≤ 1 cm (microcarcinoma), N0, M0; no extrathyroid extension	No indication for ablation
Low risk	All patients not very low risk or high risk	No consensus. Benefits are controversial. Perhaps 131-I should be administered to select patients such as those with less than total thyroidectomy; no lymph node dissection; age <18 yr; T1 > 1 cm; and T2, N0, M0, or unfavorable histology
High risk	Distant metastases or incomplete tumor resection or complete tumor resection but high risk for recurrence or mortality; tumor extension beyond the thyroid capsule or lymph node involvement	Definite 131-I ablation; use ≥3.7 GBq (100 mCi) after thyroid hormone withdrawal

Data from Cooper DS, Doherty GM, Haugen BR, et al. Management guidelines for patients with thyroid nodules and differentiated thyroid cancer. Thyroid 2006;16:109–42.

Table 3
Comparison of American Thyroid Association and European Consensus guidelines for the indications of radioiodine (131-I) treatment for locoregional disease, pulmonary metastases, bone metastases, and brain metastases

	Recommendation
Locoregional	
ATA	"Despite the apparent effectiveness of 131-I therapy in many patients, the optimal therapeutic activity remains uncertain and controversial." (Recommendation I: neither for nor against)
EC	"Treatment is based on the combination of surgery and 131-I in those with 131-uptake."
	"When complete surgical excision is not possible, external beam radiotherapy may be indicated if there is no significant radioiodine uptake within the tumor."
Pulmonary	
ATA	"Pulmonary micrometastases should be treated with radioiodine therapy, repeated every 6–12 months as long as disease continues to respond …" (Recommendation A)
	The recommendation for macronodular pulmonary metastases is similar, but the response is lower. (Recommendation B)
EC	"… 131-I administration following prolonged withdrawal treatment … every 4–8 months during the first 2 years and thereafter at longer intervals."
Bone	
ATA	"Complete surgical resection of isolated symptomatic metastases has been associated with improved survival and should be considered especially in patients <45 y.o." (Recommendation B)
	"Radioiodine therapy of iodine-avid bone metastases has been associated with improved survival and should be used." (Recommendation B)
EC	"Bone metastases should be treated by a combination of surgery whenever possible, 131-I treatment if uptake is present, and external beam radiotherapy either as resolutive treatment or as pain control."
Brain	
ATA	"Complete surgical resection of central nervous system metastases should be considered regardless of radioiodine avidity as it is associated with significantly longer survival." (Recommendation B)
	"CNS lesions that are not amenable to surgery should be considered for external beam irradiation [eg, gamma knife]." (Recommendation C)
	"If CNS metastases do concentrate radioiodine, then radioiodine could be considered." (Recommendation C)
EC	"Whenever possible they should be resected; if not resectable and non-iodine-avid, external beam radiation may provide palliation."

Data from Cooper DS, Doherty GM, Haugen BR, et al. Management guidelines for patients with thyroid nodules and differentiated thyroid cancer. Thyroid 2006;16:109–42.

Selecting a dosage of radioiodine for ablation and treatment

The recommendations and guidelines by the ATA and EC for the selection of a dosage of 131-I for ablation and treatment are noted below in

Table 4. In addition to these guidelines, the Society of Nuclear Medicine states, "A variety of approaches have been used to select the amount of administered activity. General guidelines are: For postoperative ablation of thyroid bed remnants, activity in the range of 75-150 mCi (2.75-5.5 GBq) is typically administered, depending on the RAIU and amount of residual functioning tissue present" [23,24]. The European Association of Nuclear Medicine states, "For thyroid malignancy... for patients undergoing ablation of thyroid remnant, administered activities in the range of 100-150 mCi (3,700-5,500 MBq) are usually given" [25].

Although these recommendations and guidelines are helpful, the selection of a dosage of radioiodine for ablation and treatment remains variable and

Table 4
Comparison of American Thyroid Association and European Consensus guidelines for the dosages of radioiodine (131-I) for ablation and treatment

	Recommendation
Ablation	
ATA	"The minimum activity (30–100 mCi) necessary to achieve successful remnant ablation should be chosen, particularly for low-risk patients." (Recommendation B)
	"If residual microscopic disease is suspected or documented or if there is a more aggressive tumor histology (eg, tall cell, insular, columnar cell carcinoma), then higher activities (100–200 mCi) may be appropriate." (Recommendation C)
EC	"The administered 131-I activity ... ranges between 30 mCi (1.1 GBq) (low activity) and 100 mCi (3.7 GBq) or even more (high activity)."
Locoregional	
ATA	"In the treatment of locoregional or metastatic disease no recommendation can be made about the superiority of one method of radioiodine administration over another (eg, empiric high dose versus blood or body dosimetry)." (Recommendation I: Neither for nor against)
EC	No recommendation given
Pulmonary	
ATA	"The selection of radioiodine activity ... can be empiric (100–300 mCi) or estimated by dosimetry to limit whole body retention to 80 mCi at 48 hours and 200 cGy to the red bone marrow." (Recommendation C)
EC	"An activity ranging between 3.7 and 7.4 GBq (100–200 mCi) (or higher) is administered every 4–8 months during the first 2 years and thereafter at longer intervals."
	No maximum limit for the cumulative 131-I activity
Bone	
ATA	"The radioiodine activity administered can be given empirically (150–300 mCi) or estimated by dosimetry." (Recommendation B)
EC	No recommendation given
Brain	
ATA	No recommendation given
EC	No recommendation given

Data from Cooper DS, Doherty GM, Haugen BR, et al. Management guidelines for patients with thyroid nodules and differentiated thyroid cancer. Thyroid 2006;16:109–42.

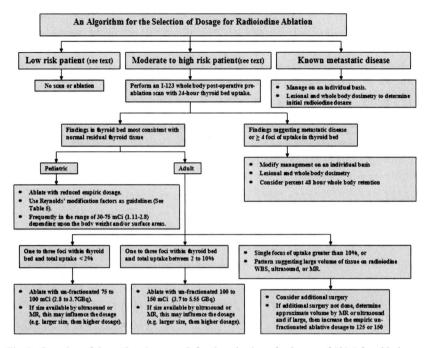

Fig. 3. Overview of the authors' approach for the selection of a dosage of 131-1 for ablation or treatment of patients who have WDTC at Washington Hospital Center. (*Modified from* Van Nostrand D. Radioiodine ablation. In: Wartofsky L, Van Nostrand D, editors. Thyroid cancer: a comprehensive guide to clinical management. 2nd Edition. Totowa (NJ): Humana Press; 2006. p. 280; with permission.)

problematic, with the dosage selected dependent upon the multiple factors listed in Box 1, and a subjective factor related to how each physician weighs each of those factors. Good prospective controlled studies are needed that compare the various empiric and dosimetric approaches, but such studies are not likely to be available in the foreseeable future.

Table 5
Reynold's modifications factors of prescribed activity for treatment for children

Factor	Body weight (kg)	Body surface area (m^2)
0.2	10	0.4
0.4	25	0.8
0.6	40	1.2
0.8	55	1.4
1.0	77	1.7

Body surface area = $0.1 \times$ (weight in kg)$^{0.67}$

From Van Nostrand D. Radioiodine treatment for distant metastases. In: Thyroid cancer: a comprehensive guide to clinical management. Wartofsky L, Van Nostrand D, editors. Totowa (NJ): Humana Press; 2006. p. 411–27; with permission; and Reynolds JC. Comparison of I-131 absorbed radiation doses in children and adults: a tool for estimating therapeutic I-131 doses in children. In: Robbins J, editor. Treatment of thyroid cancer in children. Springfield: US Department of Commerce; 1994. p. 127–35.

Box 3. Utility of a pre-ablation scan

- Demonstration of the pattern and the percent uptake of iodine in the thyroid bed or neck area that could alter the management or ablative or treatment dosage or both. Examples include
  i. A single area of significant uptake such as 10% to 30%, which suggests considering additional surgery or modifying the dosage activity of radioiodine
  ii. A single area of low uptake less than 2%, which suggest modifying the empiric dosage of radioiodine
  iii. A pattern of radioiodine uptake consistent with multiple cervical metastasis that may suggest further evaluation with MRI or high-resolution ultrasound, additional fine needle aspiration, surgery or both, or the use a larger empiric dosage of radioiodine
- Demonstration of distant metastasis that may alter the evaluation or the management of the patient before radioiodine ablation or treatment. Examples include:
  i. Focal or diffuse uptake in lung that may warrant further evaluation with CT without contrast, pulmonary function tests, dosimetry, percent 48-hour whole-body retention to determine the maximum tolerable dosage while not exceeding 80 mCi whole-body retention at 48 hours. The latter may increase or decrease dosage relative to an empiric dosage and may help minimize the potential for acute radiation pneumonitis and pulmonary fibrosis.
  ii. Focal area suggesting bone metastasis that may warrant further evaluation with CT, surgery, larger empiric prescribed activity, dosimetry, or coordination of subsequent external radiotherapy or radiofrequency ablation
  iii. Focal uptake in the head that may warrant an MR examination of the brain. If the focal area is a brain metastasis, then surgery should be considered. If radioiodine is administered, then a reduction of the empiric dosage may be warranted, and pretreatment management of the patient may be altered to include steroids, glycerol, or mannitol.

- Demonstration of altered biodistribution, such as breast uptake that may alter the management of the patient by postponing radioiodine ablation or treatment.

The pre-ablation scan can offer significant information that may modify the management of a patient before administration of the preablation dosage of radioiodine and may improve outcomes. Preablation scans do not provide important information in all cases. Nevertheless, we believe that the potential information gained and the potential for alteration of management is worth the reasonable cost and minimal inconvenience. In addition, with the use of 123-I, the potential problem and argument of "stunning" is eliminated.

Modified from Atkins F, Van Nostrand D. Radioiodine whole body imaging. In: Thyroid cancer: a comprehensive guide to clinical management. Wartofsky L, Van Nostrand D, editors. Totowa (NJ): Humana Press; 2006. p. 133–50; with permission.

Washington Hospital Center approach

For patients to be ablated with 131-I, our facility could use an empiric or a dosimetrically determined dosage depending upon the clinical circumstances (Fig. 3). If there is no evidence of metastases before the 123-I pre-ablation scan and if that scan demonstrates none of the findings in Box 3, then the patient is treated with an empiric dosage of radioiodine. For adults, we typically use 75 to 150 mCi (2.78–5.55 GBq). For pediatric patients, we use the Reynolds' modification factors shown in Table 5 [26]. These empiric dosages for children or adults may be further modified on an individual basis by one or more of the factors listed in Box 1. The adult dosage may also be modified by the thyroid bed uptake and the number and size of the area(s) of residual thyroid tissue seen on the diagnostic scan (Fig. 3); this has been discussed in more detail elsewhere [21].

If the patient had a pre-ablation scan that demonstrated one of the findings in Box 3, then the empiric dosage may be increased, whole-body dosimetry may be performed with the dosage selected as previously discussed, or the ablation or treatment may be postponed until further evaluation or treatment is performed. Further evaluation typically starts with imaging by ultrasound or MRI of the neck, CT of the chest, 18-F fluoro-2-deoxyglucose positron emission tomography scanning, and fine-needle aspiration for cytologic examination of any lesions imaged that appear suspicious. With positive cytology for cancer, additional surgical intervention would frequently be recommended.

For patients who have known metastases before the preablation scan or before the first pretreatment scan or for follow-up of patients who have elevated thyroglobulin levels or known or strongly suspected locoregional recurrence or distant metastatic disease, we perform whole-body dosimetry to help determine the MTA that the patient could receive without exceeding the MTD—the calculated 200 rads (cGy) to the blood (bone marrow). We also use the guidelines of not exceeding 80 mCi (2.96 GBq) whole-body retention at 48 hours in patients who have pulmonary metastases and 120 mCi (4.44 GBq) whole-body retention at 48 hour in all other patients. We use a low diagnostic dosage of 131-1 in the range of 1 to 2 mCi (37–74 MBq) to avoid or minimize significant potential stunning. The final treatment dosage of 131-1 is selected to not exceed the MTA and the guidelines for whole body retention. The selected dosage may be individualized and decreased based on one or more of the factors listed in Box 1.

Summary

131-I ablation and treatment remain indispensable components in the armamentarium for the management of patients who have WDTC. The dosages of 131-I can be selected by empiric or dosimetric approaches. With a thorough understanding of the various empiric and dosimetric approaches along with thoughtful consideration of the many factors that may alter the dosage of 131-I, we believe that a team that is comprised of a nuclear medicine physician (or nuclear radiologist) and an endocrinologist may select an appropriate dosage of radioiodine that is individualized for that patient's specific situation.

References

[1] Seidin SM, Marinelli LD, Oshry E. Radioactive iodine therapy effect on functioning metastases of adenocarcinoma of the thyroid. JAMA 1946;132:838–47.
[2] Beierwaltes WH, Rabbani R, Dmuchowski C, et al. An analysis of ablation of thyroid remnants with I-131 in 511 patients from 1947–1984: experience at University of Michigan. J Nucl Med 1984;25:1287–93.
[3] Schlumberger M, Challeton C, De Vathaire F, et al. Radioactive iodine treatment and external radiotherapy for lung and bone metastases from thyroid carcinoma. J Nucl Med 1996;37: 598–605.
[4] Petrich T, Widjaja A, Musholt TJ, et al. Outcome after radioiodine therapy in 107 patients with differentiated thyroid carcinoma and initial bone metastases: side effects and influence of age. Eur J Nucl Med 2001;28:203–8.
[5] Brown AP, Greening WP, McCready VR, et al. Radioiodine treatment of metastatic thyroid carcinoma: The Royal Marsden hospital experience. Br J Radiol 1984;57:323–7.
[6] Menzel C, Grunwald F, Schomburg A, et al. "High-dose" radioiodine therapy in advanced differentiated thyroid carcinoma. J Nucl Med 1996;37:1496–503.
[7] Hindié E, Melliere D, Lange F, et al. Functioning pulmonary metastases of thyroid cancer: does radioiodine influence the prognosis? Eur J Nucl Med 2003;30:974–81.
[8] Cooper DS, Doherty GM, Haugen BR, et al. Management guidelines for patients with thyroid nodules and differentiated thyroid cancer. Thyroid 2006;16:1–33.
[9] Pacini F, Schlumberger M, Drale H, et al. European consensus for the management of patients with differentiated thyroid carcinoma of the follicular epithelium. Eur J Endocrinol 2006;154:787–803.
[10] Atkins F, Van Nostrand D. Radioiodine whole body imaging. In: Wartofsky L, Van Nostrand D, editors. Thyroid cancer: a comprehensive guide to clinical management. Totowa (NJ): Humana Press; 2006. p. 133–50.

[11] McDougal R. Differentiated thyroid cancer. In: McDougal RI, editor. Management of thyroid cancer and related nodular disease. New York: Springer; 2006. p. 163–283.

[12] Van Nostrand D, Atkins F, Yeganeh F, et al. Dosimetrically determined doses of radioiodine for the treatment of metastatic thyroid carcinoma. Thyroid 2002;12:121–34.

[13] Maxon HR, Thomas SR, Hertzbert VS, et al. Relation between effective radiation dose and outcome of radioiodine therapy for thyroid cancer. N Engl J Med 1983;309:937–41.

[14] Thomas SR, Maxon HR, Kereiakes JG. In vivo quantitation of lesion radioactivity using external counting methods. Med Phys 1976;3:253–5.

[15] Benua RS, Cicale NR, Sonenberg M, et al. The relation of radioiodine dosimetry to results and complications in the treatment of metastatic thyroid cancer. AJR Am J Roentgenol 1962;87:171–82.

[16] Sgouros G. Bone marrow dosimetry for radioimmunotherapy: theoretical considerations. J Nucl Med 1993;34:689–94.

[17] Dorn R, Kopp J, Vogt H, et al. Dosimetry-guided radioactive iodine treatment in patients with metastatic differentiated thyroid cancer: largest safe dose using a risk-based approach. J Nucl Med 2003;44:451–6.

[18] Leeper R. Controversies in the treatment of thyroid cancer: The New York Memorial Hospital Approach. Thyroid Today 1982;5:1–4.

[19] Kulkarni K, Van Nostrand D, Atkins FB, et al. The frequency with which empiric amounts of radioiodine "over-" or "under-" treat patients with metastatic well-differentiated thyroid cancer. Thyroid 2006;16:1019–23.

[20] Tuttle RM, Leboeuf R, Robbins RJ, et al. Empiric radioactive iodine dosing regimens frequently exceed maximum tolerated activity levels in elderly patients with thyroid cancer. J Nucl Med 2006;47:1587–91.

[21] Van Nostrand D. Radioiodine ablation. In: Wartofsky L, Van Nostrand D, editors. Thyroid cancer: a comprehensive guide to clinical management. 2nd edition. Totowa (NJ): Humana Press; 2006. p. 611–2.

[22] Van Nostrand D. Radioiodine treatment for distant metastases. In: Wartofsky L, Van Nostrand D, editors. Thyroid cancer: a comprehensive guide to clinical management. 2nd edition. Totowa (NJ): Humana Press; 2006. p. 611–2.

[23] Society of Nuclear Medicine. Society of nuclear medicine procedure guideline for therapy of thyroid disease with iodine-131 (sodium iodide). Procedure manual, version 1.0; 2002. p. 159–64.

[24] Meier DA, Brill DR, Becker DV, et al. Procedure guideline for therapy of thyroid disease with I-131. J Nucl Med 2002;43:856–61.

[25] EANM procedure guidelines for therapy with iodine-131. Eur J Nucl Med 2003;30:BP27–31.

[26] Reynolds JC. Comparison of I-131 absorbed radiation doses in children and adults: a tool for estimating therapeutic I-131 doses in children. In Robbins J, editor. Treatment of thyroid cancer in children. Springfield: US Department of Commerce; 1994. p. 127–35.

ELSEVIER
SAUNDERS

Endocrinol Metab Clin N Am
36 (2007) 823–837

ENDOCRINOLOGY
AND METABOLISM
CLINICS
OF NORTH AMERICA

Medullary Thyroid Cancer: Monitoring and Therapy

Douglas W. Ball, MD

Johns Hopkins University School of Medicine, Suite 333,
1830 East Monument Street, Baltimore, MD 21287, USA

Overview of clinical features and natural history

Medullary thyroid cancer (MTC) accounts for 2% to 5% of cases of thyroid cancer. In the United States, there were an estimated 30,180 new cases of thyroid cancer in 2006, with 1500 deaths [1]. Although a marked increase has been observed in thyroid cancer incidence in the United States, this increase has been almost entirely accounted for by differentiated thyroid cancer (DTC), especially papillary cancer. No comparable increase has been detected in MTC [2]. In SEER data from 1973 through 2002, in the United States, patients who had MTC had a median age of 50 years at diagnosis, and there was a slight female preponderance [3]. Approximately 25% of MTC cases are inherited in one of the three disorders comprising MEN 2, all stemming from activating mutations in the ret proto-oncogene. The most common form of MEN 2 is MEN 2A, comprising MTC as the cardinal feature, pheochromocytoma in approximately 50% and hyperparathyroidism in approximately 20%, depending on the ret mutation. Familial medullary thyroid cancer is operationally defined as MTC without other hereditary endocrine tumor. Some families initially classified as having familial medullary thyroid cancer develop cases of pheochromocytoma, making this classification tentative, especially in families with fewer than eight affected members. MEN2B comprises MTC as the cardinal feature; pheochromocytoma, enteric ganglioneuromas, enlarged corneal nerves, and a marfanoid body habitus are also seen. A minority of patients who have MEN 2A develop characteristic cutaneous lichen amyloidosis or a limited form of Hirschsprung syndrome.

Supported in part by a NIH-NCI PAR-00-087, SPORE grant in Head and Neck Cancer.
E-mail address: dball@jhmi.edu

At presentation, patients who have sporadic MTC most commonly present with an isolated thyroid nodule or a palpable cervical lymph node. Diagnosis is made through a combination of fine-needle aspiration cytology and serum calcitonin. Increasingly, patients who have MTC are also being identified through detection of incidental thyroid nodules or lymph nodes, discovered in the course of carotid ultrasound, neck or chest CT or 18F-fluoro-2-deoxy-D-glucose positron emission tomography (FDG-PET) performed for another indication. A minority of patients who have MTC present with systemic manifestations of their cancer, including diarrhea, flushing, symptoms related to hypercortisolism due to ectopic adrenocorticotropin hormone production, or painful bone metastases.

Cervical lymphadenopathy is a common manifestation that occurs early in the clinical course of MTC. Moley and DeBenedetti [4] found that greater than 75% of patients who have MTC with palpable primary tumors had associated lymph node metastases. Machens and colleagues [5] reported a significantly higher rate of nodal metastasis for MTC than PTC, with a trend toward more frequent involvement of the contralateral cervical and mediastinal compartments in MTC. Cervical nodal involvement involves central and ipsilateral nodes more frequently than contralateral nodes; Scollo and colleagues [6] found that central and ipsilateral node involvement occurred in approximately 50% of patients, whereas contralateral nodes had a 25% to 30% prevalence. Contralateral and mediastinal involvement becomes common (50%–60%) when the primary tumor is locally invasive (pT4) [5]. Machens and colleagues [7] noted the strong correlation between contralateral and mediastinal nodal disease and distant metastases, arguing that the presence of adenopathy at these sites is an important marker of systemic (therefore surgically noncurable) disease.

MTC distant metastases typically occur in the mediastinum, lung, liver, abdominal lymph nodes, and bone. Clinically occult liver metastases are a leading cause of failure to achieve biochemical cure with surgery. Early in their course, these liver metastases have a miliary pattern that makes radiographic detection difficult. Even macroscopic liver metastases may be misdiagnosed as hepatic cysts based on the low-attenuation signal of these lesions as seen in typical venous-phase contrast CT. The estimated prevalence of MTC liver metastases varies depending on the technique, but hepatic arteriography shows that prevalence may be as high as 90% in some patient populations [8]. For bone involvement, MRI has proved more sensitive than conventional technetium bone scintigraphy and indicates a prevalence of approximately 75% in a population of patients who have known distant metastases at any site (versus 57% for conventional scintigraphy) [9].

Survival in MTC is intermediate between well differentiated and poorly differentiated or anaplastic thyroid cancers. In U.S. SEER data (1973–2002) reviewed by Sosa and colleagues, patients who had tumors classified as confined to the thyroid gland had a 10-year survival greater than 95%, whereas patients who had regional disease had an overall survival of 75%. Patients who had distant metastases had a 40% 10-year survival. No significant survival improvements were detectable across this 30-year interval [3]. Among the entire cohort of Swedish patients who had MTC, the overall relative survival for sporadic cases was 63% at 10 years and 50% at 20 years. Initial clinical stage remains highly predictive of future mortality even up to 20 years after diagnosis [10]. The application of two relatively new markers, calcitonin doubling time and somatic ret mutation status, to assess prognosis and select patients for clinical trials is discussed below.

Molecular pathogenesis and markers

Activating germline mutations in the ret proto-oncogene occur in virtually all patients who have inherited MEN 2, whereas somatic (tumor-specific) ret mutations are detectable in a significant fraction of sporadic MTC cases. Ret is a single-pass transmembrane receptor belonging to the tyrosine kinase superfamily. Closest neighbors in this family are fibroblast growth factor receptors and VEGF receptors. Ret binds to a set of circulating ligands, including glial-derived neurotrophic factor, in the presence of accessory proteins referred to as glial-derived neurotrophic factor receptor–alpha 1-4. Ligand binding leads to ret dimerization and to autophosphorylation of key tyrosine residues in the intracellular domain of ret, especially Tyr1062. Phosphorylated Tyr1062 and additional sites become docking residues for the adaptor molecules, including Shc, IRS1 and 2, and others, leading to activation of downstream signaling pathways, such as P-I3K-AKT and Ras-Raf-Mek-Erk. Several research groups have provided comprehensive reviews of ret signaling [11,12].

The ret gene is normally expressed in a narrow range of neural crest-derived tissues in the adult, including basal ganglia, autonomic neurons, enteric ganglia, thyroid calcitonin-producing parafollicular cells, and adrenal medullary chromaffin cells. Germline-inactivating mutations of ret are responsible for approximately 50% of cases of familial Hirschsprung disease [13]. The key role of Tyr1062 phosphorylation in ret signaling and development is illustrated by "knock-in" transgenic mice in which the Tyr1062 residue of the endogenous ret alleles was replaced by phenylalanine (which is not phosphorylatible). These knock-in mice showed marked growth retardation and had defects in enteric neurons and renal development, although this phenotype is less severe than complete ret knockout [14]. Ret is classified as a proto-oncogene because naturally occurring or experimental mutations that activate the receptor can lead to neoplastic transformation of a variety of cell types. A reasonable assumption is that activated forms of ret can transform many tissue types and that the restricted tumor and hyperplasia syndromes seen in MEN 2 reflect the limited range of tissues in which the ret promoter is normally active. A slightly different paradigm is observed in approximately 20% of cases of papillary thyroid cancer.

Here, a truncated, active form of ret is genetically rearranged as a RET-PTC oncogene so that a variety of different promoters inappropriately transcribe the mutant ret gene in thyroid epithelial cells (see [15] for review).

There is experimental evidence suggesting that ret mutations play a critical role in initiating MTC tumorigenesis. Transgenic mice bearing the M918T ret mutation characteristic of MEN2B develop diffuse and nodular C cell hyperplasia but no frank MTC by 12 months of age. In addition, these experimental mice develop pheochromocytomas and enteric ganglioneuromas [16]. In contrast to these "knock-in" results, transgenic overexpression of MEN 2A and MEN 2B forms of ret under the control of a tissue-specific calcitonin promoter does lead to frank MTC [17,18].

In human familial MTC, there is extensive literature correlating specific germline ret mutations with age-specific penetrance of cancer development and nodal metastases [19]. For the most common mutation in MEN 2A (codon 634, accounting for 68% of MEN 2 families), 50% of affected children develop at least microscopic MTC by age 10. Forty percent develop nodal metastases by age 20, with the earliest reported nodal disease at age 5 [19,20]. The codon 634 mutation has been assigned a risk category level 2, with a consensus for prophylactic thyroidectomy by age 5 [21]. The codon 918 mutation associated with the vast majority of cases of MEN 2B confers a high risk of metastatic MTC beginning in the first years of life. This mutation (along with codons 883 and 912) has been assigned a risk category level 3, indicating highest risk, and a need for prophylactic thyroidectomy in the first year of life, if possible. In contrast, patients who have several other intracellular domain codon mutations, including 768, 790, 791 804, and 891, have variably reduced penetrance and are assigned risk category 1 [2].

In sporadic MTC, a limited amount of literature suggests that the presence of somatic ret mutations, especially M918T, may confer an adverse prognosis. Somatic ret mutations have a variable prevalence in different series, ranging from 20% to 50% [22,23]. The discovery that mutation-positive and mutation-negative regions may coexist in the same sporadic MTC tumor [24] suggests that such genetically heterogeneous MTCs may not be clonally derived from a ret mutant initiating tumor cell. Data from Schilling and colleagues indicate that in spite of genetic heterogeneity within primary tumors, 76% of patients have concordant ret mutation results in all lymph nodes tested (43% all positive, 33% all negative) [25]. The presence of an M918T mutation in any specimen was a strong negative prognostic indicator for metastasis-free survival and, by trend, for overall survival. Ten-year survival was approximately 45% in M918T- positive patients versus 90% when the mutation was absent [25]. Larger-scale studies are needed to further explore this provocative finding and to validate somatic M918T mutations as a marker of high-risk disease and, potentially, of susceptibility to ret-targeted therapies.

Integrated medullary thyroid cancer monitoring: genetic and biochemical markers and imaging

Preoperative

Germline testing for ret proto-oncogene mutations is accepted as standard of care as part of the initial diagnostic work-up of MTC, even in the absence of a family history of MTC or MEN 2. Approximately 4% to 6% of family history–negative individuals are found to harbor germline mutations [26]. These mutations tend to be disproportionately clustered among the class 1 mutations listed previously, with reduced clinical penetrance compared with classic extracellular mutations, such as codon 634. Patients found to harbor cryptic germline mutations require testing for pheochromocytoma and hyperparathyroidism and family screening. In addition, surgical decision-making may be altered, based on a higher risk of bi-lobar tumors and contralateral nodal metastasis. In our institution, patients who have newly diagnosed MTC are evaluated with ret proto-oncogene testing, 24-hour urine metanephrine, or fractionated plasma metanephrine, serum calcium, calcitonin, and carcinoembryonic antigen (CEA). Calcitonin is a specific and highly sensitive biomarker for MTC and C-cell disease. Although calcitonin values in early occult MTC may merge with the upper limit of normal, the vast majority of patients who have MTC exhibit significant calcitonin elevations. European data have shown that preoperative calcitonin levels correlate with tumor size and disease stage. Calcitonin levels less than 100 pg/mL were associated with a median tumor size of 3 mm, with 98% less than 1 cm. Calcitonin levels greater than 1000 pg/mL correlated with a median tumor diameter of 2.5 cm [27]. Nodal metastasis first could be observed at basal calcitonin levels of 10 to 40 pg/mL (normal range, <10 pg/mL). Distant metastasis and extrathyroidal growth began appearing in patients who had calcitonin levels of 150 to 400 pg/mL. Node-positive patients did not achieve biochemical remission when their preoperative basal calcitonin levels exceeded 3000 pg/mL in the population reported by Machens and colleagues [28].

In parallel with calcitonin, CEA levels may provide valuable information for risk stratification in patients who have MTC. Machens and colleagues [7] have recently reported that preoperative serum CEA levels greater than 30 ng/mL in their series were incompatible with surgical remission. The rate of central and lateral lymph node involvement in these patients was 70%; this rate increased to 90% if the CEA levels were greater than 100. CEA levels greater than 100 were also associated with high rates of contralateral nodal disease and distant metastases.

The choice of preoperative imaging for patients who have MTC varies depending on hereditary status, age, and calcitonin and CEA levels. Thyroid and neck ultrasound, coupled with fine-needle aspiration (FNA), allows detection of multifocal thyroid involvement and metastasis to central and jugular chain nodes. The preoperative sensitivity of cervical ultrasound is only moderate, with 32% of patients having false-negative central neck examinations and 14% false negatives in the ipsilateral neck [29]. Ultrasound is also highly operator dependent, with many facilities lacking experience in performing nodal surveillance in thyroid cancer. Additional imaging is guided by the degree of calcitonin elevation. Neck, chest, and abdominal CT scanning are most commonly performed in preoperative staging of patients who have significant calcitonin elevations. The use of an arterial-phase contrast abdominal CT has proven useful in other neuroendocrine tumors [30] and may improve detection of macroscopic MTC liver metastases. Hepatic arteriography, though more sensitive than CT for small lesions, has not been used widely.

Postoperative

In the postoperative setting, repeat calcitonin testing is typically deferred approximately 6 weeks to allow for a postoperative nadir. Levels of CEA, elevated in approximately 30% of patients who have MTC, may reach their nadir later. A hallmark of surgical remission is an undetectable basal and pentagastrin-stimulated calcitonin. The majority of sporadic patients have persistent calcitonin elevations postoperatively, indicating residual cancer. After comprehensive lymphatic clearance along with thyroidectomy, those patients found to be node negative have a 95% chance of an undetectable basal calcitonin level. The presence of lymphadenopathy reduces the chance of calcitonin normalization to approximately 30% [6]. Recent data from the French MTC consortium show that serial postoperative calcitonin measurement can provide valuable prognostic information. At least four measurements of calcitonin over a 2- to 3-year period could provide an accurate estimate of the calcitonin doubling time in most patients, which remained relatively stable over the natural history of the disease. A calcitonin doubling time shorter than 6 months was associated with a significant risk of death in a 5-year follow-up interval (75%), whereas none of the patients who had a doubling time greater than 2 years had disease-specific mortality in follow-up. Calcitonin doubling time was a strong prognostic indicator in multivariate analyses, even when adjusted for clinical stage [31]. CEA doubling time, in general, was comparably informative to calcitonin doubling time in patients who had both markers elevated. These findings are promising because they allow detection of some high-risk individuals even at a relatively early point in their disease course, potentially before the detection of extensive stage IV disease on imaging studies. Rapid calcitonin doubling time is an indicator of progressive disease and may prompt more intensive imaging or, in some circumstances, referral of patients for clinical trials of systemic therapy.

Clinicians and patients may be frustrated with calcitonin testing because of chaotically variable swings from test to test. It is well documented, although poorly explained, that some patients have widely variable readings, whereas other patients conform more closely to a trendline [31]. Intrinsic biologic variability in calcitonin secretion is a contributing factor. Calcitonin measurement may also be hampered by the high dose hook effect, seen with some immunoradiometric assays [32]. The hook effect may be suspected when rising CEA or changing imaging findings are not accompanied by rising calcitonin. A hook effect may be confirmed by showing that the observed calcitonin reading remains similar despite serial dilution of the sample. Perhaps more insidious than the hook effect is the nonlinearity of calcitonin assays at higher levels. Consistent use of a reputable calcitonin assay with concurrent CEA testing is probably the best approach to this problem.

Germline ret mutational analysis has become an accepted standard of care in the initial work-up after diagnosis of MTC. One can anticipate two other potential uses of ret testing in monitoring patients with established MTC. An emerging class of small molecule inhibitors, described below, inhibits the tyrosine kinase activity of ret. Two critical issues have yet to be resolved regarding ret as a biomarker. First, do sporadic patients bearing the common M918T (or other) ret mutations in their tumors respond differently to small molecule inhibitors of ret? There is precedent that tumors bearing a specific ret mutation at codon 804 are markedly resistant to the kinase inhibitor zactima [33]. One might speculate that tumors bearing M918T mutations could exhibit oncogene dependence and initial sensitivity, although further mutations conferring resistance could emerge. Commercial laboratories do not offer somatic ret mutation analysis, and this remains a research test. A further application of ret analysis is to measure the effectiveness of therapy targeting ret. Clinical trials are using immunohistochemical analysis of active, phosphorylated ret in posttreatment biopsy specimens as a key biomarker to indicate whether ret is being inhibited or not. It is not clear whether posttreatment FNAs to measure ret inhibition could have a role in clinical practice.

The choice of postoperative imaging depends on prior imaging results, calcitonin and CEA levels, the presence of any symptoms, and the rationale for potential treatment. Patients who have undetectable or low calcitonin levels are unlikely to have identifiable disease on imaging. In our institution, we frequently consider periodic imaging with neck ultrasound in patients who have modest calcitonin elevations (>20 pg/mL) and more extensive imaging with higher calcitonin levels (>100–200 pg/mL). Neck ultrasound has the potential to detect recurrent or persistent lymph nodes less than 1 cm and allows efficient selection of nodes for FNA. Neck CT and MRI, exhibiting somewhat less resolution, have the capacity to image deeper structures in the neck, as does FDG-PET [34]. Mediastinal and lung metastases are detected with chest CT. Detection of hepatic metastases remains a major challenge in MTC, with a trade-off between highly sensitive/highly invasive techniques (laparoscopic biopsy and hepatic arteriography) versus a moderately sensitive/noninvasive technique (arterial phase contrast abdominal CT). Detection of bone metastases is effective with an axial MRI including cervical, thoracic, lumbar, and pelvic sequences [9]. FDG-PET seems to have utility for whole-body bone imaging [34]. Conventional technetium bone scintigraphy has proven disappointing in MTC [9].

Two imaging indications deserve mention. The first indication is selection of patients for systemic therapy clinical trials. Most MTC trials have used Recist criteria, requiring measurable disease such as lesions greater than 1 cm on spiral CT [35]. Bone lesions or other lesions without quantifiable three-dimensional measurements are not applicable. Patients who have progressive stage IV disease on imaging should be actively considered for clinical trials. The presence of moderate cervical lymphadenopathy and distant metastases could be considered advantageous in targeted therapy trials, allowing for a posttreatment biopsy to assess the degree of target inhibition. A more traditional indication of imaging is the selection of patients for potentially curative reoperation. Here the importance of imaging is to effectively rule out inoperable disease. On the other hand, the use of new imaging techniques to detect operable disease and promote curative resection has been generally ineffective [34,36]. This lack of effectiveness has frequently been attributed to the high frequency of occult liver metastases in patients who have long-standing MTC [8,37]. A more realistic surgical strategy for reoperation is described below. This strategy reserves this procedure for patients who have incomplete or inadequate primary surgery or a clear-cut intent for palliation or forestalling likely complications.

Evolving therapy of medullary thyroid cancer

Surgery

Surgical treatment of MTC has been extensively studied and reviewed, and several excellent summaries have been published [38–40]. For patients who have established, palpable sporadic MTC, the recommended procedure is total thyroidectomy with central compartment and ipsilateral modified radical neck dissection, encompassing levels II through VI. Some centers also routinely perform an initial contralateral neck dissection, whereas others select contralateral nodal dissection at a second stage, based on the predictive value of a positive contralateral central neck specimen [6], combined with postoperative calcitonin measurement and other indicators.

In the United States, a high percentage of patients who have MTC have undergone incomplete surgery as their initial operation. In SEER data (1973–2002), more patients underwent thyroidectomy without lymph node dissection (37%) than total thyroidectomy with modified radical or radical neck dissection (26%) as their initial procedure [3]. Potential explanations for this clinical practice include the initial misdiagnosis of MTC by FNA in some cases and the relatively high percentage of initial operations performed by surgeons who have limited experience with the disorder. A strong case can be made for centralized referral of MTC patients to centers of excellence. Intraoperative assessment of lymph nodes by palpation and observation is not an adequate method of assessing nodal involvement, with less than 70% sensitivity and specificity [41]. The performance of the central lymph node dissection is of critical importance because of the predilection of MTC to sites in the tracheo-esophageal groove, which may be difficult to access. An appropriate central nodal dissection entails removal of lymphatic tissue from the level of the hyoid bone to the innominate vessels and laterally to the carotid arteries [41]. It is important to emphasize the importance of local control of MTC, even in patients who have relatively advanced stage IV disease. Because even widespread MTC may be associated with long, symptom-free intervals, it is critical to obtain local control to forestall complications such as vocal cord paralysis, airway obstruction, and hemoptysis.

The role of reoperative neck surgery in MTC remains controversial. Reoperation with a curative intent is most feasible in patients who have had an inadequate initial operation. A second indication is imageable recurrent cervical metastasis. If the intent of reoperation is curative (ie, reducing the postoperative calcitonin to undetectable levels), then there is an onus on the clinician to extensively rule out distant, inoperable disease, including sensitive examinations of the liver. Moley and colleagues have shown a 25% prevalence of occult liver metastases by laparoscopic biopsy, and even higher rates have been detected by hepatic arteriography [8,42]. Palliative reoperation may be indicated if there is risk for future compression or invasion of the trachea or major vesselss.

Radiation

External-beam radiation therapy has a limited role in MTC that has been well summarized elsewhere [43]. Four nonrandomized studies support the use of adjuvant external-beam radiotherapy in postoperative patients at high risk for local recurrence, (eg, in patients who have locally invasive tumor, grossly positive surgical margins, or extensive adenopathy with extranodal extension). In this setting, adjuvant XRT may reduce the 10-year local recurrence rate by 30% to 50% [44]. External-beam radiotherapy is also useful in a palliative fashion in bone metastases. There is no role for radioiodine therapy in MTC. Targeted radiotherapy, using anti-CEA monoclonal antibodies or radiolabeled somastatin receptor ligands, is also under investigation.

Systemic therapy

Experience with single-agent or combination chemotherapy for MTC has been largely unsatisfactory, and no large-scale or phase III studies have been performed. Nocera and colleagues [45] reported a partial response rate of

15% in patients who had MTC treated with a combination of doxorubicin, streptozotocin, 5-FU, and dacarbazine. Approximately 28% of patients who had advanced MTC had partial responses in a small-scale trial of cyclophosphamide, vincristine, and dacarbazine [46]. Based on the significant mortality of stage IV MTC and the absence of effective conventional chemotherapy, a number of groups have sought targeted therapy of the disease, using the ret tyrosine kinase, angiogenic growth factors, somatatostatin receptors, CEA, the proteasome, and heat-shock proteins as principal targets.

Ret as a therapeutic target

Proof-of-principal that ret inhibition can provide useful treatment for MTC stems from several experimental studies. A dominant negative ret molecule, preserving the extracellular and transmembrane domains of the receptor but lacking the intracellular tyrosine kinase domain, was capable of inducing growth arrest and programmed cell death when overexpressed in MTC cells that expressed a native ret-activating mutation at codon 634 but had no effect in heterologous tumor cells lacking a mutant ret [47]. Neutralizing antibodies directed at activated ret (including phosphorylated Tyr1062) also inhibited growth [48]. Based on such encouraging proof-of-principal studies and on the remarkable initial responses of such small molecule inhibitors as imatinib in CML and gastrointestinal stromal tumor, a growing list of candidate inhibitors of ret have been identified and tested.

Small-molecule tyrosine kinase inhibitors (TKIs) with activity against ret include the following: RPI-1, sunitinib (SU11248), PP1 and PP2, CEP-701 and CEP-751, zactima (ZD6474), sorafenib (BAY 43-9006), XL-880, and XL-184 (see Refs. [12] and [49] for recent summaries). Other small-molecule inhibitors of ret are expected to emerge soon. Most of these agents bind to the ATP-binding pocket of ret, which is highly conserved compared with other receptor tyrosine kinases, creating the potential for multiple inhibitory targets and greater side effects. Sunitinib, zactima, sorafenib, XL-880, and XL-184 target KDR/VEGFR2, a second highly important target in MTC. It is a challenge for clinical trials to distinguish anti-Ret efficacy from activity stemming from inhibition of VEGF receptors and other targets.

Early clinical trials using TKIs targeting ret suggest that this strategy could be well tolerated and relatively effective, at least in a cytostatic fashion. Wells and colleagues reported preliminary data on a phase II trial of zactima, a multifunction TKI targeting ret (IC_{50} 100 nM), VEGFR2/KDR (IC_{50} 40 nM), and EGFR [50]. Of 15 patients who had hereditary MTC, three showed partial tumor responses, 10 showed stable disease, and two showed progressive disease. Median duration of treatment was 136 days. Twelve of 15 patients had a greater than 50% decrease in calcitonin; some patients had greater than 90% declines. Approximately half of the patients had significant declines in CEA. Side effects for this oral drug included diarrhea, nausea, skin rash, and fatigue, often necessitating dose reductions. Although this trial was not powered to distinguish responses to different ret mutations, independent in vitro work has indicated marked differences in sensitivity to this agent, with one common mutation at codon 804 highly resistant to zactima but relatively sensitive to sorafenib [33,51]. An international large scale phase II trial is evaluating the efficacy across a broader population of MTC patients.

MTC clinical trials are planned or underway for sorafenib and sunitinib. Agents earlier in the developmental pipeline have the potential to inhibit ret at subnanomolar concentrations and have significant promise for hereditary and at least some cases of sporadic MTC.

The strategy of combining targeted therapy with cytotoxic chemotherapy has had some notable successes (eg, trastuzamab plus chemotherapy in breast cancer). Targeted and cytotoxic agent pairings need to be carefully designed. Preclinical studies are beginning to examine ret inhibition in combination with cytotoxic drugs. As a single agent in MTC xenograft studies in mice, irinotecan had excellent activity with median progression-free survival of 95 days and all mice being progression free at 75 days [52]. The combination of irinotecan plus the TKI CEP-751 did not reach median progression-free survival at 135 days, with 100% of mice being progression free at 110 days, after a 30-day treatment course. CEP-751 has an IC_{50} for RET of 100 nM in the presence of serum and additional activity against VEGFR2 and TrkA [52]. Although the mechanism for the additive activity of CEP-751 and irinotecan is uncertain, the TKI in this experiment seemed to abrogate the mid-S phase arrest associated with the DNA damage response to irinotecan. Other TKIs targeting ret shared this property, although the specificity of this interaction needs further investigation [52].

Angiogenesis inhibitors

Two phase II clinical trials recently have been completed for single-agent TKIs targeting VEGF receptors 1 through 3 in thyroid cancer, including significant populations of patients who had MTC. Axitinib (AG-013736) was associated with an overall partial response rate of 20% in patients who had thyroid cancer in preliminary results. Two of 12 patients who had MTC had radiographic partial responses, and six patients had stable disease, with four patients progressing on treatment [53]. Follicular thyroid cancer has exhibited the strongest response (33% PR, 87% PR or SD). Reported side effects of this oral agent were moderate and included fatigue, hypertension, and proteinuria. The best overall response rate to Axitinib as a single agent is in renal cell carcinoma (46%), a von Hippel-Lindau and VEGF-dependent tumor [54]. A phase II study of the VEGFR inhibitor AMG-706 (Amgen, Thousand Oaks, CA) in MTC has also reached completion. It will be interesting to see if combinations of angiogenesis inhibitors and chemotherapy or other targeted agents show greater efficacy in MTC, as has been observed in colorectal cancer. Multifunction TKIs have the potential to target ret and VEGFRs, combining these two excellent targets in MTC.

Other target targeted therapies

A number of other therapeutic targets are under investigation in MTC. These investigational approaches include targeting somatostatin receptors with high-energy–emitting ligands [55], radioimmunotherapy using monoclonal antibodies to CEA [56], and proteasome inhibitors such as bortezomib, potentially targeting the AKT-Nf kappa B pathway [57]. Heat-shock protein inhibitors, such as 17-AAG and other geldanomycin derivatives, can lead to impaired protein folding and to destabilization of mutant proteins, such as activated ret [58].

Future prospects for monitoring and therapy

Activated Ret is the outstanding target for therapy in MTC, based on the relatively high prevalence of this mutated oncogene ($\sim$50% of tumors overall), a relatively specific expression pattern, and emerging proof-of-principal studies. There is an immediate need to correlate biomarkers relating to ret mutational status and ret inhibition at the tumor level, with clinical response to TKIs. There are several critical monitoring issues for patients who have MTC who fail ret inhibitor treatment: (1) Do they exhibit a "sensitive" ret mutation? (2) Is heterogeneity of ret mutations within their tumors a problem? And (3) Has ret kinase activity been effectively inhibited by the drug? Conventional Recist criteria may provide inadequate imaging guidelines for response to therapies such as ret inhibitors, which seem to be primarily cytostatic. The role of functional imaging, such as FDG-PET or DCE-MRI, has not been studied in this setting.

A further challenge will be to devise effective drug combinations that overcome the resistance associated with effective kinase inhibitors in other disorders, such as imatinib in CML and GIST, which may stem from second-site mutations or more complex adaptive mechanisms [59,60]. Understanding the tumor adaptation to ret inhibition may be helpful in developing combination strategies. It is encouraging to patients and clinicians that a variety of promising avenues is emerging for MTC.

References

[1] Jemal A, Siegel R, Ward E, et al. Cancer statistics, 2006. CA Cancer J Clin 2006;56(2): 106–30.
[2] Davies L, Welch HG. Increasing incidence of thyroid cancer in the United States, 1973–2002. JAMA 2006;295(18):2164–7.

[3] Roman S, Lin R, Sosa JA. Prognosis of medullary thyroid carcinoma: demographic, clinical, and pathologic predictors of survival in 1252 cases. Cancer 2006;107(9):2134–42.

[4] Moley JF, DeBenedetti MK. Patterns of nodal metastases in palpable medullary thyroid carcinoma: recommendations for extent of node dissection. Ann Surg 1999;229(6):880–7; [discussion: 887–8].

[5] Machens A, Hinze R, Thomusch O, et al. Pattern of nodal metastasis for primary and reoperative thyroid cancer. World J Surg 2002;26(1):22–8.

[6] Scollo C, Baudin E, Travagli JP, et al. Rationale for central and bilateral lymph node dissection in sporadic and hereditary medullary thyroid cancer. J Clin Endocrinol Metab 2003; 88(5):2070–5.

[7] Machens A, Holzhausen HJ, Dralle H. Contralateral cervical and mediastinal lymph node metastasis in medullary thyroid cancer: systemic disease? Surgery 2006;139(1):28–32.

[8] Szavcsur P, Godeny M, Bajzik G, et al. Angiography-proven liver metastases explain low efficacy of lymph node dissections in medullary thyroid cancer patients. Eur J Surg Oncol 2005;31(2):183–90.

[9] Mirallie E, Vuillez JP, Bardet S, et al. High frequency of bone/bone marrow involvement in advanced medullary thyroid cancer. J Clin Endocrinol Metab 2005;90(2):779–88.

[10] Bergholm U, Bergstrom R, Ekbom A. Long-term follow-up of patients with medullary carcinoma of the thyroid. Cancer 1997;79(1):132–8.

[11] Ichihara M, Murakumo Y, Takahashi M. RET and neuroendocrine tumors. Cancer Lett 2004;204(2):197–211.

[12] de Groot JW, Links TP, Plukker JT, et al. RET as a diagnostic and therapeutic target in sporadic and hereditary endocrine tumors. Endocr Rev 2006;27(5):535–60.

[13] Attie T, Pelet A, Edery P, et al. Diversity of RET proto-oncogene mutations in familial and sporadic Hirschsprung disease. Hum Mol Genet 1995;4(8):1381–6.

[14] Jijiwa M, Fukuda T, Kawai K, et al. A targeting mutation of tyrosine 1062 in Ret causes a marked decrease of enteric neurons and renal hypoplasia. Mol Cell Biol 2004;24(18): 8026–36.

[15] Santoro M, Melillo RM, Carlomagno F, et al. Molecular mechanisms of RET activation in human cancer. Ann N Y Acad Sci 2002;963:116–21.

[16] Smith-Hicks CL, Sizer KC, Powers JF, et al. C-cell hyperplasia, pheochromocytoma and sympathoadrenal malformation in a mouse model of multiple endocrine neoplasia type 2B. EMBO J 2000;19(4):612–22.

[17] Michiels FM, Chappuis S, Caillou B, et al. Development of medullary thyroid carcinoma in transgenic mice expressing the RET protooncogene altered by a multiple endocrine neoplasia type 2A mutation. Proc Natl Acad Sci U S A 1997;94(7):3330–5.

[18] Acton DS, Velthuyzen D, Lips CJ, et al. Multiple endocrine neoplasia type 2B mutation in human RET oncogene induces medullary thyroid carcinoma in transgenic mice. Oncogene 2000;19(27):3121–5.

[19] Machens A, Niccoli-Sire P, Hoegel J, et al. Early malignant progression of hereditary medullary thyroid cancer. N Engl J Med 2003;349(16):1517–25.

[20] Gill JR, Reyes-Mugica M, Iyengar S, et al. Early presentation of metastatic medullary carcinoma in multiple endocrine neoplasia, type IIA: implications for therapy. J Pediatr 1996; 129(3):459–64.

[21] Brandi ML, Gagel RF, Angeli A, et al. Guidelines for diagnosis and therapy of MEN type 1 and type 2. J Clin Endocrinol Metab 2001;86(12):5658–71.

[22] Hofstra RM, Landsvater RM, Ceccherini I, et al. A mutation in the RET proto-oncogene associated with multiple endocrine neoplasia type 2B and sporadic medullary thyroid carcinoma. Nature 1994;367(6461):375–6.

[23] Blaugrund JE, Johns MM Jr, Eby YJ, et al. RET proto-oncogene mutations in inherited and sporadic medullary thyroid cancer. Hum Mol Genet 1994;3(10):1895–7.

[24] Eng C, Mulligan LM, Healey CS, et al. Heterogeneous mutation of the RET proto-oncogene in subpopulations of medullary thyroid carcinoma. Cancer Res 1996;56(9):2167–70.

[25] Schilling T, Burck J, Sinn HP, et al. Prognostic value of codon 918 (ATG->ACG) RET proto-oncogene mutations in sporadic medullary thyroid carcinoma. Int J Cancer 2001; 95(1):62–6.

[26] Wohllk N, Cote GJ, Bugalho MM, et al. Relevance of RET proto-oncogene mutations in sporadic medullary thyroid carcinoma. J Clin Endocrinol Metab 1996;81(10):3740–5.

[27] Cohen R, Campos JM, Salaun C, et al. Preoperative calcitonin levels are predictive of tumor size and postoperative calcitonin normalization in medullary thyroid carcinoma. Groupe d'Etudes des Tumeurs a Calcitonine (GETC). J Clin Endocrinol Metab 2000;85(2):919–22.

[28] Machens A, Schneyer U, Holzhausen HJ, et al. Prospects of remission in medullary thyroid carcinoma according to basal calcitonin level. J Clin Endocrinol Metab 2005;90(4): 2029–34.

[29] Kouvaraki MA, Shapiro SE, Fornage BD, et al. Role of preoperative ultrasonography in the surgical management of patients with thyroid cancer. Surgery 2003;134(6):946–54.

[30] Paulson EK, McDermott VG, Keogan MT, et al. Carcinoid metastases to the liver: role of triple-phase helical CT. Radiology 1998;206(1):143–50.

[31] Barbet J, Campion L, Kraeber-Bodere F, et al. Prognostic impact of serum calcitonin and carcinoembryonic antigen doubling-times in patients with medullary thyroid carcinoma. J Clin Endocrinol Metab 2005;90(11):6077–84.

[32] Leboeuf R, Langlois MF, Martin M, et al. "Hook effect" in calcitonin immunoradiometric assay in patients with metastatic medullary thyroid carcinoma: case report and review of the literature. J Clin Endocrinol Metab 2006;91(2):361–4.

[33] Carlomagno F, Guida T, Anaganti S, et al. Disease associated mutations at valine 804 in the RET receptor tyrosine kinase confer resistance to selective kinase inhibitors. Oncogene 2004; 23(36):6056–63.

[34] de Groot JW, Links TP, Jager PL, et al. Impact of 18F-fluoro-2-deoxy-D-glucose positron emission tomography (FDG-PET) in patients with biochemical evidence of recurrent or residual medullary thyroid cancer. Ann Surg Oncol 2004;11(8):786–94.

[35] Therasse P, Arbuck SG, Eisenhauer EA, et al. New guidelines to evaluate the response to treatment in solid tumors. European Organization for Research and Treatment of Cancer, National Cancer Institute of the United States, National Cancer Institute of Canada. J Natl Cancer Inst 2000;92(3):205–16.

[36] Udelsman R, Ball D, Baylin SB, et al. Preoperative localization of occult medullary carcinoma of the thyroid gland with single-photon emission tomography dimercaptosuccinic acid. Surgery 1993;114(6):1083–9.

[37] Machens A, Dralle H. Angiography-proven liver metastases explain low efficacy of lymph node dissections in medullary thyroid cancer patients. Eur J Surg Oncol 2005;31(9):1051–2.

[38] You YN, Lakhani V, Wells SA Jr, et al. Medullary thyroid cancer. Surg Oncol Clin N Am 2006;15(3):639–60.

[39] Fleming JB, Lee JE, Bouvet M, et al. Surgical strategy for the treatment of medullary thyroid carcinoma. Ann Surg 1999;230(5):697–707.

[40] Machens A, Ukkat J, Brauckhoff M, et al. Advances in the management of hereditary medullary thyroid cancer. J Intern Med 2005;257(1):50–9.

[41] Fialkowski EA, Moley JF. Current approaches to medullary thyroid carcinoma, sporadic and familial. J Surg Oncol 2006;94(8):737–47.

[42] Tung WS, Vesely TM, Moley JF. Laparoscopic detection of hepatic metastases in patients with residual or recurrent medullary thyroid cancer. Surgery 1995;118(6):1024–9; [discussion: 1029–30].

[43] Brierly JD, Tsang RW. External radiation therapy of medullary thyroid cancer. In: Wartofsky L, Van Nostrand D, editors. Thyroid cancer: a comprehensive guide to clinical management. Totowa (NJ): Humana; 2006. p. 605–7.

[44] Brierley J, Tsang R, Simpson WJ, et al. Medullary thyroid cancer: analyses of survival and prognostic factors and the role of radiation therapy in local control. Thyroid 1996;6(4): 305–10.

[45] Nocera M, Baudin E, Pellegriti G, et al. Treatment of advanced medullary thyroid cancer with an alternating combination of doxorubicin-streptozocin and 5 FU-dacarbazine. Groupe d'Etude des Tumeurs a Calcitonine (GETC). Br J Cancer 2000;83(6):715–8.

[46] Wu LT, Averbuch SD, Ball DW, et al. Treatment of advanced medullary thyroid carcinoma with a combination of cyclophosphamide, vincristine, and dacarbazine. Cancer 1994;73(2): 432–6.

[47] Drosten M, Hilken G, Bockmann M, et al. Role of MEN2A-derived RET in maintenance and proliferation of medullary thyroid carcinoma. J Natl Cancer Inst 2004;96(16):1231–9.

[48] Salvatore D, Barone MV, Salvatore G, et al. Tyrosines 1015 and 1062 are in vivo autophos-phorylation sites in ret and ret-derived oncoproteins. J Clin Endocrinol Metab 2000;85(10): 3898–907.

[49] Santoro M, Carlomagno F. Drug insight: small-molecule inhibitors of protein kinases in the treatment of thyroid cancer. Nat Clin Pract Endocrinol Metab 2006;2(1):42–52.

[50] Wells SYY, Lakhani V, Hou J. A phase II trial of ZD6474 in patients with hereditary metastatic medullary thyroid cancer. Journal of Clinical Oncology 2006;24(18S):5553.

[51] Carlomagno F, Anaganti S, Guida T, et al. BAY 43-9006 inhibition of oncogenic RET mutants. J Natl Cancer Inst 2006;98(5):326–34.

[52] Strock CJ, Park JI, Rosen DM, et al. Activity of irinotecan and the tyrosine kinase inhibitor CEP-751 in medullary thyroid cancer. J Clin Endocrinol Metab 2006;91(1):79–84.

[53] Kim SRL, Cohen EE, Cohen RB. A phase II study of axitinib (AG-013736), a potent inhibitor of VEGFRs, in patients with advanced thyroid cancer. J Clin Oncol 2006;24(8S): Abstract 5529.

[54] Larkin JM, Eisen T. Kinase inhibitors in the treatment of renal cell carcinoma. Crit Rev Oncol Hematol 2006;60(3):216–26.

[55] Bodei L, Handkiewicz-Junak D, Grana C, et al. Receptor radionuclide therapy with 90Y-DOTATOC in patients with medullary thyroid carcinomas. Cancer Biother Radiopharm 2004;19(1):65–71.

[56] Chatal JF, Campion L, Kraeber-Bodere F, et al. Survival improvement in patients with medullary thyroid carcinoma who undergo pretargeted anti-carcinoembryonic-antigen radioimmunotherapy: a collaborative study with the French Endocrine Tumor Group. J Clin Oncol 2006;24(11):1705–11.

[57] Mitsiades CS, McMillin D, Kotoula V, et al. Anti-tumor effects of the proteasome inhibitor bortezomib in medullary and anaplastic thyroid carcinoma cells in vitro. J Clin Endocrinol Metab 2006;91(10):4013–21.

[58] Cohen MS, Hussain HB, Moley JF. Inhibition of medullary thyroid carcinoma cell prolifer-ation and RET phosphorylation by tyrosine kinase inhibitors. Surgery 2002;132(6):960–6; [discussion: 966–7].

[59] Agaram NP, Besmer P, Wong GC, et al. Pathologic and molecular heterogeneity in imatinib-stable or imatinib-responsive gastrointestinal stromal tumors. Clin Cancer Res 2007;13(1): 170–81.

[60] Ritchie E, Nichols G. Mechanisms of resistance to imatinib in CML patients: a paradigm for the advantages and pitfalls of molecularly targeted therapy. Curr Cancer Drug Targets 2006; 6(8):645–57.

ELSEVIER
SAUNDERS

Endocrinol Metab Clin N Am
36 (2007) 839–853

ENDOCRINOLOGY
AND METABOLISM
CLINICS
OF NORTH AMERICA

Thyroid Cancer Molecular Signaling Pathways and Use of Targeted Therapy

Priya Kundra, MD[a], Kenneth D. Burman, MD[a,b],*

[a]*Endocrine Sections, Washington Hospital Center, Georgetown University Medical Center,*
110 Irving Street, NW, Washington, DC 20010, USA
[b]*Department of Medicine, Georgetown University, 4000 Reservoir Road NW, Washington,*
DC 20007, USA

Thyroid cancer is the most prevalent endocrine neoplasia diagnosed each year in approximately 25,690 new individuals in the United States alone [1]. The development of new treatment modalities for thyroid cancer is crucial because of the lack of effective therapies for tumors that prove to be resistant to radioiodine and thyroid-stimulating hormone (TSH)–suppressive therapy. Although considered untreatable in the past, over the past several years, a large number of new compounds have been developed that target pathways activated in progressive thyroid cancers, several of which have progressed into clinical trials. This review focuses on agents targeted to inhibit critical pathways in thyroid tumorigenesis or progression, with an effort to include agents with different but often overlapping mechanisms of action (Table 1).

Ras-directed therapy

Ras represents a family of small guanosine triphosphate (GTP)–binding proteins (G proteins) that are essential signaling molecules downstream of many cell surface receptors. Activation of Ras results in a cascade of signaling activity, primarily through the Raf-Mek-Erk cascade that regulates a wide variety of cellular functions, including cell cycle progression, proliferation, motility, and apoptosis. Constitutive activation of Ras, by mutations or by activation of one of its upstream regulators, and activation of its downstream effector, BRAF, are the most common oncogenic events

---

* Corresponding author. Endocrine Sections, Washington Hospital Center, Georgetown University Medical Center, 110 Irving Street, NW, Washington, DC 20010.
E-mail address: kenneth.burman@medstar.net (K.D. Burman).

0889-8529/07/$ - see front matter © 2007 Elsevier Inc. All rights reserved.
doi:10.1016/j.ecl.2007.06.001   *endo.theclinics.com*

Table 1
Open trials for thyroid cancer

Therapeutic target	Action	Compound name	Status
Raf and tyrosine kinase	Inhibitor	Sorafenib	Recruiting: Phase II Trial of BAY 43-9006 in Patients with Advanced Anaplastic Carcinoma of the Thyroid, Phase II Study of Sorafenib (BAY 43-9006) in Patients with Metastatic Medullary Thyroid Carcinoma
Tyrosine kinase	Inhibitor	Gleevec, Imatinib	Recruiting: Phase II Trial Evaluating Gleevec (Imatinib Mesylate Formerly Known as STI571) in Patients with Anaplastic Thyroid Cancer, Phase I/II Study to Evaluate the Efficacy and Toxicity of Imatinib Mesylate in Combination with Dacarbazine and Capecitabine in Medullary Thyroid Carcinoma
Tyrosine kinase	Inhibitor	Sunitinib	Recruiting: Phase II Study of Sunitinib Malate in Patients with Iodine I 131-Refractory Unresectable Well-Differentiated Thyroid Cancer or Medullary Thyroid Cancer
Tyrosine kinase, vascular endothelial growth factor, epidermal growth factor receptor	Inhibitor	Vandetanib	Recruiting: Phase II Study to Assess the Monotherapy in Locally Advanced or Metastatic Medullary Thyroid Cancer
Tyrosine kinase and vascular endothelial growth factor 1, 2, and 3	Inhibitor	Axitinib	Recruiting: Pivotal Phase 2 Study of the Anti-Angiogenesis Agent AG-013736 In Patients with 131I-Refractory Metastatic or Unresectable Locally Advanced Papillary, Follicular, or Hürthle-Cell Thyroid Cancer Who Are Also Refractory to, or Intolerant of, or Have Clinical Contraindication to Doxorubicin Treatment

(continued on next page)

Table 1 (*continued*)

Therapeutic target	Action	Compound name	Status
Tubulin-binding protein	Inhibition of angiogenesis	Combretastatin A4	Recruiting: Phase II Trial of Combretastatin A-4 Phosphate (CA4P) in Advanced Anaplastic Carcinoma of the Thyroid
unknown	Inhibition of angiogenesis	Lenalidomide	Recruiting: Phase II Trial of REVLIMID (Lenalidomide) for Therapy of Radioiodine-Unresponsive Papillary and Follicular Thyroid Carcinomas
Heat shock protein	Inhibitor	17-AAG	Recruiting: Phase II Trial of 17-Allylaminogeldanamycin (17-AAG) in Advanced Medullary and Differentiated Carcinoma of the Thyroid
Histone deacetylase	Inhibitor	FR901228	Recruiting: Phase II Study of Single Agent Depsipeptide (FK228) in Radioiodine (RAI)-Refractory Metastatic Non-Medullary (Papillary, Follicular, and Hürthle Cell Variants) Thyroid Carcinoma
DNA methylation	Inhibition	Decitabine	Recruiting: Phase II Study of Decitabine in Patients with Metastatic Papillary Thyroid Cancer or Follicular Thyroid Cancer Unresponsive to Radioiodine
Proteasome	26S proteasome inhibition	Bortezomib	Recruiting: Phase II Study of Bortezomib in Metastatic Papillary Thyroid Carcinoma or Follicular Thyroid Cancer
Topoisomerase	Inhibition	Irinotecan	Recruiting: Phase II Trial of Irinotecan for Treatment of Metastatic Medullary Thyroid Cancer
PPAR-γ	Agonist	Rosiglitazone	Recruiting: Pilot Study of Rosiglitazone in Patients with Incurable Differentiated Thyroid Cancer

Data from National Institute of Health, ClinicalTrials.gov. Available at: clinicaltrials.gov. Accessed June 2007. This information is subject to change, and more current information can be obtained from clinicaltrials.gov.

in human cancers, including thyroid cancer. Activating mutations in N-RAS are particularly common in follicular carcinomas and in papillary cancers that maintain a follicular architecture (ie, follicular variant of papillary cancer [FVPC]) [2]. Activation of RAS by means of oncogenic rearrangements involving RET (eg, RET/PTC) and NTRK tyrosine kinase receptors is common in papillary thyroid cancers, particularly when related to radiation exposure or in children. Activation of this cascade by means of mutations in BRAF (V600E) or, more rarely, through translocations involving BRAF is particularly common in papillary thyroid cancers with typical or tall-cell papillary architecture in adults [3]. Taken together, activation of this pathway through oncogenic events occurs in approximately 70% of all thyroid cancers; therefore, the tyrosine kinase-Ras-Raf-MEK pathway represents an important potential therapeutic target for thyroid cancer [4]. After a series of intermediate events involving Grb proteins and Shc, Ras binds to GTP, becomes activated, and initiates downstream signaling events. One key step in this process is the membrane association of Ras, a step that places Ras in proximity to its upstream activators. This step requires post-translational modification of the Ras proteins by farnesylation [5]. Farnesylation of Ras proteins is necessary for their activity and is catalyzed by a family of enzymes called farnesyl protein transferases (FPTases). Thus, FPTases represent a potential therapeutic target for inhibiting Ras-mediated signaling in cancer cells.

Manumycin, a natural product of streptomyces, has been shown to possess antineoplastic properties through inhibition of FTPase activity. In vitro, manumycin reduces cell growth and survival of six anaplastic thyroid cancer (ATC) cell lines as a solitary agent and in a cooperative manner with paclitaxel, doxorubicin, or cisplatin, agents with a modest antitumor effect in ATC [6]. The combination of manumycin plus paclitaxel was further tested in vivo, where it inhibited growth and angiogenesis in a mouse xenograft model of ATC [7]. Manumycin has not been evaluated in clinical trials because of toxicity in animal models; however, other FTPase inhibitors, such as R115777 (Tipifarnib) and SCH66336 (Lonafarnib), are being studied alone and in combination for other malignancies.

Another approach to inhibition of Ras-Raf-MEK signaling is to block Raf kinase activity. This is particularly attractive for thyroid cancer, in which BRAF is commonly mutated and activated. Bay 43-9006 (Sorafenib, Nexavar; Bayer Pharmaceuticals, Wayne, New Jersey) is a biaryl urea compound that targets all the Raf kinases as well as a panel of tyrosine kinase receptors—vascular endothelial growth factor receptor (VEGFR)-2 (KDR), VEGFR-3 (Flt-4), Flt-3, platelet-derived growth factor receptor (PDGFR)-B, and KIT—at nanomolar concentrations in vitro [8]. More recently, Carlomagno and colleagues [8] also showed that BAY 43-9006 was able to inhibit RET signaling and in vitro and in vivo growth of RET-transfected fibroblasts and thyroid cells that express RET/PTC oncogenes. Bay 43-9006 also blocked the growth of xenograft tumors that were derived from a medullary thyroid cancer (MTC) cell line with endogenous expression of a mutant RET common for this disease. In phase I studies, partial responses were identified in several patients with thyroid cancer treated with Bay 43-9006, which has subsequently led to several phase II clinical trials of patients with metastatic PTC and ATC. Although the data from these studies are not yet published, it is important to note that this compound has been approved for use in patients with renal cell carcinoma in the United States. This is of interest from a mechanistic view, because renal cell cancer rarely is associated with BRAF mutations, suggesting that the mechanism of action for BAY 43-9006 in these patients is not through its effects on Raf kinase activity but may be attributable to effects on tyrosine kinase receptors, such as VEGFR and PDGR. Detailed target validation studies have not yet been reported, however.

Tyrosine kinase inhibitors

Receptor tyrosine kinase (RTK) inhibitors are the most commonly over-expressed receptors in thyroid cancers. Genetic rearrangements resulting in the expression of chimeric proteins involving the tyrosine kinase domain of RET are common in radiation-related and sporadic papillary thyroid cancer. Overexpression of other RTKs, including vascular endothelial growth factor (VEGF), mesenchymal epithelial transition factor (CMET), epidermal growth factor (EGF), and many others, has been identified. Thus, inhibition of tyrosine kinase receptor signaling, specifically or using less specific approaches, represents a logical alternative for thyroid cancer.

Several growth factors are involved in the process of angiogenesis in malignant tumors; among them, VEGF seems to be particularly important in thyroid cancer. Higher levels of VEGF have been associated with occurrence of metastasis and also with a worse prognosis in thyroid cancer [9]. Construction of the 293 embryonic kidney cell line that expresses soluble VEGFR-1 was inoculated at a site remote to where an FTC-133 follicular thyroid cancer cell tumor transplant was conducted [10]. Tumor was inhibited in 70.37% of cases compared with the control. Immunohistochemical analysis of microvessel densities in treated tumor demonstrated robustly suppressed intratumor angiogenesis. Application of VEGF monoclonal antibody to block VEGF function was performed intraperitoneally twice weekly in xenografted nude mice with papillary thyroid cancer [11], FTC-133 cells [12], and ARO-81 [13]. These studies illustrated that VEGF was produced by the follicular thyroid cancer cell line and stimulated angiogenesis and thyroid cancer cell growth. This stimulation can be blocked by monoclonal antibody A.4.6.1, however. VEGF antagonism seems to be a promising modality for thyroid carcinoma.

Epidermal growth factor receptor (EGFR), which is encoded by the c-erb proto-oncogene, is a transmembrane cell-surface glycoprotein consisting of an extracellular ligand-binding domain, a transmembrane domain, and an intracellular domain with intrinsic tyrosine kinase activity. Dimerization of EGFR after the binding of the ligand results in transphosphorylation of this receptor and subsequent activation of several downstream signal transduction pathways, including the mitogen-activated protein kinase (MAPK) and phosphatidylinositol-3' kinase signaling pathways, which are involved in promoting cellular proliferation and survival. Gefitinib (Iressa, ZD1839) is an orally active EGFR tyrosine kinase inhibitor that blocks EGFR signal transduction pathways. Schiff and colleagues [14] showed that five of six (KAT-4, K18, C643, HTH, and ARO) ATC cell lines expressed EGFR by Western blot analysis, with the exception of DRO cells. In addition, gefitinib given at a dose of 150 mg/kg was able to suppress EGFR activation for 24 to 48 hours in a nude mouse model of thyroid cancer. Furthermore, an dimethyl thiazolyl diphenyl tetrazdium salt (MTT) assay showed that gefitinib at a dose of 12 μmol/L caused near-total growth inhibition. Gefitinib at a dose of 22 μmol/L induced a rate of apoptosis greater than 80%. A subsequent study by Nobuhara and colleagues [15] showed that EGFR was universally expressed in anaplastic cancer cell lines. Furthermore, specific EGFR stimulation with EGF showed significant phosphorylation of ERK1/2 and Akt and resulted in marked growth stimulation in an ATC cell line, which highly expressed EGFR. This EGFR-transmitted proliferation effect of the cancer cell line was completely inhibited by gefitinib. Growth of xenografts inoculated in mice was inhibited in a dose-dependent manner using oral gefitinib. These findings had prompted a phase II trial of gefitinib in patients with iodine-refractory locally advanced or metastatic thyroid cancer.

Another agent, ZD6474 (Vandetanib), has been shown to be an inhibitor of the VEGFR-2 (flk-1/KDR) tyrosine kinase. It also inhibits the EGFR and TIE-2, however, and Carlomagno and colleagues [16] showed that it had inhibitory activity toward RET/MEN2B, and RET/PTC3 in vitro and in vivo. Targeting RET oncogenes with ZD6474 might offer a potential treatment strategy for medullary and papillary carcinomas. Sunitinib (sutent) is a selective orally administered RTK inhibitor that targets PDGFR, VEGFR, and fms-related tyrosine kinase 3 (FLT3). Kim and colleagues [17] recently showed that sunitinib inhibits phosphorylation of the synthetic tyrosine kinase substrate peptide E4Y by RET/PTC3 in a dose-dependent manner. There are currently phase II trials of sunitinib in thyroid cancer and phase II trials of vandetanib in MTC.

Kim and colleagues [18] reported on a preclinical study of AEE788, a dual inhibitor of EGFR and VEGFR. AEE788 was able to inhibit the proliferation and induce apoptosis of ATC cell lines in vitro. AEE788, alone or in combination with paclitaxel, given to athymic nude mice bearing subcutaneous ATC xenografts inhibited the growth of ATC xenografts by 44% and 69% and showed an increase in apoptosis of tumor cells by six- and eightfold, respectively. Immunofluorescence showed the inhibition of EGFR autophosphorylation on the tumor cells as well as the inhibition of VEGFR-2 autophosphorylation on tumor endothelium. Concurrent inhibition of EGFR and VEGFR tyrosine kinases seems to be a promising anticancer strategy for ATC. Another new agent, PTK787/ZK222584 (PTK/ZK), a specific blocker of VEGFR tyrosine kinases, could inhibit the growth of poorly differentiated thyroid cancer. Schoenberger and colleagues [19] showed that treatment with PTK/ZK induced a 41.4% reduction in tumor volumes after 4 weeks of oral treatment in mice that were implanted with human follicular thyroid tumor xenografts. PTK/ZK might serve as a useful drug for advanced thyroid neoplasms.

RPI-1, a 2-indolinone Ret tyrosine kinase inhibitor, has been investigated on cells that express RET C634 oncogenic mutants in the MEN2A syndrome. Cuccuru and colleagues [20] discovered that in NIH3T3 cells expressing the Ret mutant, Ret protein and tyrosine phosphorylation were undetectable after 24 hours of RPI-1 treatment. In human MTC TT cells, RPI-1 inhibited proliferation, Ret tyrosine phosphorylation, and Ret protein expression. In mice, oral daily RPI-1 inhibited the tumor growth of TT xenografts by 81%. In addition, RPI-1 may be able to inhibit cell growth of Ret/ptc1-driven signaling. Another agent, pyrazolopyrimidine inhibitor (PP1), has been shown to induce RET/PTC and RETMEN2A/RETMEN2B oncoprotein destruction [21]. After PP1-mediated dephosphorylation, RET oncoproteins are rapidly targeted to proteosomal destruction [22]. Yet another pyrazolopyrimidine (PP2) has been shown to block the enzymatic activity of isolated RET kinase and RET/PTC1 oncoprotein [23]. Furthermore, CEP-701 and CEP-751, two indolocarbazole derivatives, can inhibit RET in MTC cells [24]. These compounds inhibit RET phosphorylation in a dose-dependent manner and block growth of MTC cells in culture. These agents may be useful in the future by inhibiting RET and blocking the growth of MTC cells.

A single preclinical study of ATC with imatinib mesylate (Gleevec), another tyrosine kinase inhibitor, prompted off-label use in some patients. Podtcheko and colleagues [25] studied the effect of Gleevec on ATC cell lines highly expressing c-ABL ARO (mutated p53) and FRO (undetectable p53). These cell lines showed marked inhibition of cell growth after treatment with STI571 (Gleevec). Fluorescent-activated cell sorting analysis revealed that Gleevec increased the fraction of FRO and ARO cells in S and G2/M phases, respectively, indicating induction of S and G2/M transition arrest. These changes were accompanied by inhibition of c-ABL phosphorylation/activation. Growth of FRO cells implanted into immunocompromised mice was significantly inhibited by Gleevec. Dziba and Ain [26] showed that Gleevec did not have any discernible antineoplastic activity against ATC, however. Gleevec had no constitutive kinase activity against nine ATC cell lines. There is currently a phase II trial of Gleevec in ATC.

Antiangiogenic compounds

Combrestatin A4 (CA4P), derived from the African willow and a tubulin-binding protein, has been shown to possess direct antineoplastic activity against thyroid cancer cells as well as unique vascular targeting properties. CA4P had generated substantial interest because it was found to produce a durable response in a single patient with ATC in a phase I clinical trial [27]. Dziba and colleagues [28] evaluated CA4P cytotoxicity in four ATC cell lines injected in nude mice. Significantly lower tumor weights were observed in animals treated with CA4P compared with vehicle. Although there is a phase II trial for this agent with ATC, the delay in reporting results suggests less dramatic responses.

Thalidomide has been shown to have antiangiogenic properties, although the mechanism by which growth inhibition on new vessels occurs is not fully understood. Preliminary results of a phase II trial of thalidomide monotherapy in patients with rapidly progressive iodine-unresponsive distant metastasis from papillary and follicular thyroid carcinoma suggest antitumor activity [29]. In 20 patients, there was a greater than 50% response rate, with durability of at least 8 months in 30% of the responders. Further evaluation of a thalidomide derivative, lenalidomide, with less toxicity is under evaluation in a phase II trial.

Apoptosis-inducing compounds

Aplidine is a second-generation didemnin isolated from the Mediterranean tunicate *Aplidium albicans* that inhibits protein and DNA synthesis and induces apoptosis and a G1 cell-cycle arrest in cancer cells. The antiproliferative properties of aplidine may result from its binding to several key enzymes, including elongation factor 1-α, ornithine decarboxylase, and palmitoyl protein thioesterase 1, with the latter being involved in the lipidation process of several signaling proteins. In addition, aplidine was shown to inhibit flt-1 gene expression encoding VEGFR-1, to decrease VEGF secretion, and to induce apoptosis in cancer cells as well as blocking matrix metalloproteinase (MMP) production by endothelial cells. Straight and colleagues [30] have shown that aplidine reduces growth of ATC xenografts in nude mice. This was associated with increased levels of the apoptosis-related proteins polyadenosylribose polymerase 85 and caspase 8. Aplidine treatment was associated with lost or reduced expression of several angiogenesis genes, including VEGF.

KP372-1, an Akt inhibitor, has been recognized as an agent that may be useful for thyroid cancer by inducing apoptosis. Akt is highly phosphorylated in thyroid cancer cells [31]. In addition, KP372-1 inhibited Akt kinase activity, phosphorylation of Akt, and downstream targets of Akt in thyroid cancer cell lines WRO and NPA187.

Integrin ligase (ILK), a focal adhesion serine-threonine protein kinase, is a potential target for ATC. ILK mediates cell growth and survival signals and is overexpressed in several cancers. QLT0267, an ILK inhibitor, has been shown to inhibit cell growth and induce apoptosis in the NPA187, DRO, and K4 cell lines. Tumor volumes in mice treated with QLT0267 were reduced compared with controls [32]. Growth arrest in vitro and in vivo suggests that ILK is a potential target for ATC.

Early preclinical studies suggested increased cyclooxygenase-2 (COX-2) expression in thyroid carcinomas. When activated, COX-2 inhibits apoptosis and enhances angiogenesis. A phase II clinical trial with celecoxib, 400 mg administered twice daily, in patients with radioiodine-refractory metastatic differentiated thyroid cancer resulted in 23 of 25 patients with progressive disease, 1 with a partial response, and 1 with disease stabilization [33]. COX-2 is likely not a useful therapeutic target.

Matrix metalloproteinases inhibitor(s)

MMPs are an important class of enzymes involved in tumor progression. The novel application of marimastat, an inhibitor of MMPs, failed to prevent progression of follicular thyroid carcinoma after embolization of metastasis in seven patients compared with controls [34].

Hsp90 inhibitor(s)

Hsp90 protein is a chaperone that stabilizes growth factor receptors and signaling molecules. Inhibition of Hsp90 leads to Raf-1 depletion and consequent inhibition of MAPK MEK 1/2 phosphorylation and to degradation of Akt, causing reduced cell signaling and cell growth and leading to cell death. 17-Allylamino-17-demethoxygeldanamycin (17-AAG) is the first Hsp90 inhibitor to enter clinical studies. It is derived from the benzoquinoid ansamycin antibiotic geldanamycin, an agent with potent antitumor activity. In cancer cells, Hsp90 is a part of a complex with enhanced activity and high affinity for 17-AAG at approximately 100-fold that of normal cells. Braga-Basaria and colleagues [35] incubated NPA, WRO, and ARO cells with 17-AAG in vitro. Western blot analysis demonstrated that NPA cells were most resistant to 17-AAG–induced cytotoxicity, had the lowest levels of Hsp90, and were the only cells with persistent levels of Akt. WRO and ARO cells that were sensitive to 17-AAG–induced cell death did not undergo apoptosis, suggesting that cancer cells may have a reduced apoptotic response to 17-AAG. The sensitivity of thyroid cancer cells to 17-AAG is likely related to Hsp90 levels rather than to the histologic subtype. In addition, Marsee and colleagues [36] found that inhibition of Hsp90 with 17-AAG reduces PTC1 protein levels and increases radioiodide accumulation in thyroid cells. The increased accumulation was unrelated to sodium-iodide symporter (NIS) expression and likely resulted from decreased iodide efflux by means of a PKA-independent mechanism. More recently, Elisei and colleagues [37] showed that 17-AAG prolonged the retention time of ^{131}I in NIS-transfected FRO-19 tumor cells. Currently, there is a phase II trial of 17-AAG in advanced thyroid cancer.

Histone deacetylase inhibitor(s)

Histone deacetylase inhibitors are a heterogeneous group of structurally dissimilar compounds whose precise mechanism of action has yet to be elucidated. Histone deacetylases cause compaction of the nuclear chromatin and are primarily associated with transcriptional repression of genes controlling cellular growth and differentiation. The different types of histone deacetylase inhibitors seem to share the ability to alter the chromatin structure of the 2% of the human genome regulating growth, differentiation, and apoptosis. Some of the drugs with histone deacetylase activity studied in thyroid cancer include depsipeptide (FK228) and suberoylanilide hydroxamic acid (SAHA). FK228 is a cyclic peptide that was first isolated as a fermentation product of *Chromobacterium violaceum*. Several studies have demonstrated that FK228 induces growth arrest in thyroid cancers. Kitazono and colleagues [38] studied the effects of FK228 on follicular and ATC cell lines. Growth curves and cytotoxicity profiles using the MTT assay demonstrated that a nanomolar concentration of FK228 (1 ng/mL) was optimal for inhibiting thyroid cancer cell growth with minimal toxicity. FK228 increased expression of thyroglobulin and NIS in all four cell lines as well as increasing ^{125}I uptake, confirming the functional effects of NIS upregulation. Currently, there are phase II trials of FK228 in recurrent or metastatic thyroid cancer. SAHA is another histone deacetylation inhibitor with preclinical activity in poorly differentiated cancer and ATC. Cell lines treated with SAHA exhibited growth arrest and enhancement of apoptosis with histone acetylation [39]. In a phase I trial of 73 patients with cancer, of whom 6 had thyroid cancer (4 with papillary cancer, 1 with Hürthle cancer, and 1 with medullary cancer), 1 patient with papillary cancer had a partial response and 2 others showed disease stabilization for more than 37 months; 1 of the 3 evaluated with radioactive iodine showed increased uptake in tumor metastasis [40]. This particular agent warrants further investigation in the near future.

DNA methylation inhibitor(s)

5-Azacytidine and 5-aza-2′-deoxycytidine (5-azadeoxycytidine) are compounds that are incorporated into DNA and are able to inhibit methylation. In thyroid cancer, hypermethylation of the NIS gene promoter has been demonstrated and treatment with 5-azacytidine restores NIS expression, resulting in enhanced iodide uptake in some cell lines [41]. Currently, a phase II trial of 5-azadeoxycytidine or decitabine is available for metastatic papillary or follicular thyroid cancer.

Proteasome inhibitor(s)

PS-341 (bortezomib) is a selective inhibitor of the 26S proteasome. Inhibition of the 26S proteasome in cancer cell cultures is related to growth arrest, inhibition of angiogenesis, and enhanced radiosensitivity and chemo-sensitivity. Currently, there is a phase II trial of bortezomib in metastatic thyroid cancer.

Topoisomerase inhibitor(s)

A topoisomerase inhibitor, irinotecan, has recently been shown to have inhibitory growth effects on MTC alone or in combination with CEP-751 and cetuximab. Strock and colleagues [42] showed that in TT xenografts, iri-notecan caused complete remission of the xenograft tumors, with a median duration of approximately 70 days. CEP-51 in combination with irinotecan caused complete remission of the TT xenografts for more than 130 days. Furthermore, irinotecan in combination with cetuximab (monoclonal antibody against EGFR) showed that cetuximab potentiated the in vitro antiproliferative and proapoptotic effects of irinotecan. Cetuximab, irinote-can, and cetuximab/irinotecan resulted in 77%, 79%, and 93% in vivo inhi-bition of tumor growth, respectively [43]. Currently, there is a phase II trial of irinotecan in MTC.

Peroxisome proliferator activated receptor-γ agonist(s)

Peroxisome proliferator activated receptor-γ (PPAR-γ) is one of three iso-forms of PPAR, and regulates cellular growth and differentiation. The effects of PPAR-γ agonists on cancer cells include growth inhibition, induction of ap-optosis, and redifferentiation. Recent studies have examined the effects of PPAR-γ agonist treatment in a series of thyroid cancer cell lines. Ohta and col-leagues [44] found that in four PPAR-γ–positive papillary thyroid cancer cell lines, treatment with troglitazone (10 μmol/L) and rosiglitazone (10 μmol/L) inhibited growth and stimulated apoptosis by means of the c-myc pathway; there was no effect on growth or apoptosis in the PPAR-γ–negative thyroid cancer cell lines. In vivo studies with tumor xenografts in nude mice resulted in significant growth inhibition when troglitazone treatment was initiated. Martelli and colleagues [45] showed that transfection of wild-type PPAR-γ cDNA into the PPAR-γ–negative papillary thyroid cancer cell line resulted in a significant growth inhibitory effect when ciglitazone treatment was initi-ated. The growth inhibitory effects of ciglitazone in these experiments seemed to be related to cell cycle arrest mediated by p27. Flow cytometry analysis of ciglitazone-treated cells showed a significant increase in the percentage of cells undergoing apoptosis. Currently, there is a clinical trial of rosiglitazone in ad-vanced or metastatic thyroid cancer.

Gene therapy

The use of suicide-inducing genes has been widely employed in the field of gene therapy. In general, the most prevalent approaches feature gene transfer of prodrug-activating enzymes in combination with the application of prodrugs, which, in turn, are converted into suicide-inducing agents. The most commonly used example is based on gene transfer of herpes simplex type 1 thymidine kinase (HSV-TK) with concomitant application of ganciclovir (GCV). The HSV-TK/GCV system has also been applied to MTC gene therapy. Recently, Jiang and colleagues [46] analyzed the potential of HSV-TK/GCV treatment using the calcitonin promoter/enhancer system to restrict expression to thyroid tumor cells selectively. The application of adenoassociated virus vectors as gene delivery tools allowed selective killing of TT and human medullary thyroid cancer (hMTC) cells as MTC models. In ATC, two patients received intralesional injections of a retroviral vector carrying the interleukin (IL)-2 gene and the HSV-TK gene, followed by GCV [47]. The result was an increase in T-helper type I cytokines and local tumor necrosis. This approach has not yet been used in patients but is a consideration for the future.

Loss of expression of the p53 tumor suppressor gene seems to be an important step in the transformation of differentiated thyroid cancers to anaplastic tumors. Nagayama and colleagues [48] showed that adenovirus-mediated wild-type p53 gene introduction may decrease the malignant potential of ATC cell lines and restore responsiveness to standard chemotherapeutic agents in vitro and in vivo.

Several trials have been conducted with radiolabeled monoclonal anti-Carcinoembryonic antigen (CEA) antibodies in patients with MTC. In two separate studies conducted at the same institution, two different types of ^{131}I-labeled murine anti-CEA antibodies, NP-4 or MN-14 F(ab)2, were administered to a total of 18 patients with advanced MTC. Half of the 14 evaluable patients had evidence of antitumor effects lasting up to 26 months [49]. Dendritic cells, which are derived from bone marrow antigen-presenting cells, have been used for cancer immunotherapy to present tumor-associated antigens, thereby generating tumor-specific immunity. In vitro, dendritic cells pulsed with autologous medullary tumor lysates are able to evoke a cytotoxic T-cell response [50]. Clinical studies of the immunotherapeutic strategy are ongoing in MTC. In one report, autologous dendritic cells pulsed with calcitonin and CEA were administered to 7 patients with disseminated MTC [51]. One patient demonstrated a partial response that continued with slightly longer than 1 year of follow-up, whereas 2 others had mixed responses. This approach may show some promise, but further clinical trials are warranted.

In summary, several agents are currently being tested in vitro, in xenograft models, and in clinical studies that target thyroid molecular signaling and cancer cell biology. The pathways involved include but are not limited to the Ras pathway, VEGF and EGF receptors and antibodies, angiogenesis inhibitors, tyrosine kinase inhibitors, heat shock protein inhibitors, demethylating agents, histone deacetylase inhibitors, and gene therapy. Each of these targeted approaches holds promise for our future ability to treat patients with thyroid cancer unresponsive to traditional therapy.

References

[1] American Cancer Society Web site 2005.
[2] Zhu Z, Gandhi M, Nikiforova MN, et al. Molecular profile and clinical-pathologic features of the follicular variant of papillary thyroid carcinoma. An unusually high prevalence of ras mutations. Am J Clin Pathol 2003;120:71–7.
[3] Xing M. BRAF mutations in thyroid cancer. Endocr Relat Cancer 2005;12:245–62.
[4] Kondo T, Ezzat S, Asa SL. Pathogenetic mechanisms in thyroid follicular-cell neoplasia. Nat Rev Cancer 2006;6:292–306.
[5] Sarlis NJ, Gourgiotis L. Molecular elements of apoptosis-regulating pathways in follicular thyroid cells: mining for novel therapeutic targets in the treatment of thyroid carcinoma. Curr Drug Targets Immune Endocr Metabol Disord 2004;4:187–98.
[6] Yeung SC, Xu G, Pan J, et al. Manumycin enhances the cytotoxic effect of paclitaxel on anaplastic thyroid carcinoma cells. Cancer Res 2000;60:650–6.
[7] Xu G, Pan J, Martin C, et al. Angiogenesis inhibition in the in vivo antineoplastic effect of manumycin and paclitaxel against anaplastic thyroid carcinoma. J Clin Endocrinol Metab 2001;86:1769–77.
[8] Carlomagno F, Anaganti S, Guida T, et al. BAY 43-9006 inhibition of oncogenic RET mutants. J Natl Cancer Inst 2006;98(5):326–34.
[9] Tuttle RM, Fleisher M, Francis GL, et al. Serum vascular endothelial growth factor levels are elevated in metastatic differentiated thyroid cancer but not increased by short-term TSH stimulation. J Clin Endocrinol Metab 2002;87(4):1737–42.
[10] Ye C, Feng C, Wang S, et al. SFLT-1 gene therapy of follicular thyroid carcinoma. Endocrinology 2004;145:817–22.
[11] Bauer AJ, Aptel A, Terrell R, et al. Systemic administration of vascular endothelial growth factor monoclonal antibody reduces the growth of papillary thyroid carcinoma in a nude mouse model. Ann Clin Lab Sci 2003;33:192–9.
[12] Hung CJ, Zarnegar R, Ginzinger DG, et al. Expression of vascular endothelial growth factor-C in benign and malignant thyroid tumors. J Clin Endocrinol Metab 2003;88:3694–9.
[13] Bauer A, Terrell R, Doniparthi K, et al. Vascular endothelial growth factor monoclonal antibody inhibits growth of anaplastic thyroid cancer xenografts in nude mice. Thyroidology 2002;12:953–61.
[14] Schiff B, McMurphy AB, Jasser SA, et al. Epidermal growth factor receptor (EGFR) is overexpressed in anaplastic thyroid cancer, and the EGFR inhibitor Gefitinib inhibits the growth of anaplastic thyroid cancer. Clin Cancer Res 2004;10:8594–602.
[15] Nobura Y, Onoda N, Yamashita Y, et al. Efficacy of epidermal growth factor receptor-targeted molecular therapy in anaplastic thyroid cancer cell lines. Br J Cancer 2005;92:1110–6.
[16] Carlomagno F, Vitagliano D, Guida, et al. ZD6474, an orally available inhibitor of KDR tyrosine kinase activity, efficiently blocks oncogenic RET kinases. Cancer Res 2002;62:7284–90.
[17] Kim D, Jo YS, Jung HS, et al. An orally administered multitarget tyrosine kinase inhibitor, SU11248, is a novel potent inhibitor of thyroid oncogenic RET/papillary thyroid cancer kinases. J Clin Endocrinol Metab 2006;91(10):4070–6.
[18] Kim S, Schiff BA, Yigitbasi OG. Targeted molecular therapy of anaplastic thyroid carcinoma with AEE788. Mol Cancer Ther 2005;4(4):632–40.
[19] Schoenberger J, Grimm D, Kossmehl P, et al. Effects of PTK787/ZK222584, a tyrosine kinase inhibitor, on the growth of a poorly differentiated thyroid carcinoma: an animal study. Endocrinology 2004;145(3):1031–8.

[20] Cuccuru G, Lanzi C, Cassinelli G, et al. Cellular effects and antitumor activity of RET inhibitor RPI-1 on MEN2A-associated medullary thyroid carcinoma. J Natl Cancer Inst 2004;96(13):1006–14.

[21] Kundra P, Burman K. Molecular pathogenesis of endocrine cancers. In: Molecular basis of cancer. 3rd edition. in press.

[22] Carniti C, Perego C, Mondellini P, et al. PP1 inhibitor induces degradation of RETMEN2A and RETMEN2B oncoproteins through proteosomal targeting. Cancer Res 2003;63: 2234–43.

[23] Carlomagno F, Vitagliano D, Guida T, et al. Efficient inhibition of RET/papillary thyroid carcinoma oncogenic kinases by 4-amino-5-(4-chloro-phemyl)-7-(t-butyl)pyrazolo[3,4-d]pyrimidine (PP2). J Clin Endocrinol Metab 2003;88(4):1897–902.

[24] Strock C, Park JI, Rosen M, et al. CEP-701 and CEP-751 inhibit constitutively activated RET tyrosine kinase activity and block medullary thyroid carcinoma cell growth. Cancer Res 2003;63:5559–63.

[25] Podtcheko A, Ohtsuru A, Tsuda S, et al. The selective tyrosine kinase inhibitor, ST1571, inhibits growth of anaplastic thyroid cancer cells. J Clin Endocrinol Metab 2003;88(4): 1889–96.

[26] Dziba J, Ain K. Imatinib mesylate (Gleevec; ST1571) monotherapy is ineffective in suppressing human anaplastic thyroid carcinoma cell growth in vitro. J Clin Endocrinol Metab 2004; 89(5):2127–35.

[27] Dowlati, Robertson K, Cooney M, et al. A phase I pharmokinetic and translational study of the novel vascular targeting agent combretastatin A-4 phosphate on a single-dose intravenous schedule in patients with advanced cancer. Cancer Res 2002;62:3408–16.

[28] Dziba J, Marcinek R, Venkataraman G, et al. Combretastatin A4 phosphate has primary antineoplastic activity against human anaplastic thyroid carcinoma cell lines and xenograft tumors. Thyroidology 2002;12(12):1063–70.

[29] Ain K, Lee C, Williams K, et al. Phase II trial of thalidomide for therapy of radioiodine-unresponsive papillary and follicular thyroid carcinomas and medullary thyroid carcinomas: preliminary results [abstract]. Cancer Invest 2002;21(suppl 1):38.

[30] Straight A, Oakley K, Moores R, et al. Aplidin reduces the growth of anaplastic thyroid cancer xenografts and the expression of several angiogenic genes. Cancer Chemother Pharmacol 2006;57:7–14.

[31] Mandal M, Younes M, Swan EA, et al. The Akt inhibitor KP372-1 suppresses Akt activity and cell proliferation and induces apoptosis in thyroid cancer cells. Br J Cancer 2005;92: 1899–905.

[32] Younes M, Kim S, Yigitbasi OG, et al. Integrin-linked kinase is a potential therapeutic target for anaplastic thyroid cancer. Mol Cancer Ther 2005;4(8):1146–56.

[33] Mrozek, Kloos RT, Ringel MD, et al. Phase II study of celecoxib in metastatic differentiated thyroid carcinoma. J Clin Endocrinol Metab 2006;91(6):2201–4.

[34] Smit J, van Tol KM, Hew JM, et al. Marimastat therapy as adjuvant to selective embolization in skeletal metastases of differentiated thyroid carcinoma. Clin Endocrinol 2001;55: 421–2.

[35] Braga-Basaria M, Hardy E, Gotfried R, et al. 17-Allylamino-17-demethoxygeldanamycin activity against thyroid cancer cell lines correlates with heat shock protein 90 levels. J Clin Endocrinol Metab 2004;89(6):2982–8.

[36] Marsee D, Venkateswaran A, Tao H, et al. Inhibition of heat shock protein 90, a novel RET/PTC1-associated protein, increases radioiodide accumulation in thyroid cells. J Biol chem 2004;279(42):43990–7.

[37] Elisei R, Vivaldi A, Ciampi R, et al. Treatment with drugs able to reduce iodine efflux significantly increases the intracellular retention time in thyroid cancer cells stably transfected with sodium iodide symporter complementary deoxyribonucleic acid. J Clin Endocrinol Metab 2006;91(6):2389–95.

[38] Kitazono M, Robey R, Zhan Z, et al. Low concentrations of the histone deacetylase inhibitor, depsipeptide (FR901228), increase expression of the Na+/I− symporter and iodine accumulation in poorly differentiated thyroid carcinoma cells. J Clin Endocrinol Metab 2001; 86(7):3430–5.

[39] Mitsiades CS, Poulaki V, McMullan C. Novel histone deacetylase inhibitors in the treatment of thyroid cancer. Clin Cancer Res 2005;11(10):3958–65.

[40] Kelly W, O'Connor OA, Heaney ML, et al. Phase I study of an oral histone deacetylase inhibitor, suberoylanilide hydroxamic acid, in patients with advanced cancer. J Clin Oncol 2005;23:3923–31.

[41] Venkataraman G, Yatin M, Marcinek R, et al. Restoration of iodide uptake in dedifferentiated thyroid carcinoma: relationship to human Na+/I− symporter gene methylation status. J Clin Endocrinol Metab 1999;84:2449–57.

[42] Strock J, Park JI, Rosen DM, et al. Activity of Irinotecan and the tyrosine kinase inhibitor CEP-751 in medullary thyroid cancer. J Clin Endocrinol Metab 2006;91(1):79–84.

[43] Kim S, Prichard CN, Younes MN, et al. Cetuximab and Irinotecan interact synergistically to inhibit the growth of orthotopic anaplastic thyroid carcinoma xenografts in nude mice. Clin Cancer Res 2006;12(2):600–7.

[44] Ohta K, Endo T, Haraguchi K, et al. Ligands for peroxisome proliferator-activated receptor gamma inhibit growth and induce apoptosis of human papillary thyroid carcinoma cells. J Clin Endocrinol Metab 2001;86:2170–7.

[45] Martelli M, Iuliano R, Le Pera I, et al. Inhibitory effects of peroxisome proliferator-activated receptor gamma on thyroid carcinoma cell growth. J Clin Endocrinol Metab 2002;87: 4728–35.

[46] Jiang S, Altmann A, Grimm D, et al. Tissue-specific gene expression in medullary thyroid carcinoma cells employing calcitonin regulatory elements and AAV vectors. Cancer Gene Ther 2001;8:469–72.

[47] Barzon, Pacenti M, Taccaliti A, et al. A pilot study of combined suicide/cytokine gene therapy in two patients with end-stage anaplastic thyroid carcinoma. J Clin Endocrinol Metab 2005;90:2381–4.

[48] Nagayama Y, Yoloi H, Takeda K, et al. Adenovirus-mediated tumor suppressor p53 gene therapy for anaplastic thyroid carcinoma in vitro and in vivo. J Clin Endocrinol Metab 2000;85:4081–6.

[49] Juweid M, Sharkey RM, Behr T, et al. Radioimmunotherapy of medullary thyroid cancer with iodine-I131-labeled anti-CEA antibodies. J Nucl Med 1996;37:905–11.

[50] Bachleitner-Hofmann T, Stift A, Friedl J, et al. Stimulation of autologous antitumor T-cell responses against medullary thyroid carcinoma using tumor lysate-pulsed dendritic cells. J Clin Endocrinol Metab 2002;87:1098–104.

[51] Schott M, Seissler J, Lettmann M, et al. Immunotherapy for medullary thyroid carcinoma by dendritic cell vaccination. J Clin Endocrinol Metab 2001;86:4965–9.

ELSEVIER
SAUNDERS

Endocrinol Metab Clin N Am
36 (2007) 855–871

ENDOCRINOLOGY
AND METABOLISM
CLINICS
OF NORTH AMERICA

Index

Note: Page numbers of article titles are in **boldface** type.

A

Ablation, in radioiodine treatment,
807–808. See also *Radioiodine ablation.*
laser thermal, for thyroid nodules, 728
radiofrequency, for bone metastases,
of thyroid cancer, 694–695
for thyroid nodules, 729

Acropachy, thyroid, in Graves' disease, 620

Adenoma, of pituitary, thyroid-stimulating
hormone–secreting, 625
of thyroid, 740–742
follicular, 747–749
Hürthle cell type, 747,
749–750
toxic, 621
treatment of, 644–645

Adenopathy. See *Lymphadenopathy.*

β-Adrenergic receptor blockade, for
thyrotoxicosis, 638
pregnancy and, 648
nonthyroidal illness syndrome and,
665

Age-metastasis-extent of disease-size of
tumor (AMES) classification, of
thyroid cancer, 808
in children, 784

Agranulocytosis, thionamides causing,
637–638

Alkaline phosphatase (ALP), in bone
physiology, 675, 677–678, 686

American Association of Clinical
Endocrinologists (AACE), papillary
thyroid cancer guidelines of, 756–758,
761–762, 764–769

American Joint Commission on Cancer
(AJCC), on cancer staging systems,
758, 808–809

American Thyroid Association (ATA), on
radioiodine treatment, 807, 813–814
dosages, 816–818

indications/recommendations,
814–817
on thyroid cancer, in children,
779–780, 782–784
papillary thyroid cancer guidelines of,
756–758, 761–769

Amiodarone, nonthyroidal illness syndrome
and, 665

Amiodarone-induced thyrotoxicosis (AIT),
624–625, 633
treatment of, 639, 645–646

Anaplastic thyroid cancer, fine-needle
aspiration of, 746–748

Angiogenesis inhibitors, for medullary
thyroid cancer, 833–834

Antiangiogenic compounds, for thyroid
cancer, 841, 845–846

Antibody(ies), thyroglobulin, as thyroid
function test, 589–591
in thyroid cancer, in children,
788–793
thyroid nodules and, 720–721

"Apathetic" hyperthyroidism, 629

Apoptosis-inducing compounds, for thyroid
cancer, 846–847

Appendages, hypothyroidism impact on,
601

Autoimmune hepatitis, chronic,
hypothyroidism related to, 597
nonthyroidal illness syndrome
and, 664

Autoimmune thyroiditis, fine-needle
aspiration of, 741–742

B

Benign aspirates, of thyroid, 740–744

Biliary cirrhosis, primary, nonthyroidal
illness syndrome and, 664

Moving?

Make sure your subscription moves with you!

To notify us of your new address, find your **Clinics Account Number** (located on your mailing label above your name), and contact customer service at:

E-mail: elspcs@elsevier.com

800-654-2452 (subscribers in the U.S. & Canada)
407-345-4000 (subscribers outside of the U.S. & Canada)

Fax number: 407-363-9661

Elsevier Periodicals Customer Service
6277 Sea Harbor Drive
Orlando, FL 32887-4800

*To ensure uninterrupted delivery of your subscription, please notify us at least 4 weeks in advance of move.